AF804544

The Urban Book Series

Editorial Board

Margarita Angelidou, Aristotle University of Thessaloniki, Thessaloniki, Greece

Fatemeh Farnaz Arefian, The Bartlett Development Planning Unit, UCL, Silk Cities, London, UK

Michael Batty, Centre for Advanced Spatial Analysis, UCL, London, UK

Simin Davoudi, Planning & Landscape Department GURU, Newcastle University, Newcastle, UK

Geoffrey DeVerteuil, School of Planning and Geography Cardiff University, Cardiff, UK

Jesús M. González Pérez, Department of Geography, University of the Balearic Islands, Palma (Mallorca), Spain

Daniel B. Hess, Department of Urban and Regional Planning, University at Buffalo, State University, Buffalo, New York, USA

Paul Jones, School of Architecture, Design and Planning University of Sydney, Sydney, NSW, Australia

Andrew Karvonen, Division of Urban and Regional Studies, KTH Royal Institute of Technology, Stockholm, Stockholms Län, Sweden

Andrew Kirby, New College Arizona State University, Phoenix, AZ, USA

Karl Kropf, Department of Planning, Headington Campus, Oxford Brookes University, Oxford, UK

Karen Lucas, Institute for Transport Studies, University of Leeds, Leeds, UK

Marco Maretto, DICATeA, Department of Civil and Environmental Engineering, University of Parma, Parma, Italy

Ali Modarres, Tacoma Urban Studies, University of Washington Tacoma, Tacoma, WA, USA

Fabian Neuhaus, Faculty of Environmental Design, University of Calgary, Calgary, AB, Canada

Steffen Nijhuis, Architecture and the Built Environment, Delft University of Technology, Delft, The Netherlands

Vitor Manuel Aráujo de Oliveira, Porto University, Porto, Portugal

Christopher Silver, College of Design, University of Florida, Gainesville, FL, USA

Giuseppe Strappa, Facoltà di Architettura, Sapienza University of Rome, Rome, Roma, Italy

Igor Vojnovic, Department of Geography, Michigan State University, East Lansing, MI, USA

Claudia Yamu, Department of Spatial Planning and Environment, University of Groningen, Groningen, Groningen, The Netherlands

Qunshan Zhao, School of Social and Political Sciences, University of Glasgow, Glasgow, UK

The Urban Book Series is a resource for urban studies and geography research worldwide. It provides a unique and innovative resource for the latest developments in the field, nurturing a comprehensive and encompassing publication venue for urban studies, urban geography, planning and regional development.
The series publishes peer-reviewed volumes related to urbanization, sustainability, urban environments, sustainable urbanism, governance, globalization, urban and sustainable development, spatial and area studies, urban management, transport systems, urban infrastructure, urban dynamics, green cities and urban landscapes.It also invites research which documents urbanization processes and urban dynamics on a national, regional and local level,welcoming case studies, as well as comparative and applied research.
The series will appeal to urbanists, geographers,planners, engineers, architects, policy makers, and to all of those interested in a wide-ranging overview of contemporary urban studies and innovations in the field. It accepts monographs, edited volumes and textbooks.

Indexed by Scopus!.

More information about this series at http://www.springer.com/series/14773

Miguel A. Montoya • Aleksandra Krstikj
Johannes Rehner • Daniel Lemus-Delgado
Editors

COVID-19 and Cities

Experiences, Responses, and Uncertainties

Springer

Editors
Miguel A. Montoya
School of Architecture, Art and Design
Tecnológico de Monterrey
Guadalajara, Mexico

Aleksandra Krstikj
School of Architecture, Art and Design
Tecnológico de Monterrey
Ciudad de Mexico, Mexico

Johannes Rehner
Institute of Geography, Pontificia
Universidad Católica de Chile
Santiago, Chile

Daniel Lemus-Delgado
School of Social Science and Government
Tecnológico de Monterrey
Guadalajara, Mexico

ISSN 2365-757X ISSN 2365-7588 (electronic)
The Urban Book Series
ISBN 978-3-030-84133-1 ISBN 978-3-030-84134-8 (eBook)
https://doi.org/10.1007/978-3-030-84134-8

© The Editor(s) (if applicable) and The Author(s), under exclusive license to Springer Nature Switzerland AG 2021
This work is subject to copyright. All rights are solely and exclusively licensed by the Publisher, whether the whole or part of the material is concerned, specifically the rights of translation, reprinting, reuse of illustrations, recitation, broadcasting, reproduction on microfilms or in any other physical way, and transmission or information storage and retrieval, electronic adaptation, computer software, or by similar or dissimilar methodology now known or hereafter developed.
The use of general descriptive names, registered names, trademarks, service marks, etc. in this publication does not imply, even in the absence of a specific statement, that such names are exempt from the relevant protective laws and regulations and therefore free for general use.
The publisher, the authors, and the editors are safe to assume that the advice and information in this book are believed to be true and accurate at the date of publication. Neither the publisher nor the authors or the editors give a warranty, expressed or implied, with respect to the material contained herein or for any errors or omissions that may have been made. The publisher remains neutral with regard to jurisdictional claims in published maps and institutional affiliations.

This Springer imprint is published by the registered company Springer Nature Switzerland AG
The registered company address is: Gewerbestrasse 11, 6330 Cham, Switzerland

Preface

The pandemic caused by COVID-19 has had a multidimensional impact on all spheres of societal organization and has dramatically challenged the role of cities. The virus expansion revealed vulnerabilities in urban systems, even in developed countries. While waiting for a vaccine to arrive, the most effective way of containing the virus has been social distancing and lockdowns, a paradox in a highly interconnected and interdependent world in which cities are the main contact nodes. Cities have responded in different ways, with some achieving notable results in containing the pandemic.

Cities are centers of innovation and development and can play a decisive role in the battle against the disease by developing protocols, vaccines, and treatments. Besides this, cities are the principal tool to revive the economy since they concentrate sectors that are human capital intensive, but they also concentrate informal work that is particularly vulnerable to a crisis like this. In this context, the big question is: what is and what could be the role of a city in this historical moment? Faced with mounting vulnerability and increasing uncertainties, how should we plan a city's resilience to this crisis and those of the future? How did cities respond around the globe? There is an urgent need to rethink urban systems in terms of service capacity, resource depletion, and economic relations to plan the efficient, effective, and equitable city of tomorrow. We believe that a broad revision of experiences from different cities, especially cities in China and Latin America, can provide a base for the necessary multidisciplinary analysis of the COVID-19 implications that can inform future action.

In this context, a group of four academics from the Pontificia Universidad Catolica de Chile and Tecnologico de Monterrey (Mexico) set out to edit a book on COVID-19 and cities that could contribute with discussions on experiences, responses, and uncertainties faced by cities in Latin America and Asia in times of a new pandemic. The collaboration was framed by a consortium of 12 universities from Latin America and Fudan University (FLAUC), where Pontificia Universidad Catolica de Chile and Tecnologico de Monterrey have been founding members since 2017.

The process of organizing the edited book started in June 2020 when a call was launched for chapter abstract proposals. We received a total of 31 abstracts by the end of July, from which 23 chapters were selected by the editors in the first review, as proposals that best fit the book's concept. By the end of August, we received the first full text versions of the chapters. In September, we conducted a second blind peer review of the chapters, where all the authors who participated in the book reviewed at least two chapters different from their own. In this process, some collaborations were rejected, thus the final number of contributed chapters that were accepted came to 17. In October, feedback was sent to the authors of the accepted chapters and the revised chapters were received in early November. In parallel, in September 2020, the book proposal was sent to Springer Nature. We received feedback from two anonymous reviewers of the editorial house, and after two rounds of reviews, the book was accepted to be published in early 2021.

We are grateful to many people for their support in creating this book. Our utmost gratitude goes to the authors of the chapters for their diligent work in preparing their own manuscript and revising them with consideration to received feedback, for reviewing chapters from other colleagues in the best peer spirit, and assertively communicating thoughts on different topics. It is important to acknowledge the support of the School of Architecture, Art and Design (EAAD) of the Tecnológico de Monterrey (Mexico), particularly Dean Dr. Roberto Iñiguez. This book is part of the initiative of the Tec de Monterrey's Observatory of Cities, where cities are analyzed and compared to understand the territorial conditions that determine the quality of life. Dr. Alfredo Hidalgo, the director of the Observatory and associate dean of the School of Architecture, Art and Design, has played a fundamental part in this effort, and this book could not have been produced without his support and encouragement. Rossana Valdivia, the executive coordinator of the Observatory, has also helped us a great deal to disseminate the findings of this book. The editing process of the book has benefited from the funds provided by the Observatory of Cities. Finally, we appreciate all the logistics and research of the staff at the School of Architecture, Art and Design at Tec de Monterrey, in particular, S. Raúl Silva and David Roque.

The editors also wish to thank the Center for Sustainable Urban Development (CEDEUS) and the Institute of Geography and the Center for Asian Studies of the Pontificia Universidad Catolica de Chile for their support. We are especially grateful to the Fudan Development Institute at Fudan University in Shanghai, China, in particular to Dr. Zhang Yi, Executive Vice Dean, and Dr. Chen Yinzhang, General Secretary, for their support in creating this research and collaboration network between Latin America and Asia. Finally, we thank our families for their support and patience, especially during our long hours of absence.

Guadalajara, Mexico Miguel A. Montoya
Ciudad de Mexico, Mexico Aleksandra Krstikj
Santiago, Chile Johannes Rehner
Guadalajara, Mexico Daniel Lemus-Delgado

Contents

Contributors

David Arboleda Universidad de los Andes, Cundinamarca, Colombia

Ana Laura Azparren Almeira Facultad de Ciencias Sociales, Universidad de Buenos Aires, Buenos Aires, Argentina

Stefania Biondi Tecnológico de Monterrey, Escuela de Arquitectura, Arte y Diseño, Querétaro, Mexico

Giaime Botti Department of Architecture and Built Environment & Centre for Sustainable Energy Technologies (CSET), University of Nottingham, Ningbo, China

Sofía Boza Faculty of Agricultural Sciences and Institute of International Studies, University of Chile, Santiago, Chile

Carlos Cerda School of Social Sciences and Government, Tecnológico de Monterrey, Guadalajara, Mexico

Ali Cheshmehzangi Department of Architecture and Built Environment & Centre for Sustainable Energy Technologies (CSET), University of Nottingham, Ningbo, China

Carlos Cobreros Tecnológico de Monterrey, Escuela de Arquitectura, Arte y Diseño, Querétaro, Mexico

Moises Gerardo Contreras Ruiz Esparza Instituto de Ingeniería, Universidad Nacional Autónoma de México, Mexico City, México

Rafael de Souza Salomão Architect and Urbanist, Campinas, SP, Brazil

Roberto L. do Carmo University of Campinas, São Paulo, Brazil

Rodrigo Durán López Universidad Anáhuac México, Naucalpan, Mexico

Ana Paula Emídio Universidade Federal de Minas Gerais, Belo Horizonte, Brazil

Mariana Flores-García Tecnológico de Monterrey, Escuela de Arquitectura, Arte y Diseño, Querétaro, Mexico

Giovanna Gastaldo Cifoni Architect and Urbanist, Campinas, SP, Brazil

Miguel Angel Gil Robles Jönköping International Business School, Jönköping University, Jönköping, Sweden

Emanuele Giorgi Tecnologico de Monterrey, School of Architecture, Art and Design, Chihuahua, Mexico

Ana Maria Girotti Sperandio Faculty of Civil Engineering and Architecture, University of Campinas, Campinas, SP, Brazil

Tommaso Gravante Centro de Investigaciones Interdisciplinarias en Ciencias y Humanidades, Universidad Nacional Autónoma de México, Ciudad de México, México

Mariana Hase Ueta University of Campinas, São Paulo, Brazil

Hisako Koura Graduate School of Arts and Design, Kobe Design University, Kobe, Japan

Aleksandra Krstikj School of Architecture, Art and Design, Tecnológico de Monterrey, Ciudad de Mexico, Mexico

Salvador Leetoy Escuela de Humanidades y Educación, Tecnologico de Monterrey, Guadalajara, Mexico

Daniel Lemus-Delgado School of Social Sciences and Government, Tecnológico de Monterrey, Guadalajara, Mexico

Evgenia Likhovtseva Trinity College Dublin, Dublin, Ireland

Eugenio Mangi Department of Architecture and Built Environment & Centre for Sustainable Energy Technologies (CSET), University of Nottingham, Ningbo, China

Lucía Martín López Tecnologico de Monterrey, School of Architecture, Art and Design, Querétaro, Mexico

Ana Luíza Matos de Oliveira FLACSO, São Paulo, Brazil

Mariana Maya Tecnológico de Monterrey, Escuela de Arquitectura, Arte y Diseño, Querétaro, Mexico

Miguel A. Montoya School of Architecture, Art and Design, Tecnológico de Monterrey, Guadalajara, Mexico

Elsa N. Ontiveros-Ortíz Tecnológico de Monterrey, Escuela de Ciencias Sociales y Gobierno, Querétaro, Mexico

Elsa A. Pérez-Paredes División de Ciencias Sociales, Licenciatura en Políticas y Proyectos Sociales, Universidad Abierta y a Distancia de México, México City, México

Johannes Rehner Institute of Geography, Pontificia, Universidad Católica de Chile, Santiago, Chile

Yuan Ren School of Social Development and Public Policy, Institute of Population Research, Fudan University, Shanghai, China

Beatriz Alejandra Sanchez-Jimenez Instituto Mexicano del Seguro Social, Centro Medico Nacional La Raza, Mexico City, Mexico

Augusto F. J. Schmidt University of Campinas, São Paulo, Brazil

Erick Tjong World Bank, Washington, DC, USA

Angela Alessandra Torezan Silingardi Architect and Urbanist, Safety Engineer, Campinas, SP, Brazil

Francisco Valderrey Tecnologico de Monterrey, Monterrey, Mexico

Meng Wang Department of Public Administration, Zhejiang University of Finance and Economics, Hangzhou, China

Niklas W. Weins University of Campinas, São Paulo, Brazil

Andrés Zambrano Universidad de los Andes, Cundinamarca, Colombia

About the Editors

Miguel A. Montoya has a Ph.D. in applied economics at the Universidad Autonoma de Barcelona, Spain. He is tenure professor in the Tecnologico de Monterrey. He is part of the Mexican Academy of Sciences, National Council for Technology and Science (CONACYT-Mexico), and Academy of International Business, among others. He has published articles in academic journals and book chapters, and he has participated in different academic conferences. He is coeditor of two Cambridge University Press books, *Mexican Multinationals: Building Multinationals in Emerging Markets* (2018) and *Innovations for the Middle of the Pyramid in Emerging Economies* (2021), and he also edited *China and Latin America Paths to Overcoming the Middle-Income Trap* (2018) for Fudan Development Institute (China). Dr. Montoya teaches courses on international economics and business at Tecnologico de Monterrey and, as a visitor professor, at Darla Moore School of Business (University of South Carolina, USA), ESAN (Peru), Universidad de San Francisco de Quito (Ecuador), Instituto Ortega y Gasset (Spain), Burdeaux School of Business, and Montpellier Business School (France). He is a founding member of the Fudan-Latin America University Consortium (FLAUC).

Johannes Rehner is a full professor at the Institute of Geography at the Pontificia Universidad Católica de Chile and a member of the Center for Asian Studies (CEAUC). He studied geography at Ludwig-Maximilians-Universität Munich, Germany, where he also obtained his Ph.D. (Dr. Oec. Publ.) in 2003. He worked at Ludwig Maximilians-Universität in Munich as a researcher and teacher (Wiss. Mitarbeiter) from 1998 to 2003, and as assistant professor (Wiss. Assistant) from 2003 to 2007. Between 2009 and 2017, he was associate professor at the Institute of Geography, Pontificia Universidad Católica de Chile, and since 2018, he has been a professor at this University. In 2019, he assumed the role of deputy director of the Institute of Geography. He also served as director of the Center for Asian Studies, Pontificia Universidad Católica de Chile (2016–2020), and as a consultant to the United Nations ECLAC in Santiago de Chile (2008–2014). He participates in various international collaborations such as: the FLAUC network (led by Fudan University, China), cooperation with the University of Heidelberg (Germany) in the field of natural resource governance and risk, an international research project on responsible research and innovation in salmon farming with the Western Norwegian University of Applied Sciences, and, in the past, a project with the Victoria University of Wellington (New Zealand) on ethical value chains. His main research topics are economic geography, Asian studies, and sustainable urban development, and he participated in several research projects: as associate researcher at the Center for Sustainable Urban Development (CEDEUS; FONDAP No. 15110020; funded by the Research Council of Chile Conicyt; 2013–2022), as principal investigator of a project on the local impacts of the export boom and the global crisis in Chile, and as principal investigator of a project on trade relations between Chile and Asia. He has published numerous articles, book chapters, and a book in the field of economic geography, relations between Latin America and Asia, urban economics, and sustainable development.

Aleksandra Krstikj is a full-time research professor in the School of Architecture, Art and Design at Tec de Monterrey. She is leading the national research group "Sustainable Territorial Development," where she organizes a monthly research seminar and coordinates research projects. She has a master's degree in architectural engineering from the Kyoto Institute of Technology and a doctorate from the Osaka University's School of Engineering. Her research focuses on sustainable land use, spatial equity, and urban conservation of historic centers, with a total of 10 years' research experience. She has active research collaborations with researchers from Design University Kobe (Japan), University of Colorado Boulder (USA), Zhejiang University of Finance and Economics (China), and UNAM (Mexico). She has published her work in the best international scientific journals such as *Habitat International* and the Journal of Asian Architecture and Building Engineering. Dr. Krstikj is a member of the National System of Researchers of Mexico and the Architectural Institute of Japan. Dr. Krstikj is coordinating the cluster Urbanism in the framework of Tec's Think Tank Post Covid-19 focused on recovery and urban development post COVID-19.

Daniel Lemus-Delgado has a Ph.D. in Trans-Pacific International Relations, University of Colima, México. He is a member of the National System of Researchers, level II (period 2018–2021). He participates in the Pacific Economic Cooperation Council (Mexico Section), the International Studies Association, the Mexican Network for International Development Cooperation, and the Fudan Latin America University Consortium. At the present, he is an international associate researcher for the period 2020–2022 at Fudan University. Also, he is a professor in the School of Social Sciences and Government, Tecnologico de Monterrey. His research includes foreign policy, international cooperation for development, and regional innovation systems focused on East Asia.

Chapter 1
COVID-19, Resilience, and Cities: A Conceptual Introduction

Aleksandra Krstikj, Johannes Rehner, Daniel Lemus-Delgado, and Miguel A. Montoya

> The impacts of the responses to COVID-19, as with historical responses to public health crises such as Ebola (in 2014), H1N1 (in 2009) or SARS (in 2003) – or even further back historically, the cholera pandemics in cities (for example in London and New York in the mid-19th century) – are filtering through to the built environment design, planning and building processes. (Gupte & Mitlin, 2020, p. 10)

The COVID-19 pandemic exposed many of the structural weaknesses of the contemporary world and accentuated already existing risks, such as social inequity and exclusion, the digital divide within countries, and some tendencies toward nationalism and authoritarianism. In many institutional settings it became even more evident that the economic and social systems do not protect the quality of human life but rather tend to deepen income gaps and heighten the risks of unforeseen events for the well-being of the majority. Nevertheless, cities have often played a crucial role as an integrating spatial system in the development of mankind.

The restrictions imposed to prevent the spread of SARS-Cov2 had a huge impact on global economic growth. As noted by the World Bank (2020a): "COVID-19 has triggered a global crisis like no other – a global health crisis that, in addition to an enormous human toll, is leading to the deepest global recession since the Second World War." The outbreak mainly affected the poorest and most vulnerable people

A. Krstikj (✉)
School of Architecture, Art and Design, Tecnológico de Monterrey, Ciudad de Mexico, Mexico
e-mail: sandra.krstik@tec.mx

J. Rehner
Institute of Geography, Pontificia, Universidad Católica de Chile, Santiago, Chile

D. Lemus-Delgado
School of Social Science and Government, Tecnológico de Monterrey, Guadalajara, Mexico

M. A. Montoya
School of Architecture, Art and Design, Tecnológico de Monterrey, Guadalajara, Mexico
e-mail: mmontoya@tec.mx

© The Author(s), under exclusive license to Springer Nature Switzerland AG 2021
M. A. Montoya et al. (eds.), *COVID-19 and Cities*, The Urban Book Series,
https://doi.org/10.1007/978-3-030-84134-8_1

on the planet and pushed millions of people into poverty. In 2020, after decades of constant progress in reducing extreme poverty, this type of poverty increased. According to the World Bank (2020b), the COVID-19 crisis drove more than 88 million people into extreme poverty. Additionally, the economic slowdown had a deep impact on businesses and jobs. The micro, small, and medium enterprises, mostly in the developing world, experienced intense pressure to survive. At the same time, the pandemic highlighted the need for an effective, accessible, and affordable health care system. Furthermore, at the height of the lockdown, more than 160 countries had required different forms of school closures that affected at least 1.5 billion students and their opportunities to learn and improve their hopes for a better future (Blake & Wadhwa, 2020). Finally, gender gaps may widen as a result of the pandemic, reversing decades of progress made by women. However, how we respond to COVID-19 can help strengthen our ability to cope with risks and shocks in the future. This pandemic is also a unique opportunity to rethink how cities can be more sustainable, inclusive, and resilient spaces.

History shows that cities can innovate and change profoundly in response to disasters or after suffering an intense crisis such as a pandemic. In many cases, cities evolve to become improved urban systems, as literature based on the resilience perspective suggests (e.g., Cheshmehzangi, 2020). For instance, sewage systems, garbage disposal arrangements, public parks, urban zoning plans, and even the regulation of agriculture within urban areas were often introduced or upgraded as a response to catastrophic episodes of the spread of a disease (Brinkley & Vitiello, 2013). The current COVID-19 pandemic has been described as "the greatest challenge that humankind has faced since the Second World War" (Chakraborty & Maity, 2020). In the context of this extraordinary year, researchers are recalling the capacities of cities to respond and improve their internal structures and are engaging in discussions on how the experiences of managing the current COVID-19 pandemic may change cities (Klaus, June 2020; 2020a; 2020b).

The pandemic has opened a new debate about some of the most challenging issues of city planning and management: density and physical proximity between people in the urban space, poor housing conditions, urban poverty and inequality, lack of public policies for mitigation and crisis control, deficient access to urban public services, to name a few. According to Gupte and Mitlin (2020, p. 2) the debate is "fueling a misinterpretation of the nature of social relationships that produce and sustain agglomeration." They warn against short-cut arguments that link density with virus propagation in a straightforward manner and urge for consideration of the systemic nature of urban conglomerations that demands analysis of the context and circumstances of transmission, overcrowding, lack of services, etc., rather than solely population density (Gupte & Mitlin, 2020, p. 9). On the other hand, the mere concentration of a population and close interactions that are fundamental to urban life require rapid responses from both governmental management and civil daily praxis to adapt the urban system to the current stress brought about by COVID-19.

Recent literature has increasingly addressed the specific link between urbanization and emerging infectious diseases (Connolly et al., 2020; Wolf, 2016). The booming interest in topics that link space, society, and the pandemic has led to special issues in journals such as *Urban Studies, Cities,* and the *Journal of Urban*

Management, as well as from disciplinary fields like geography (Aalbers et al., 2020; Rose-Redwood et al., 2020; Spark & Anguelov, 2020). Besides socioeconomic impacts, challenges to managing the crisis and related governance issues, impacts on transportation and urban design, and environmental effects have been addressed in the first few months of the pandemic (Sharifi & Khavarian-Garmsir, 2020). Nevertheless, while significant research has been produced on air and water quality and meteorological parameters, the remaining aspects are still underexplored (Sharifi & Khavarian-Garmsir, 2020). The book "Covid-19 and Cities" addresses the gap in the academic literature on the particular role of cities in facing the current pandemic, especially concerning their adaptation to the pandemic and long-term impacts from a resilience and sustainability perspective – a field that still needs conceptual development and empirical inputs (Allam & Jones, 2020; Cohen, 2020; Corburn et al., 2020).

The concept of resilience is helpful to address the topics of how cities face disasters and how they adapt or evolve into more resistant systems. We refer to an evolutionary concept of resilience that goes beyond the understanding of resilience as a capacity of a system to bounce back to its initial state after an external shock, or to absorb external pressure without losing its functionality and stability, as discussed for instance by Beilin and Wilkinson (2015), Davoudi (2012), and Folke (2006). Instead, we rely on the evolutionary understanding of resilience (Brunetti et al., 2019; Davoudi, 2012) that focuses on how a system evolves in response to external shock: *"Hence, resilience involves a dynamic process of `bouncing forward´, which provides for the adaptation and constant reinvention needed to innovate and to do new things"* (Shaw, 2012, p. 309). Recent studies have shown that evolutionary resilience has gained importance among diverse understandings of resilience, being particularly important in the field of urban planning (Chelleri & Baravikova, 2021). Such a concept also implies a paradigm shift as it challenges any linear assumption, common in planning theory and praxis (Shaw, 2012, p. 311).

Currently, and from a mid-term perspective, cities are facing several profound crises as an immediate impact that is likely to result in cities retroceding in terms of development indicators, eroding progress achieved over the last few decades. The simultaneous crises caused by COVID-19 are calling for a critical reflection on the structural foundations of cities and creating the necessity for the generation of a broad citizen debate on many aspects of city management, such as urban planning, care and responsibility for vulnerable people, community-oriented development, environmental challenges, and the global nature of certain crises that demands international cooperation. This crisis is also an opportunity to think about possible political action focused on the common good, the right to the city, and new economic proposals for the transformation of the capital–labor relationship, emphasizing activities that guarantee the right to a good life. While urban spaces are aiming for more sustainable development in the twenty-first century, perspectives like the ecological footprint and social integration have become key aspects of urban design and policy; nevertheless, the current pandemic requires social distancing and thus implicitly promotes individual mobilization and many practices that tend to be excluding, challenging established scenarios and opportunities for sustainability.

Furthermore, the immediate responses to the pandemic generate expectations that communication technologies, artificial intelligence, and home-office arrangements will probably alter the world of labor more quickly than previously expected. Impacts on urban design and the built environment in cities are also expected (Megahed & Gonheim, 2020) but are yet to be identified.

This book aims to share experiences of how cities are facing and responding to the pandemic crisis; in what possible directions cities could evolve as a consequence of this traumatic experience; what strategies are implemented by which agents, individuals, and groups; what institutional and structural ruptures and developments can be observed; and what kind of practices seem successful or promising, and relate those lessons to inputs for facing uncertainties in future sustainable urban development.

The Starting Point (and Beyond)

On December 31, 2019, the Wuhan Municipal Health Commission informed the WHO about an outbreak of 27 cases of a disease similar to pneumonia that originated in the seafood market of the city (World Health Organization, 2020a). On January 5, 2020, the Chinese government announced the origin of a new type of coronavirus, different from SARS or MERS (Wang et al., 2020). Some days later, President Xi affirmed that the epidemic was: "fast-spreading and very difficult to prevent and control." As a consequence, the new virus was the most critical health problem in the history of the People's Republic of China (Zheng, 2020). On January 22, the authorities imposed a strict quarantine that confined more than 40 million residents of the Hubei Province for several weeks (Graham-Harrison & Kuo, 2020). Among other measures, train and plane travel were canceled and the city's highways and roads were closed (Yu & Li, 2020). Soon, the same measures taken in Wuhan were repeated throughout China.

On January 30, 1 month after the new virus was officially reported by the Chinese authorities, the World Health Organization (WHO) declared the new coronavirus a global emergency (World Health Organization, 2020b). On the same day, 170 deaths and 7711 cases in China were reported (Chinese Center for Disease Control and Prevention, 2020). The new illness was called 'Coronavirus Disease 2019' (COVID-19) by the World Health Organization, and the virus that causes it was called 'Severe Acute Respiratory Syndrome Coronavirus 2' (SARS-CoV-2) (Roser et al., 2020).

Six months after the official recognition of the new outbreak, the problem caused by COVID-19 was considered a global crisis. On June 1, 6.12 million cases of infection and 372,418 deaths caused by COVID-19 were confirmed worldwide (European Centre for Disease Prevention and Control, 2020). According to the WHO, by December 2020, a cumulative total of about 70 million cases and more than 1.5 million deaths had been reported since the start of the outbreak. Because SARS-CoV-2 was a new virus, people had no immunity to it. Thus, compared to the closely related coronaviruses SARS and MERS, the outbreak of COVID-19 is much more serious due to its high virulence (Deng, 2020). The rapid spread into a pandemic is a result of growing globalization, mainly propelled through urban conglomerates. The epicenter of the new disease had moved from China, Korea, and Japan, where the first cases appeared, to Europe and the USA, and later spread worldwide, exceeding the international community's capacity to contain the outbreak. This was followed by different waves that devastated societies all around the world.

Images of paralyzed cities, empty squares, closed schools and universities, canceled religious services, stationary public transport, closed airports, and suspended non-essential economic activities displayed the vulnerability of societies. Hundreds of millions of people in Asia, Europe, and the Americas were confined due to unprecedented large-scale lockdowns. Emblematic cities such as Rome, Madrid, New York, London, Mexico City, and Lima were brought to a standstill to cut the chain of transmission of the virus. By March 2020, more than 90 countries or territories and 3.9 billion people worldwide had been asked or ordered by their governments to stay at home to prevent the spread of the deadly COVID-19 disease (Sandford, 2020). The frenetic and pulsating twenty-first-century cities in which the lives of millions of people converged, turned cold, deserted, empty, and desolate. The virus revealed the structural weaknesses of cities.

The extraordinary speed of scientific advances made it possible to decipher the genetic sequence of the virus quickly, clarifying the track of its mutations as it spread (John Hopkins University, 2020). Additionally, it was soon possible to recognize the characteristics of the virus, its forms of contagion, the way to contain its spread, the most vulnerable populations, and symptoms and development of the new disease. It soon became clear that without a vaccine and effective treatment for the disease, returning to pre-COVID-19 conditions and ways of social interaction was impossible. An effective vaccine was considered the best option for ending the pandemic (Lurie et al., 2020), and after roughly a year, by the end of 2020, vaccinations had started in some countries. In the first trimester of 2021, several countries achieved important progress in massive vaccination campaigns, hoping for effective results.

Unleashing Multiple Crises

As the new disease spread to countries with weaker health systems, the direct and indirect impact of the pandemic was more profound. Highly unequal cities with weak social protection networks revealed that the virus had socially unequal effects, impacting more dramatically families in overcrowded living conditions, informal workers, and households with no financial reserves to rely on. The experiences of outbreaks in different cities showed the difficulties related to effective confinement, since people gradually started to return to daily activities. Disgruntled citizens of Berlin, for example, turned to public protests against coronavirus curbs (Manancourt, 2020). It became evident that citizens played a critical role in containing the virus.

The impact of COVID-19 then goes far beyond a health crisis, as we can identify three different crises generated simultaneously by the pandemic. Firstly, there is the health crisis that directly affected the functioning of urban systems. In many countries, health systems have been stifled by budget constraints and privatization of the medical sector. This situation is present both in some developed countries, such as Italy and Spain, and in developing nations, such as Chile, Ecuador, and Mexico. In most cases, the social protection system, worn down over the years by policies that privileged the maximization of economic benefit over general welfare, showed extreme gaps. The world watched with sadness and incredulity at the tragic scenes of overflowing hospitals with a lack of sufficient personnel, insufficient protection material, and a lack of palliative drugs, which resulted in their incapacity to save the most vulnerable. In some cities, such as New York, Madrid, and Milan, the growth of infections was so rapid that doctors could not properly care for the sick and many people died without even being able to get proper hospital treatment.

Nevertheless, these direct health impacts are often distributed unevenly within the cities. Urban inequality translates into diverse groups of people being affected differently by the pandemic: in New York City, for example, richer neighborhoods in Manhattan showed the lowest per capita rates of COVID-19 infection; meanwhile poorer neighborhoods, particularly in Queens, had the highest rates. Belonging to the African-American community increases the probability of infection several times over compared to the white population (Dobkin & Gottehrer-Cohen, 2020). While all cities display some level of inequality, the outbreak probably exacerbated the existing gaps (Gupte & Mitlin, 2020, p. 2), not only due to different levels of exposure, and thus the probability of getting ill, but also as health service inequities influence the possibilities of overcoming the virus, correlating with income strata and ethnic group or race. Therefore, the health crisis is deeply altering the way urban societies work and live together. Important impacts on intra-metropolitan travel frequency have also been observed (e.g., for Hong Kong by Zhang et al., 2021).

The second crisis is economic. According to the International Monetary Fund (IMF), COVID-19 generated a deep recession in the world economy. The forecast made in October 2020 estimated a global growth of −4.4% in 2020 and warned about the adverse impact on low-income households, jeopardizing the significant progress made in reducing extreme poverty in the world since the 1990s (IMF, 2020). The growth projection for 2020 in the United States was −4.3%; the Euro Area, −8.3%; the UK, −9.8%; Japan, −5.3%; Russia, −4.1%; Brazil, −5.8%; Mexico, −9%; India, −10.3%; the Middle East and Central Asia, −4.1%; the ASEAN, −5 to 3.4%; and the Sub-Saharan Africa, −3%. China could have a marginal growth of 1.9% (IMF, 2020). The necessary lockdowns have had an obvious impact on economic activities although there is a recent discussion on possibilities to mitigate such adverse effects (Rahman et al., 2020). While vaccine approvals have raised hopes of a shift in the pandemic, the possibilities of new waves and the emergence of new variants of the coronavirus generate exceptional uncertainty about the future of the global economy. The International Monetary Fund projected that the world economy will grow by 5.5% 2021 and 4.2% in 2022 (IMF, 2020).

Behind this stark macroeconomic data, the pandemic has meant that millions, especially of informal workers, need to expose themselves to risk through working on the streets to survive. Precarious contracts and lack of social protection leave many of them without alternatives. Social distancing can never prevent all contagions, but individuals can play a critical role in slowing the spread of the coronavirus (Pearls, 2020). However, in Latin American countries, where many people work in the informal economy, responding to the request for social distancing to contain the spread of the virus was an impossible task. Thus, the harsh reality of the economic precariousness in many urban areas prevented efficient virus containment among the most vulnerable sectors of the population.

Severe impact on income and livelihoods, especially of the poor, have already been observed (Gupte & Mitlin, 2020, p. 12). Linkages between the magnitude of the pandemic impacts and different spheres of informality in Latin America have also been well reported (Duque Franco et al., 2020). Recent studies at the Center for Urban Sustainable Development in Chile (CEDEUS) also show how socio-spatial segregation in Santiago de Chile is linked to precarious work, concentrating on workers with an uncertain contractual situation and informal employment in poorer areas that have an infrastructural deficit and can be considered a periphery. In these neighborhoods, a higher percentage of workers engage in low qualification service jobs. Such conditions are typical for big cities in Latin America and the impact of the pandemic on the labor market are likely to be greater for low-qualified, informal, and unprotected jobs, thus potentially increasing inequity considerably (Weller, 2020). Marginalized neighborhoods suffer a greater economic impact from the lockdowns as their income completely relies on their day-to-day presence on the streets. Therefore, the economic impact of lockdowns, without comprehensive support measures, is deepening the social divide in Latin-American metropolises. Providing food security and public health to poor neighborhoods became critical in some cities and is accounting for almost two-thirds of the community-oriented emergency initiatives in Latin America, as reported by Duque Franco et al. (2020, p. 535).

The third crisis is political, reflected both in the domestic issues of each country and in international politics. Political regimes have been questioned regarding their ability to manage the crisis, with fissures abounding between supporters and opponents of governments, such as that of Bolsonaro in Brazil, Trump in the United States, Modi in India, and López Obrador in Mexico. These cases have highlighted the impossibility of reaching the minimum political agreements that would allow the assumption of a state policy to face the health crisis, stop the contagion, and reactivate the economy. In some cases, leaders of countries have adopted a "hands-off" policy, even discouraging citizens from following public health measures taken in other countries (Blackburn & Ruyle, 2020). With these "policies" corresponding in fact to the activities of the nation-state, it meant that on many occasions it fell to governors of sub-national entities or mayors to enforce proper measures. In the context of the previous pandemic (SARS), there have been claims that different approaches to urban governance are needed to face the challenges that emerging infectious diseases put on global cities, particularly highlighting the role of local governance (Keil & Ali, 2007).

Another way in which the political crisis caused by COVID-19 manifests itself is in the international system. The pandemic exacerbated the crisis in the multilateral system and increased tensions and brutal competition between the two main world economies, the United States and China. Our global governance system, based on states and multilateral organizations, proved unable to establish minimum international cooperation. The response of many national governments was authoritarianism that sought to centralize political decisions. In turn, a considerable failure of multinational and supranational organizations is their inability to order a collective response to the crisis, privileging the internal positions of each country while many countries withdrew and decreed the closure of borders unilaterally. To fill such a void, calls have been made for strengthening network-based governance models linking cities and communities (Bai et al., 2020).

The pandemic is indisputably a global crisis; however, the main areas affected are cities, but cities are also places where solutions to challenges are sought. Thus, thinking about cities is a fundamental task to secure the future of humanity. It is possible to affirm that we are living in an unprecedented historical moment, characterized by generalized global unemployment that slowed down the dynamics of cities. The huge political and economic governance system gap that COVID-19 amplified must be remedied by cities and citizens. The great challenge is to build or consolidate a guarantor state in a stage of advanced participatory democracy, new governance, and international action for solidarity and cooperation, to overcome the COVID crisis. For this to be possible, it is essential to think about actions from the viewpoint of city development. Cities have the capacity to generate resources, contribute knowledge, and create technological innovations to overcome the current crisis.

Resilience as a Unifying Concept

The concept of resilience is used in many disciplines, but there is no common definition recognized by all scholars. In these definitions, distinct factors are emphasized, but all of them point in general to the constant ability of an individual, community, or system, to adapt to any sort of disturbance so that these entities can continue to operate, or rapidly recuperate its ability to function, during and after stress (National Research Council, 2011). The general idea of resilience addresses the question of how a system deals with external shocks or exceptional pressures. In this book, we assume the idea of resilience as proposed by Paton (2006, p. 7) concerning "how well people and societies can adapt and change reality and capitalize on the new possibilities." In the context of the pandemic, it is of special interest how cities, as complex systems, not only manage an emergency but also evolve in response to such a crisis. The quote opening this introductory chapter announces the historical experiences of improving structural urban elements due to a health crisis.

Thus, relying on the idea of "resilience" appears to be the obvious choice when discussing urban system challenges and responses to crises from different disciplines and with diverse theoretical and empirical approaches.

Labels like "urban resilience," "climate resilience," "governance for resilience," and several other varieties of the "resilience" concept became *en vogue* at the beginning of the new millennium, replacing, in part, or complementing the concept of "sustainability." Urban resilience has often been used to discuss and manage cities' adaptation to climate change and disaster risk management, but more recently, urban resilience has been conceptually developed into a perspective on very different challenges of cities, closely linked to sustainability (Chelleri et al., 2015). Therefore, concepts like "sustainability" and "resilience" are both bearing the risk of becoming a buzzword of inaccurate academic use and serving political discourses, sometimes even those of ideologically contradicting purposes (Davoudi, 2012). The concept of resilience, however, has the advantage of being politically relevant, as "much of the appeal of the term lies in it being sufficiently malleable to cut across the so-called 'grey area' between academic, policy and practice discourse" (Shaw, 2012). Moreover, resilience has been increasingly gaining importance in urban governance, since it allows for consideration of the complexity and multidisciplinary nature of city planning and management. Nevertheless, "urban resilience" is often applied and used in a very similar manner as general "human development" issues or "sustainable development," based on indicators that are supposed to enhance resilience rather than evaluating the adaptation/transformation itself (e.g., see recent papers on *Urban Resilience and Covid*, Chen & Quan, 2021). "Resilience" and "sustainability" should be understood as different but complementary concepts (Elmqvist et al., 2019), especially regarding their overall goals, although there is no clear consensus about how these two concepts relate in detail (Chelleri & Baravikova, 2021).

We consider "resilience" a helpful concept since it possesses the virtue to be sufficiently open to allow for contributions from very different disciplines and perspectives, as long as a clear distinction between different meanings is made. Different traditions of understanding resilience in several academic disciplines and different historical moments have been described, referring to central concepts, such as "recovery," "return," or "bouncing back" vs. "absorption" or "adaptation" vs. "transition/transformation" (Simone et al., 2021, p. 2). Frequently, a simple distinction between three main concepts of resilience is used in the context of urban planning, reflected in the following major perspectives:

1. An "engineering" perspective on resilience referring to "the ability of a system to return to an equilibrium or steady-state after a disturbance" (Davoudi, 2012), where the recovery time is the critical indicator of resilience.
2. An "ecological" tradition in resilience is understood as "the magnitude of the disturbance that can be absorbed before the system changes its structure" (Davoudi, 2012). A rather early conceptual contribution by Adger (2000, p. 349) points out that such an ecology-based concept of resilience, oriented to stability and the understanding of resilience as a buffer able to absorb external shocks,

constitutes a certain contradiction to the idea of the transformation and evolution of complex systems – a criticism that is addressed by the following perspective.

3. An "evolutionary" perspective, also preferred in this book, includes the capacity for change and transformation in response to intense disturbances, as a key element of urban resilience (Simone et al., 2021). When understood as a capacity for evolving, resilience can be an important input for achieving more sustainable cities, as it can contribute to the transformation of urban systems for more equitable, inclusive, and just societies. Evolutionary resilience can be defined as follows:

> In this perspective, resilience is not conceived of as a return to normality, but rather as the ability of complex socio-ecological systems to change, adapt, and, crucially, transform in response to stresses and strains. (Davoudi, 2012, p. 302)

Some major criticism has focused on the observation that resilience concepts derived from the ecological and/or engineering understanding tend to be conservative in the sense of "bouncing back" and recovery of a previous state, thus not being able to properly conceptualize the system's capacity to change and possibly improve. Applying an evolutionary perspective offers the possibility to systematically include the perspective of transformation and analyze how systems adapt and consequently evolve. It has to be recognized that the current interpretation of socio-ecological systems (SES) also considers the aspect of learning, renewal, reorganization, innovation, and development aftershocks as turning points, and thus include the perspective of transformation that produces fundamental and nonlinear progressive changes addressing multiple risks (Folke, 2006; Meerow & Newell, 2019). On the other hand, Brunetti et al. (2019) refer to "territorial resilience as an emerging concept capable of aiding the decision-making process of identifying vulnerabilities and improving the transformation of socio-ecological and technological systems (SETSs)." They conceive urban and territorial resilience as the co-evolutive property of a system, where the emphasis is upon urban planning, anticipatory approaches, recognizing pre-existing governance models, historical interaction of communities, and risks. By dedicating more attention to the temporal aspects, transformation can also be seen as the last stage, after recovery and adaptation (Chelleri et al., 2015), bearing the most long-term implications. An evolutionary perspective is, furthermore, offering the possibility to consider extraordinary events as well as transformations that occur under long-term micro-pressures.

The perspective of evolutionary resilience offers the possibility of a critical approach to the concept of the evolution of a system in the sense that while a system is becoming more resistant, it does not necessarily mean it is also improving – at least not all of the elements of a system. Evolutionary perspectives necessarily consider the possibility of causing damage to certain parts of the system (remembering the principle of "selection") and thus also offer the possibility to consider often neglected trade-offs in the resilience discussion (Chelleri et al., 2015). Resilience can also conflict with sustainability goals (Elmqvist et al., 2019). This is a critical issue when using resilience to define public policy; the improvement of an urban system by damaging certain parts of society is not acceptable, and not only from a sustainability perspective. Furthermore, scale and space are critical issues from this viewpoint: "addressing resilience on one scale alone may lead to an erosion of adaptive capacities at another" (Chelleri et al., 2015, p. 194). What could be considered an improvement in terms of urban resilience has yet to be critically discussed. In this context, the concept of "resilience resistance" has also been used to refer to the process of developing "barriers to change, flexibility, and adaptability through implementation" (Shamsuddin, 2020, p. 1); by discussing an evolutionary process such barriers can be properly considered in theoretical terms.

Another field of major criticism targets the translation of resilience into policy and development programs, identifying conceptual misunderstandings as well as practical shortcomings. For instance, the frequent dominance of checklist-like approaches to resilience, which are trying to guide urban policy, mostly become technical and reductionist. A more systematical approach to analyzing resilience policies is necessary (Meerow & Newell, 2019). Such critique is pleading for an integrated, holistic approach, respecting different types of knowledge and experiences available within the urban system, and thus applying resilience in a meaningful, context-specific manner (Weichselgartner & Kelman, 2015). Furthermore, it has been stated that resilience policies tend to be a technical, external, top-down approach, rather than a concept able to rely on social relations within a certain place. These authors, therefore, propose the use of resourcefulness rather than resilience (MacKinnon & Driscoll, 2012). The technological approach has also been questioned, as it is not necessarily contributing to more inclusive cities and thus may have fewer positive impacts for disadvantaged urban residents (Gupte & Mitlin, 2020, p. 2). It also fails to recognize different types of knowledge. Urban resilience is expected to rely strongly on local and traditional knowledge, an "evolutionary" perspective helps to address these shortcomings at least in theoretical terms.

Academic literature on the concept of resilience, experienced accelerated growth since the beginning of the millennium, emphasizing the transformational or, as we prefer, the evolutionary understanding of resilience; a recent growing interest in urban resilience has also been observed (Meerow & Newell, 2019; Sharifi, 2020; Wang et al., 2018). In general, cities have been considered more resilient if they are inclusive, integrated, flexible, resourceful, robust, redundant, and reflective (Simone et al., 2021, pp. 3–4). Such studies build links between structural elements and resilience, but also frequently use relational or community approaches to discuss their importance for resilience. For instance, in the context of the structural argument, it has been stated that there is considerable evidence for a positive influence of urban design features on climate change adaptation (Sharifi, 2019). On the other hand, social conflicts are also related to such elements on the local scale, possibly limiting resilience in other regards. Others focus on economic resilience, understanding it mainly as the capacity to bounce back ("destination recovery"), and discussing the current pandemic from the experience of Macao, which shows how certain structural elements, in combination with some institutional framework characteristics, foster recovery (McCartney et al., 2021). Some scholars argue that most attention in resilience literature "has been paid to infrastructural, institutional, and environmental aspects at the expense of social and economic dimensions" (Sharifi, 2020).

From a network and system analysis approach to urban governance, there is an understanding of cities as a complex adaptive system, where collaboration in networks is considered a crucial factor in building resilience (Bixler et al., 2020; Shi et al., 2021). Reviews of studies on urban community resilience initiatives in the context of COVID-19 also highlight that resilience builds strongly on "social capital" and focuses on how governance processes in such community-based initiatives are organized, proposing to go beyond the classical top-down vs. bottom-up dichotomy (Fransen et al., 2021).

Faced with the threats of COVID-19, this network perspective becomes particularly relevant as local institutions and the underlying values, such as proximity, community, social inclusion, human security, and well-being, are transforming into key aspects in facing the challenges posed by the new coronavirus. For instance, it has been identified that civil society, through different organizations, responded to marginalized neighborhoods in a very significant way, although it has been mostly limited to food security and the provision of health services (Duque Franco et al., 2020, p. 523). Nevertheless, there are persisting major gaps in "assessing resilience against socio-economic and health risks (e.g., economic recession and pandemics such as COVID-19)" (Sharifi, 2020).

The resilience approach has experienced a certain recovery, after serious criticism in the last few years, being considered particularly relevant to study situations such as the COVID-19 pandemic (Shamsuddin, 2020). From this perspective, a variety of questions emerge, such as: how to move from the crowded city to a city that reflects a sustainable balance; how to harmonize the city with nature and the territory; how to make the city an inclusive space where respect for human rights dominates; how to place life and care for people at the center; how to make healthy cities; how to establish true human security; and how to change the logic of production, consumption, and abuse of resources, among others. The pandemic opens up the opportunity to rethink the urban system, putting people at the center of development.

The alleged lack of a clear or unique definition of what resilience means, and how this lack makes it difficult to transform the academic concept of resilience into clear guidelines for planning praxis (Shamsuddin, 2020), is not a critical issue from the perspective of this book. We present a recompilation of different experiences in a variety of cities and fields of action, proposing an overview from the perspective of resilience in the sense of inquiring how such experiences can nurture proposals for better, more sustainable cities, and can thus build resilience. This is not limited to a certain type of action, nor do we aim for a diagnostic procedure or a set of tools for action (as proposed by Wardekker et al., 2020). Such a set of tools is particularly helpful when the concept of resilience, as often is the case, relates to the quest for preparing urban systems for the likely future occurrence of well-known disasters (e.g., earthquakes) or crises (e.g., a financial market crisis) based on previous experiences and adaptation to such events (Shamsuddin, 2020). The current pandemic displays the need for resilience in the sense of making a system healthy, functional, and prepared for an unknown and unexpected crisis in the long term.

Although each chapter in this book uses a different conceptual and empirical approach to resilience, chosen by the authors, several mutual questions are addressed that analyze different cities confronting the COVID-19 pandemic. Therefore, in a transversal manner, the questions tackled throughout the book are the following:

- Are the immediate reactions to the emergency looking for short-term mitigation of impacts? Is it possible to identify "lessons learned" and what mid- or long-term implications can be expected?
- To what degree and by which means do the described processes, measures, or politics aim to recover a previous state of the urban system, or do they look for different development pathways along which the city can evolve?
- What kind of innovation or profound restructuring has been observed or can be proposed? Are these allowing for relevant and long-lasting improvements as a response to the pandemic?
- Through which specific interactions, among what type of individuals and organizations, and by what kind of decision, can such improvements be achieved?
- Can the study provide proposals for improving urban resilience?
- How do the topics analyzed respond or relate to the overall goals of urban sustainability?

To answer these questions, the authors discuss extensive evidence from Asian and Latin American regions with the intention of broadening our view of how the concepts and ideas are embodied in realities that go beyond the Western experience. If the abilities of people and communities revolve around their capacity to be resilient also implies historical and cultural factors framed by unique contexts, addressing this issue from Latin American and Asian realities can enrich our perspective on the relationship between cities, resilience, uncertainties, and risks as a consequence of the emergence of a pandemic. On the other hand, the contrasts in the management to contain the first expansion of the first waves of COVID-19 in Asian countries, such as China, Korea, and Japan, contrasted significantly with the experience of the Latin American countries.

Experiences, Responses, and Uncertainties: The Structure of This Book

The first part of this book is dedicated to the analysis of underlying mechanisms derived from urban planning that are framing the experiences of cities during the COVID-19 pandemic. The part examines some of the main gaps revealed in the way we build cities and construct our city life, sharing experiences from Japan, China, Mexico, Colombia, and Brazil. The chapter by *Eugenio Mangi* et al. focuses on a comparative analysis of gated communities in Shanghai (China) and Bogotá (Colombia) to investigate weaknesses and patterns of urban resilience against the current COVID-19 outbreak, descending from the functional and spatial organization of these residential settlements. The study highlights differences and commonalities under the typo-morphological point of view concerning the containment norms implemented by the institutions in the two contexts, as well as to the provision and quality of outdoor space and facilities, which strengthen the settlements' resilience. In the third chapter of this book, *Girotti Sperandio* et al. review the practical examples of tactical urbanism from cities such as Bogotá (Colombia), Berlin (Germany), Seattle (USA), Oakland (USA), and urban community gardens in Brazil, as potential tools for promoting social engagement and developing healthier and more equitable cities. *Aleksandra Krstikj* et al., in the fourth chapter, discuss the spatial equity in the distribution of urban services, such as parks and local shops, as a crucial condition for the community's resilience during large-scale lockdowns. Two case studies from Atizapán de Zaragoza (Mexico) and Yinchuan (China) are presented that reflect local equity issues and offer a regional perspective for future sustainability in planning. The fifth chapter by *Yuan Ren* analyzes the relations between population density and risk concentration in megacities in China and suggests implementing scientific and rational population mobility management to optimize epidemic prevention, strengthen risk management, and improve urban functioning. The critical tools for this task are found in the adoption of dynamic adjustments based on timely multi-level risk assessments, standardized mobility management according to the rule of law, and better utilization of big data and technological innovations to implement accurate tracing, tracking, and epidemic prevention. Finally, the sixth chapter is a commentary by *Hisako Koura* on the implications of the socioeconomic crisis, brought about by COVID-19, on the urban transformation of Japan. The shifts in working style, density control, and mobility, prompted by the pandemic, are discussed in a search for an alternative planning approach that can better support the ongoing processes of urban and rural transformation under the conditions of smart shrinkage. These shifts are reviewed as opportunities that can use local diversity to improve regional redundancy. An interactive process between the regional framework and local initiatives is proposed for strategic management of developments with local identification, with a focus on the Kansai metropolis. Therefore, starting from the urban shrinkage issues in Japan, via the population mobility patterns in China, to the empirical analysis of efficiencies in urban form and functions in the emerging regions of Latin America, the part provides an overview of the diverse challenges of urban transformation that were opened by unsustainable development. The works in this part set the base for an integral planning strategy with one goal – developing the urban resilience of cities under the condition of multifaceted (and often unpredictable) crises.

The second part of this book is dedicated to the current and future responses of cities to the pandemic, considering the long-lasting effects of emergency measures on equality, poverty, and urban health. The part examines concrete strategies for alleviating the suffering of the most vulnerable groups that are affected the most by amplifying multiple crises. In this part, the chapter by *Ana Luíza Matos de Oliveira* and *Ana Paula Emídio* examines how pre-existing urban inequalities and vulnerabilities have shaped the spread of COVID-19, and discusses the long-lasting effects of the pandemic on poverty and inequality in Latin America. The chapter raises issues for future public policy interventions to fulfill sustainable development objectives and reviews the challenges faced by the region to reach the 2030 Agenda targets amidst the new scenario. The following chapter, by *Carlos Cobreros* et al., focuses on the challenges of domestic confinement through biophilic design and user experience. Relying on ethnographic mixed methods and a compilation of case studies analyzed from the biophilic design perspective, the chapter offers a re-thinking of domestic space as an opportunity to improve the quality of life under confinement conditions. The chapter by *Salvador Leetoy* and *Tommaso Gravante* analyzes the importance of ethics of care in the conception of citizenship, apropos the COVID-19 pandemic in Latin America. Through a discussion of the resurgence of grassroots soup kitchen initiatives, the authors open a critical discussion of collective action and participatory publics to review the notions of care, otherness, and emotions, as three quintessential concepts to challenge dominant instrumentality in Latin American policies. The authors propose the integration of citizenship and ethics of care as a strategy for agency formation in public spaces by considering "care" as a key civic participation element. The tenth chapter of this book, written by *Ana Laura Azparren*, reviews the impact of the coronavirus in the informal settlements of the Autonomous City of Buenos Aires, with a focus on the implementation of public policies and the work developed by community organizations to deal with the social, health, and economic consequences of the pandemic in these neighborhoods. Identifying the lack of access to drinking water, poor living conditions in housing, and high levels of overcrowding as the main culprits for the greatest amount of infection, the author discusses the government response in developing specific public policies to alleviate the effects of the pandemic and highlights the importance of the care work done by community organizations for the sustainability of life in these neighborhoods. The chapter by *Sofía Boza* tackles the problem of food demand and supply in cities threatened by COVID-19 related stay-at-home orders. She reviews the responses of Shanghai, Mexico City, and Santiago between December 2019 and August 2020 and identifies efforts to adapt to the new scenario, such as increasing sanitation in stores or delivery services. Finally, Chap. 12 of this book by *Lucía Martín López* and *Rodrigo Durán López* uses a typological analysis of nursing homes for the elderly to reveal how strong infection prevention and control programs impact the management of the space. The authors clarify how the management of space is vital to protect both residents and healthcare personnel. Through a study of parameters, such as density, social distancing, sectors, and ventilation, the authors identify types of nursing homes that may have the least propagation of COVID-19, depending on their spatial structure. Thus, by focusing on efficiency, equity, and social engagement responses in the functioning of essential urban systems, such as food provision, sanitary infrastructure, and care facilities for the most vulnerable, the second part of this book indicates the failures in core urban and architectural programs to protect the vulnerable and offers useful strategic solutions for adaptation and strengthening of resilience.

Finally, the third part of this book focuses on the yet unknown; the uncertainties derived from the struggle with COVID-19 and how to rebuild cities better. The part's goal is to review challenges and opportunities in building resilience through innovation, under the condition of multiple crises and an unclear future. The chapter by *Emanuele Giorgi* et al. evaluates the significance of architectural interventions as a driving force for rebuilding the image of urban areas, with an aesthetic endowment, in several case studies in China, where cultural tourism plays an important role. The results provide insights on economic impact, cultural heritage preservation, strengthening of communitarian participation, integration with the local social context, and environmental and biodiversity protection, which chart a road map to the economic recovery of cities through a multidisciplinary approach. In the fourteenth chapter of this book, by *Miguel A. Gil-Robles* and *Beatriz Alejandra Sanchez-Jimenez*, city governance and resilience in the case of Mexico City are analyzed as critical factors to manage the emergency. Through a multilevel framework of city governance and resilience, the authors find that the reactions from the largest healthcare organization in Mexico (IMSS) and the federal and the local governments differ in different dimensions, leading to confusion and contradictory strategies. The findings clarify the urgent need for a better understanding of city governance and resilience which calls for communication and collaboration between government levels. Chapter 15, by *Augusto F. J. Schmidt* et al., discusses the building strategies and resilience in China and Brazil through analysis of the inequitable access to water. The discussion brings about different elements to understand health and vulnerability as integrated with socioeconomic intersectionalities and argues that long-term investment in access to water and sanitary infrastructure helps to build more resilient cities. The study points out the importance of taking into consideration a multi-level approach in designing public policies to prepare for unforeseen crises and building resilience, one that considers inequalities, education, healthcare, access to water and sanitation, and urban and regional mobility, among other factors. The sixteenth chapter, by *Carlos Cerda Dueñas* and *Daniel Lemus-Delgado*, analyzes, from a historical perspective, the evolution of cities in the international arena to rethink how the cities can be a relevant international actor to impulse the International Development Cooperation. The traditional role of cities in the architecture of IDC was reviewed to show that cities are not newcomers on the international scene, since they took an important path before their internationalization process. The authors conclude with a series of recommendations on how cities can contribute to the development path considering the new environment caused by the pandemic. The chapter by *Evgenia Likhovtseva* examines the changing patterns of international student migration, due to COVID-19, in the USA, UK, Australia, Sweden, and China, and their effect on urban and city development. By comparative analysis, the author finds that Chinese cities, especially the more international cosmopolitan hubs like Shanghai or Beijing, were able to present themselves as "safe" places, while the rest of the world struggled with the pandemic. With the national university sector strengthened by returning international students, the author discusses the potential benefit for emerging economies of the Global South, by promoting regional student mobility and wider cooperation. At the end, the final chapter of this part, written by *David Arboleda* and *Andrés Zambrano*, analyzes the effect of COVID-19 on the economic and health indicators of Bogotá, and the responses of the local government to soften the economic shock. The importance of designing policies that are adapted to the local context and complement existing strategies at the national level was highlighted, and the implementation of ambitious local programs that would be too difficult to execute nationally was encouraged. The authors conclude that the benefits derived from having ample fiscal space due to the good performance of previous administrations allow financing these programs with a sustainable debt. Hence, by reviewing innovations from architectural, urban, organizational, and managerial aspects of cities, the third part of this book provides a valuable guidebook to city rebuilding, with a strong focus on resilience enhancement on the local and global scales.

References

Aalbers, M. B., Beerepoot, N., & Gerritsen, M. (2020). Editorial: The geography of the COVID-19 pandemic. *Tijdschrift voor Economische en Sociale Geografie, 111*(3), 201–204.

Adger, W. N. (2000). Social and ecological resilience: Are they related? *Progress in Human Geography, 24*(3), 347–364.

Allam, Z., & Jones, D. S. (2020). On the coronavirus (COVID-19) outbreak and the smart city network: Universal data sharing standards coupled with artificial intelligence (AI) to benefit urban health. *Monitoring and Management. Healthcare, 8*(1), 46. https://doi.org/10.3390/healthcare8010046

Bai, X., Nagendra, H., Shi, P., & Liu, H. (2020). Cities: Build networks and share plans to emerge stronger from COVID-19. *Nature, 584*, 517–520.

Beilin, R., & Wilkinson, C. (2015). Introduction: Governing for urban resilience. *Urban Studies, 52*(7), 1205–1217.

Bixler, R. P., Lieberknecht, K., Atshana, S., Zutz, C. P., Richter, S. M., & Belaire, J. A. (2020). Reframing urban governance for resilience implementation: The role of network closure and other insights from a network approach. *Cities, 103*(2020), 102726.

Blackburn, C., & Ruyle, L. (2020, May 27). How leadership in various countries has affected COVID-19 response effectiveness. *The Conversation*. https://theconversation.com/how-leadership-in-various-countries-has-affected-covid-19-response-effectiveness-138692. Accessed Aug 2020.

Blake, P., & Wadhwa, D. (2020, December 14). 2020 year in review: The impact of COVID-19 in 12 charts. *World Bank*. https://blogs.worldbank.org/voices/2020-year-review-impact-covid-19-12-charts. Accessed Jan 2021.

Brinkley, C., & Vitiello, D. (2013). From farm to nuisance: Animal agriculture and the rise of planning regulation. *Journal of Planning History, 13*(2). https://doi.org/10.1177/1538513213507542

Brunetti, G., Ceravolo, R., Barbieri, C. A., Borghini, A., de Carlo, F., Mela, A., Beltramo, S., Longhi, A., de Lucia, G., Ferraris, S., Pezzoli, A., Quagliolo, C., Salata, S., & Voghera, A. (2019). Territorial resilience: Toward a proactive meaning for spatial planning. *Sustainability, 11*, 2286. https://doi.org/10.3390/su11082286

Chakraborty, I., & Maity, P. (2020). COVID-19 outbreak: Migration, effects on society, global environment and prevention. *Science of the Total Environment, 728*, 138882. https://doi.org/10.1016/j.scitotenv.2020.138882

Chelleri, L., & Baravikova, A. (2021). Understandings of urban resilience meanings and principles across Europe. *Cities, 108*. https://doi.org/10.1016/j.cities.2020.102985

Chelleri, L., Waters, J. J., Olazabal, M., & Minucci, G. (2015). Resilience trade-offs: Addressing multiple scales and temporal aspects of urban resilience. *Environment and Urbanization, 27*(1), 181–198. https://doi.org/10.1177/0956247814550780

Chen, X., & Quan, R. (2021). A spatiotemporal analysis of urban resilience to the COVID-19 pandemic in the Yangtze River Delta. *Natural Hazards, 106*, 829–854. https://doi.org/10.1007/s11069-020-04493-9

Cheshmehzangi, A. (2020). *The city in need: Urban resilience and city management in disruptive disease outbreak events*. Springer.

Chinese Center for Disease Control and Prevention. (2020). *Tracking the epidemic: National health commission update*. http://weekly.chinacdc.cn/news/TrackingtheEpidemic.htm. Accessed Aug 2020.

Cohen, M. J. (2020). Does the COVID-19 outbreak mark the onset of a sustainable consumption transition? *Sustainability: Science, Practice and Policy, 16*(1), 1–3. https://doi.org/10.1080/15487733.2020.1740472

Connolly, C., Keil, R., & Ali, S. H. (2020). Extended urbanisation and the spatialities of infectious disease: Demographic change, infrastructure and governance. *Urban Studies*. https://doi.org/10.1177/0042098020910873

Corburn, J., Vlahov, D., Mberu, B., Riley, L., Teixeira Caiaffa, W., Faiz Rashid, S., Ko, A., Patel, S., Jukur, S., Martínez-Herrera, E., Jayasinghe, S., Agarwal, S., Nguendo Yongsi, B., Weru, J., Ouma, S., Edmundo, K., Oni, T., & Ayad, H. (2020). Slum health: Arresting COVID-19 and improving Well-being in urban informal settlements. *Journal of Urban Health, 97*, 348–357. https://doi.org/10.1007/s11524-020-00438-6

Davoudi, S. (2012). Resilience: A bridging concept or a dead end? *Planning Theory & Practice, 13*(2), 299–307.

Deng, C. X. (2020). The global battle against SARS-CoV-2 and COVID-19. *International Journal of Biological Sciences, 16*(10), 1676–1677. https://doi.org/10.7150/ijbs.45587

Dobkin, J., & Gottehrer-Cohen, Z. (2020, April 13). The very unequal impact of COVID-19 on NYC neighborhoods. *Gothamist*. https://gothamist.com/news/very-unequal-impact-covid-19-nyc-neighborhoods. Accessed Aug 2020.

Duque Franco, I., Ortiz, C., Samper, J., & Millan, G. (2020). Mapping repertoires of collective action facing the COVID-19 pandemic in informal settlements in Latin American cities. *Environment & Urbanization, 32*(2), 523–546. https://doi.org/10.1177/0956247820944823

Elmqvist, T., Andersson, E., Frantzeskaki, N., McPhearson, T., Olsson, P., Gaffney, O., Takeuchi, K., & Folke, C. (2019). Sustainability and resilience for transformation in the urban century. *Nature Sustainability, 2*(4), 267–273. https://doi.org/10.1038/s41893-019-0250-1

European Centre for Disease Prevention and Control. (2020). *Covid-19 data*. https://www.ecdc.europa.eu/en/covid-19/data. Accessed Aug 2020.

Folke, C. (2006). The emergence of a perspective for social-ecological systems analysis. *Global Environmental Change, 16*, 253–267.

Fransen, J., Peralta, D. O., Vanelli, F., Edelenbos, J., & Olvera, B. C. (2021). The emergence of urban community resilience initiatives during the COVID-19 pandemic: An international exploratory study. *The European Journal of Development Research, 2021*. https://doi.org/10.1057/s41287-020-00348-y

Graham-Harrison, E., & Kuo, L. (2020, March 19). China's coronavirus lockdown strategy: Brutal but effective. *The Guardian*. https://www.theguardian.com/world/2020/mar/19/chinas-coronavirus-lockdown-strategy-brutal-but-effective. Accessed Aug 2020.

Gupte, J., & Mitlin, D. (2020). COVID-19: What is not being addressed. *Environment & Urbanization*, 1–18. https://doi.org/10.1177/0956247820963961

https://www.bloomberg.com/news/articles/2020-03-06/how-the-coronavirus-could-change-city-planning

International Monetary Fund. (2020, October). *World Economic Outlook*. https://www.imf.org/en/Publications/WEO/Issues/2020/09/30/world-economic-outlook-october-2020. Accessed Nov 2020.

John Hopkins University. (2020, April 2). *The role of genomic sequencing in combating COVID-19*. https://hub.jhu.edu/2020/04/02/sequencing-genome-sars-cov-2/. Accessed Aug 2020.

Keil, R., & Ali, H. (2007). Governing the sick city: Urban governance in the age of emerging infectious disease. *Antipode, 39*(5), 846–873.

Klaus, I. (June 2020). San Francisco Bay Area: Everything must change. In A. Fernández de Losada and H. Abdullah (Eds.). Cities on the Frontline: Managing the Coronavirus Crisis (CIDOB report # 05, 53-58). Barcelona: Center for International Affairs. ISSN: 2564-9078

Klaus, I. (2020a) The Post-Pandemic Urban Future Is Already Here. https://www.citylab.com/design/2020/04/coronavirus-urban-planning-cities-architecture-history/609262/ Accessed Aug 2021.

Klaus, I. (2020b) Pandemics Are Also an Urban Planning Problem. https://www.citylab.com/design/2020/03/coronavirus-urban-planning-global-cities-infectious-disease/607603/ Accessed Aug 2021.

Lurie, N., Saville, M., Hatchett, R., & Halton, J. (2020). Developing Covid-19 vaccines at pandemic speed. *New England Journal Medical, 382*, 1969–1973. https://doi.org/10.1056/NEJMp2005630

MacKinnon, D., & Driscoll Derickson, K. (2012). From resilience to resourcefulness: A critique of resilience policy and activism. *Progress in Human Geography, 37*(2), 253–270.

Manancourt, V. (2020, August 1). Thousands protest against coronavirus measures in Berlin. *Politico*. https://www.politico.com/news/2020/08/01/thousands-protest-against-coronavirus-measures-in-berlin-390021. Accessed Oct 2020.

McCartney, G., Pinto, J., & Liu, M. (2021). City resilience and recovery from COVID-19: The case of Macao. *Cities, 112*(2021), 103130.

Meerow, S., & Newell, J. P. (2019). Urban resilience for whom, what, when, where, and why? *Urban Geography, 40*(3), 309–329. https://doi.org/10.1080/02723638.2016.1206395

Megahed, N. A., & Ghoneim, E. M. (2020). Antivirus-built environment: Lessons learned from Covid-19 pandemic. *Sustainable Cities and Society, 61*.

National Research Council. (2011). *Building community disaster resilience through private-public collaboration*. National Academy of Science.

Paton, D. (2006). Disaster resilience: Building capacity to co-exist with natural hazards and their consequences. In D. Paton & D. Johnston (Eds.), *Disaster resilience: An integrated approach* (pp. 3–10). Charles C. Tomas Publisher.

Pearls, T. (2020, March 13). Social distancing: What it is and why it's the best tool we have to fight the coronavirus. *The Conversation*. https://theconversation.com/social-distancing-what-it-is-and-why-its-the-best-tool-we-have-to-fight-the-coronavirus-133581. Accessed Aug 2020.

Rahman, A., Zaman, N., Asyharic, A. T., Al-Turjmand, F., Bhuiyane, Z. A., & Zolkiplia, M. F. (2020). Data-driven dynamic clustering framework for mitigating the adverse economic impact of Covid-19 lockdown practices. *Sustainable Cities and Society, 62*.

Roser, M., Ritchie, H., & Ortiz-Ospina, E. (2020). Coronavirus disease (COVID-19) – Statistics and research. *Our World in Data*. https://ourworldindata.org/coronavirus. Accessed Aug 2020.

Rose-Redwood, R., et al. (2020). Geographies of the COVID-19 pandemic. *Dialogues in Human Geography, 10*(2), 97–106.

Sandford, A. (2020, April 3). Coronavirus: Half of humanity now on lockdown as 90 countries call for confinement. *Euronews*. https://www.euronews.com/2020/04/02/coronavirus-in-europe-spain-s-death-toll-hits-10-000-after-record-950-new-deaths-in-24-hou. Accessed Aug 2020.

Shamsuddin, S. (2020). Resilience resistance: The challenges and implications of urban resilience implementation. *Cities, 103*, 102763. https://doi.org/10.1016/j.cities.2020.102763

Sharifi, A. (2019). Urban form resilience: A meso-scale analysis. *Cities, 93*, 238–252. https://doi.org/10.1016/j.cities.2019.05.010

Sharifi, A. (2020). Urban resilience assessment: Mapping knowledge structure and trends. *Sustainability 2020, 12*(15), 5918. https://doi.org/10.3390/su12155918

Sharifi, A., & Khavarian-Garmsir, A. R. (2020). The COVID-19 pandemic: Impacts on cities and major lessons for urban planning, design, and management. *Science of the Total Environment, 749*, 142391.

Shaw, K. (2012). "Reframing" resilience: Challenges for planning theory and practice. *Planning Theory & Practice, 13*(2), 308–333.

Shi, Y., Zhai, G., Xu, L., Zhou, S., Lu, Y., Liu, H., & Huang, W. (2021). Assessment methods of urban system resilience: From the perspective of complex adaptive system theory. *Cities, 112*, 103141.

Simone, C., Iandolo, F., Fulco, I., & Loia, F. (2021). Rome was not built in a day. Resilience and the eternal city: Insights for urban management. *Cities, 110*, 103070. https://doi.org/10.1016/j.cities.2021.103070

Sparke, M., & Anguelov, D. (2020). Contextualising coronavirus geographically. *Transactions of the Institute of British Geographers, 45*, 498–508.

Wang, C., Horby, P. W., Hayden, F. G., & Gao, G. F. (2020). A novel coronavirus outbreak of Global Health Concern. *The Lancet, 395*(10223), 470–473. https://doi.org/10.1016/S0140-6736(20)30185-9

Wang, L., Xue, X., Zhang, Y., & Luo, X. (2018). Exploring the emerging evolution trends of urban resilience research by Scientometric analysis. *International Journal of Environmental Research and Public Health, 15*(10), 2181. https://doi.org/10.3390/ijerph15102181

Wardekker, A., Wilk, B., Brown, V., Uittenbroek, C., Mees, H., Driessen, P., … Runhaar, H. (2020). A diagnostic tool for supporting policymaking on urban resilience. *Cities, 101*, 102691.

Weichselgartner, J., & Kelman, I. (2015). Geographies of resilience: Challenges and opportunities of a descriptive concept. *Progress in Human Geography, 39*(3), 249–267.

Weller, J. (2020). *La pandemia del COVID-19 y su efecto en las tendencias de los mercados laborales. Documentos de Proyectos* [COVID-19 pandemic and its effects over labor markets' tendencies]. UN; CEPAL.

Wolf, M. (2016). Rethinking urban epidemiology: Natures, networks and materialities. *International Journal of Urban and Regional Research, 40*(5), 958–982.

World Bank. (2020a, June 8). *COVID-19 to plunge global economy into worst recession since World War II.* https://www.worldbank.org/en/news/press-release/2020/06/08/covid-19-to-plunge-global-economy-into-worst-recession-since-world-war-ii. Accessed Aug 2020.

World Bank. (2020b). *Poverty and shared prosperity 2020: Reversals of fortune.* https://openknowledge.worldbank.org/bitstream/handle/10986/34496/211602ov.pdf. Accessed Jan 2021.

World Health Organization. (2020a, January 12). *Novel coronavirus – China.* https://www.who.int/csr/don/12-january-2020-novel-coronavirus-china/en/. Accessed Aug 2020.

World Health Organization. (2020b, July 31). *Rolling updates on coronavirus disease (COVID-19).* https://www.who.int/emergencies/diseases/novel-coronavirus-2019/events-as-they-happen. Accessed Aug 2020.

Yu, X., & Li, N. (2020). How did Chinese government implement unconventional measures against COVID-19 pneumonia? *Risk Management Healthcare Policy, 13*, 491–499. https://doi.org/10.2147/RMHP.S251351

Zhang, N., Jia, W., Wang, P., Dung, C. H., Zhao, P., Leung, K., Su, B., Cheng, R., & Li, Y. (2021). Changes in local travel behaviour before and during the COVID-19 pandemic in Hong Kong. *Cities, 112*, 103139.

Zheng, W. (2020, February 23). *Coronavirus is China's fastest-spreading health crisis, Xi Jinping says.* South China Morning Press. https://www.politico.com/news/2020/02/23/coronavirus-china-health-crisis-116957. Accessed Aug 2020.

Part I
Experiences

Chapter 2
COVID-19, Gated Communities, and Urban Resilience: A Comparative Analysis Between China and Colombia

Eugenio Mangi, Ali Cheshmehzangi, and Giaime Botti

Introduction

The current COVID-19 pandemic has put people's lives and countries' economies under unprecedented pressure worldwide. Responses by governments have been similar, although with a varying degree of intensity, and generally based on rigid norms of social distancing and movement control that have been mostly implemented in urban areas. Consequently, considering that most of the world's population lives in cities, the concept of urban resilience against this kind of event arises as a fundamental paradigm to ensure how societies "survive, adapt, and grow" despite chronic stresses and acute shocks (100 Resilient Cities, n.d.).

Throughout history, cities have been partially shaped according to principles of hygiene and epidemic control and mitigation, as various plagues have consistently been associated with the city and the negative aspects of urban life (Engelmann et al., 2018). All the most remarkable urban reforms of the nineteenth century, from the transformation of Paris started by Georges E. Haussmann (Barnes, 2006; Frioux, 2013) or the foreign settlements in the Chinese treaty port cities (Cookson Smith, 2011; Esherick, 1999) and the African colonies (Bigon, 2016; Swanson, 1977), to the outcomes of the City Beautiful movement in the USA (Lopez, 2012) or Francisco Pereira Passos' work in Rio de Janeiro (Benchimol, 1990), have always featured a hygienist background. Thus, it can be affirmed that the morphological organization of the built-up environment plays a pivotal role in addressing, preventing, and mitigating chronic stresses affecting the city, such as a widespread epidemic. Temporary

E. Mangi (✉) · A. Cheshmehzangi · G. Botti
Department of Architecture and Built Environment, University of Nottingham Ningbo China, Ningbo, China

Centre for Sustainable Energy Technologies (CSET), University of Nottingham Ningbo China, Ningbo, China
e-mail: eugenio.mangi@nottingham.edu.cn

© The Author(s), under exclusive license to Springer Nature Switzerland AG 2021

M. A. Montoya et al. (eds.), *COVID-19 and Cities*, The Urban Book Series,
https://doi.org/10.1007/978-3-030-84134-8_2

constructions, provisional re-use and adaptation of existing structures realized at the architectural scale, may provide immediate relief (Wainwright, 2020), but, when it comes to the urban dimension, these solutions appear more complex and their implementation difficult.

This chapter addresses the problem of COVID-19 city resilience from the perspectives of urban design and morphology, by establishing a case study-based comparative analysis of a specific type of residential settlement, the gated community, in two different contexts, China and Colombia. The selection is based on the significant differences in the urban morphologies of the two contexts, including the way in which these compounds are designed, their scale, and how they define the urban structure and the cityscape. By drawing this comparison, the chapter investigates how gated communities in the two cities coped with the current pandemic, highlighting weaknesses and traits of resilience arising from their morphology and also in relation to the regulations, restrictions, and social norms implemented during this time (Cundinamarca, 2020; Xinhua, 2020). More specifically, it focuses on the scale of the communities, their spatial organization, and their connections and relations with the rest of the urban fabric. Furthermore, the chapter evaluates the presence of facilities for residents and commercial services and how they localize within or around the compounds, as well as the provision, use, and quality of green and outdoor spaces. Finally, all these considerations allow a critical assessment of the resilience of these residential settlements in facing the current public health threat and other comparable events that may arise in the future.

Methods and Rationale

The research is based on the empirical analysis and comparison of case studies of gated communities in China and Colombia, and specifically in the urban areas of Shanghai and Bogotá. The comparative study provides us with solid grounds for a discussion on the position of gated communities in both contexts and how they have developed differently in these two countries. The reasons for undertaking this comparative study are threefold: firstly, the authors have established a research track record and have first-hand experience in investigating residential settlements and enhancing resilience in these contexts (Cheshmezangi & Butters, 2016). Secondly, Shanghai in China and Bogotá in Colombia can be considered, with due respect to differences in terms of scale, history and institutional arrangements, the economic and financial centers, and development benchmarks of their respective countries over the last 20–30 years (Jiang & Waley, 2020; Montoya Garay, 2018; Walcott & Pannell, 2006; Wu, 2003). Shanghai, with 24.2 million inhabitants recorded in 2018 (Shanghai Municipal People's Government, 2019), was designated in 1992 by the then supreme Communist Party leader Deng Xiaoping, as the Dragon's Head of China, to underline the need for an acceleration in the economic transition of the country and the city's role in the development of the Yangtze River Delta area by attracting foreign investments through the Special Economic Zones or SEZ (Deng, n.d.). Developed with the renowned PuDong District, Shanghai has transformed into a global financial city in less than two decades. The growth has been extensive, with a tangible impact on urban patterns and the development of relatively dense living environments. This enhanced a progressive integration of the city into the world economy and boosted its transformation into an international financial hub and logistics center in the last decades (Chen, 2009). Bogotá is the capital of Colombia and its financial and economic center, with a higher GDP per capita than other major cities. It is also the largest city in the country with 7.4 million recorded inhabitants, one million of which were added in the last two decades, although the highest growth rate (in triple digits) happened during the 1950s and 1960s when positive demography and mass migration from the countryside transformed the city to "modernly planned and singularly developed, partly ordered and partly arbitrary" (Saldarriaga Roa, 2000, p. 30). Thirdly, gated compounds have been largely adopted in both contexts in the last decades, even though the historical, social, economic, and political background behind their widespread diffusion in the two countries is different, as well as the way they structure the urban morphology and characterize the cityscape.

The introverted residential area, with diverse grades of enclosure type, was a constant pattern in Chinese urban planning throughout the pre-1949 era, the Socialist planned economy system, and the post-1978 open policy period. This can be related to several reasons that span from the hierarchical and centralized organization of the social structure during the feudal monarchy era to the strict political and personal control imposed during the Socialist period through the adoption of the work units or *danwei* system (Qian, 2014; Xu & Yang, 2009). However, it is only in the late 1990s, after the implementation of two milestone economic reforms, that the contemporary residential gated communities started to radically transform the morphology and landscape of Chinese cities. On the one hand, the introduction in 1994 of the decentralized tax-sharing system featured a progressive economic devolution through the separation of central and local governments' fiscal systems. Among other measures, this reform allowed the local administrations to retain the revenues from leasing state-owned land to developers. Those revenues were successively employed to finance public projects aimed at achieving higher local GDP rates while shaping "the Chinese land-driven growth machine" (Wu, 2015, p. 79). On the other hand, the 1998 housing reform (State Council, 1998) transformed the house provision from a welfare assignment of the work units in the state-planned economy to a commodity asset under the market-oriented system and boosted the real estate industry to become the major economic sector that pushed the national growth in the last 30 years. In Colombia, a country traditionally marked by political violence and high crime rates, gated communities found a fertile ground, as in other Latin American countries, as a response to 'fear' (Caldeira, 2001), but have also been favored by planning regulations and pushed by real estate developers, who sold a successful product to people yearning for security and social distinction (Borsdorf et al., 2007; Cabrera Laverde, 2013; Coy & Pöhler, 2002; Hidalgo, 2004; Janoschka & Borsdorf, 2004; Lozano Triviño, 2014; Mendoza Jaramillo, 2016). While the present chapter deals with this urban form, it does not neglect the fact that a large part of the contemporary urban territory in Colombia, as well as in other Latin American countries, falls within the category of 'informal city' (Torres Tovar, 2007). Here, not only are basic needs and services systematically denied, but also the current pandemic has hit harder, although community-driven actions have sometimes been successful (Sims, 2020).

A series of selection criteria have been defined to identify comparable case studies in the two cities. In this way, it is possible to highlight some recurring typo-morphological traits that, together with the application of the specific containment measures adopted in each context, can play a role (or not) in coping with the COVID-19 pandemic and consequently enhance (or not) the urban resilience of this residential type in Shanghai and Bogotá. The first parameter taken into consideration is the construction period and the consumer target. The analyzed gated communities have generally been built in the last two decades for upper middle-income residents. In this way, the study focuses on mature and established developments with a stable population whose spatial and functional solutions have been adopted by later communities (for China: Chen & Thwaites, 2013; Rowe et al., 2016). Then, the settlements' locations have been the second criterion for the selection of the case studies. The investigation analyzes compounds located outside the central areas of the two cities to identify the recurring functional and typo-morphological patterns and to avoid the specificities that normally characterize the infill residential projects in the downtown areas, especially in these two cities with their rich historical backgrounds. As shown in Fig. 2.1, the Shanghai communities are comprised of neighborhoods located in between the Middle and the Outer Ring Road, where a progressive process of urbanization took place during the first decade of the twenty-first century due to the implementation of the 1999–2020 Shanghai Masterplan (He, 2015). In Bogotá, most of the surveyed communities are located in different sectors of the North-Northeastern parts of the city (the localities of Usaquén and Suba), which have been hugely developed during the last decades and are where the wealthiest residents tend to live.[1] However, a few of the communities are also in the more central locality of Teusaquillo, on the strategic axis of the Avenida 26, the avenue linking the city center with the airport (see Fig. 2.2).

Two other features considered during the selection of the case studies, which show substantial differences between the two contexts, have been the presence of dedicated outdoor spaces, public facilities, and the variety of residential building types within the compounds. In gated communities, the quality and the extension of the green areas and amenities for residents' exclusive use are essential elements that influence the housing price and the popularity of the real estate operation (Breitung,

[1] In Colombia, the DANE (National Department of Statistics) classifies the population into six socio-economic levels ("estratos," "layers" literally) according to the quality of the city-blocks in which they live, from 1 (very low) to 6 (high). This classification is used, among other things, to set different fees for public utilities. From this perspective, overall, the whole city of Bogotá appears segmented by an invisible socio-economic gradient, with most level 1 neighborhoods in the Southern and Westernmost localities, middle-class settlements in the center, and a predominance of levels 5 and 6 in the North.

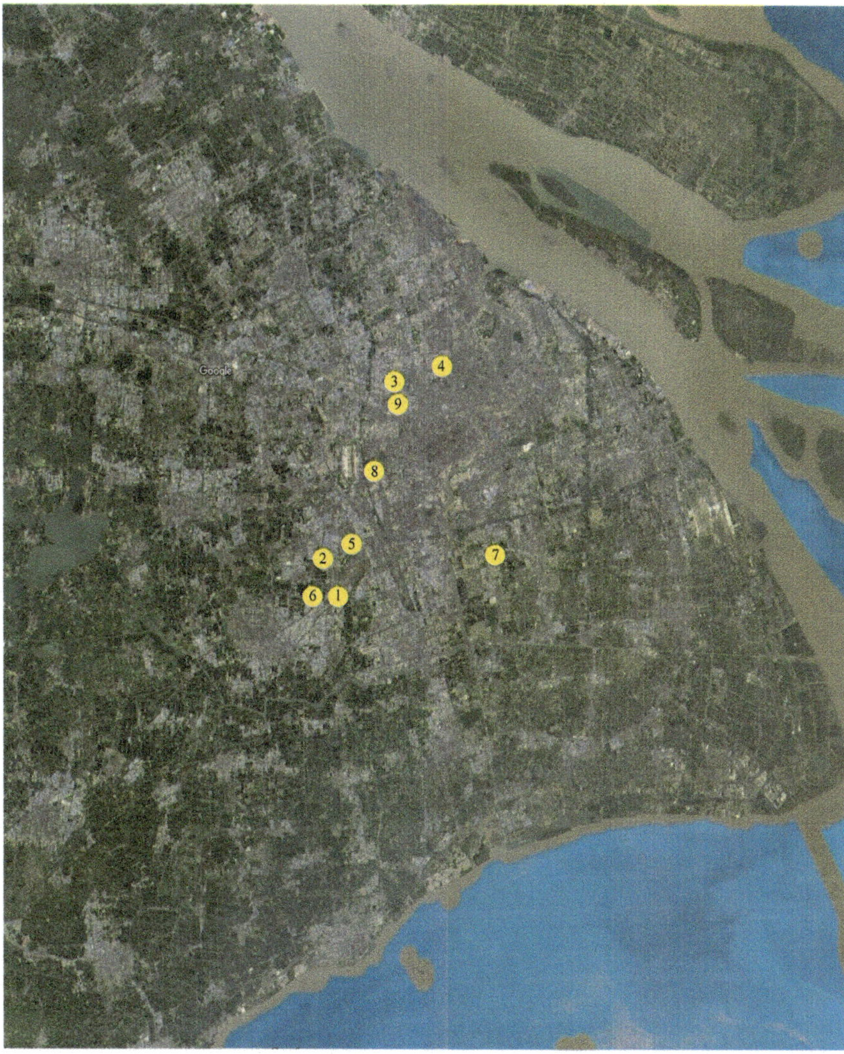

Fig. 2.1 Location of the communities in Shanghai
Source: Authors' edition based on Google Earth map. 1 – Capital of New Hongqiao; 2 – Zhicheng Huayuan; 3 – Qingshui Yi Yuan; 4 – Baoli residential community (North phase); 5 – Beishangwan; 6 – Langting Shangjun Hongjun/Langting Shangjun Yuting/Yiting Garden; 7 – Zhonghai Yujingxian Villas; 8 – Zhonghai Ziyu Haoting; 9 – Greenland Haiyuguanyuan

2013; Mendoza, 2015; Miao, 2003; Xiao et al., 2017; Wu et al., 2014). The variety of building types are: low, consisting of villas and row houses, and medium- and high-rise, which are generally very common in Chinese compounds but are rare in the Colombian ones that tend to feature a single typology. Finally, in China, gated communities developed in the twenty-first century are usually the result of a single

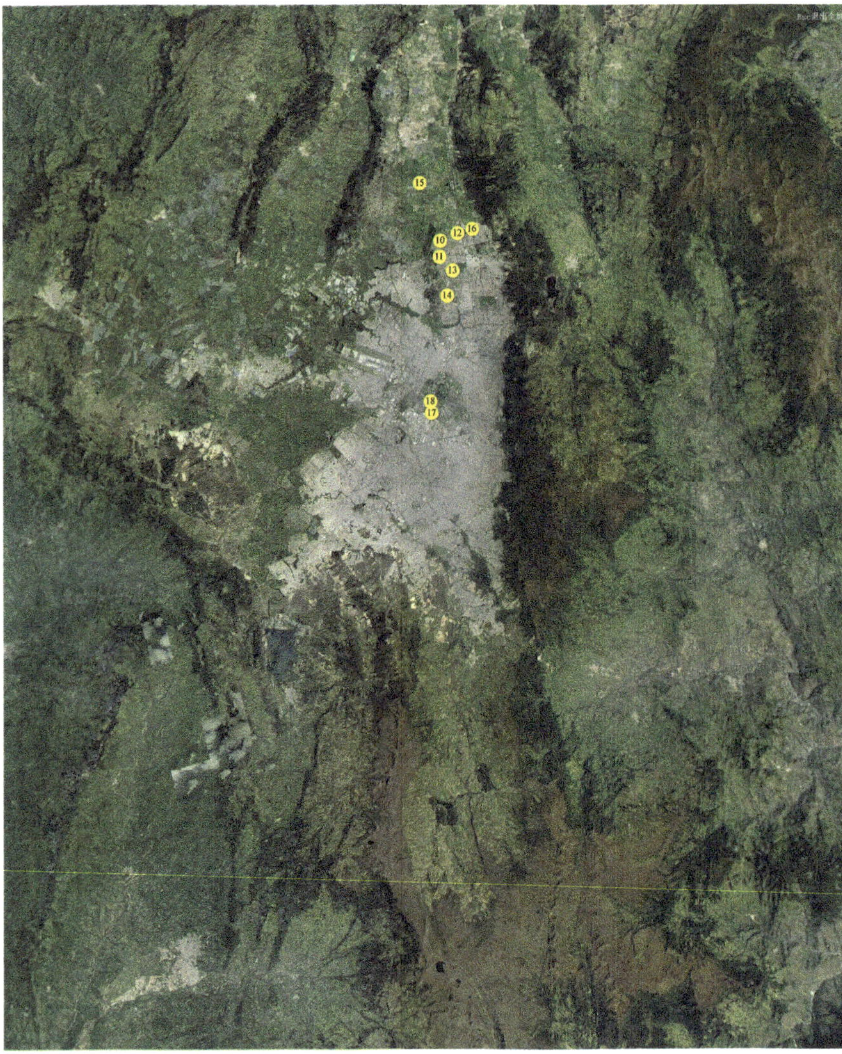

Fig. 2.2 Location of the communities in Bogotá
Source: Authors' edition based on Google Earth map. 10 – La Arborada de San José; 11 – Conjunto Residencial Del Monte; 12 – Tejares del Norte I; 13 – Parque Central Colina 1; 14 – Refugio de Gratamira; 15 – Hacienda San Sebastian; 16 – Urbanización Maranta; 17 – Conjunto Residencial Loira Real; 18 – Conjunto Residencial Avenida Parque

intervention, encompassing a whole city block of a large size, between 300 and 500 meters per side (about 15 hectares or even more), bound by wide arterial roads (Kan et al., 2017) and which can be defined as a superblock (Monson, 2008) or megaplot (Lee, 2013). In Colombia, because of the structure of land ownership and regulations, compounds are a much smaller size. In Bogotá, they have been limited to four hectares since 1979 not to fragment the urban fabric too much, while the maximum size of the "*supermanzanas*" ("superblock") has been limited to five hectares since 2004 (Lozano Triviño, 2014, p. 41).

The overlapping of these criteria has led to the selection of a sample of nine gated communities in Shanghai and Bogotá that constitute the basis of our comparative study (Tables 2.1 and 2.2). Each selected case study has been empirically investigated through aerial and street view pictures and, when available, through the dedicated real estate websites.[2] In this way, it has been possible to determine qualitative data, such as building type, functional program, provision of green space for the residents, location, number of pedestrian and vehicular entrances, and type of border. The approximate calculation of quantitative data, like the area of the compounds, their floor area ratio (F.A.R.), and the green ratio, has been defined through an accurate redraw operation of the communities carried out by intern research students (Fig. 2.3).

City Resilience in Facing the Pandemic

In this section, we briefly explain how cities are affected during the pandemic. This is generally addressed through resilience enhancement and the preparedness that leads to better management of the city during such crisis or emergency situations. The vulnerabilities of cities during the pandemic are multifaceted, and hence, require comprehensive solutions (Cheshmehzangi, 2020). Some of these vulnerabilities could be addressed with adaptive planning (Alterman, 1988) and some could be addressed through quality urban planning and design. The latter is what we focus on in terms of evaluating the gated communities that suggest prevention measures in multiple contexts. In this regard, we can highlight how the city's resilience could then be supported or enhanced through the preparedness of urban systems and related institutional factors.

The main document, developed by 100 Resilient Cities (n.d.), suggests three areas that should be addressed from the infrastructural development point of view. These (1) provide and enhance protective natural and man-made assets; (2) ensure continuity of critical services; and (3) provide reliable communication and mobility. The city should then have the ability to restore itself through a process (Admiraal & Cornaro, 2019) that indicates the level of resilience it has against the adversities caused by an outbreak. For instance, the network between multiple domains suggests critical progress in managing the city when facing the outbreak (Admiraal & Cornaro, 2018; Ban, 2012; Cheshmehzangi, 2020; Hajer & Dassen, 2014). Therefore, in the literature, we can find the term 'resilience' often related to the conceptualization of policies (Alexander, 2013; Sanchez et al., 2018; Vogel & Henstra, 2015) or related to the multidisciplinary perspective of resilience conception itself

[2] No site visit could take place due to the COVID-19 pandemic prevention regulations and travel restrictions in place in the two countries at the time of writing.

Table 2.1 Quantitative and qualitative data of the case studies in Shanghai

	Name of the community	Location	Area (m^2)	Year of construction	Number of households	Floor area ratio (F.A.R.)	Max. building height (m)	Green area ratio	Building type	Facilities
1	Capital of New Hongqiao	Songjiang District	303,482	2012	1615	0.8	50	40%	High-rise	Pool/garden/shops
							15 (villas)		Villas	
2	Zhicheng Huayuan	Songjiang District	300,000	2004	2604	1.4	55	35%	High-rise	Kindergarten/garden/gym/shop
							15 (row houses)		Row houses	
3	Qingshui Yi Yuan	Jiading District	270,000	2005	2094	1.3	60	35%	High-rise	Pool/garden/shops
							21		Medium rise	
							15 (villas)		Villas	
4	Baoli residential community (north phase)	Jiading District	200,000	2010	1181	1.8	70	35%	High-rise	Pool/garden/shops
							15 (villas)		Villas	
5	Beishangwan	Songjiang District	190,000	2008	2514	1.5	60	50%	High-rise	Gym/garden/shops
							15 (row houses)		Row houses	
6	Langting ShangjunHongjun/Langting Shangjun Yuting/Yiting garden	Songjiang District	49,846	2010	1092	0.86	40	45%	High-rise	Sports equipment/garden/shops
							15 (row houses)		Row houses	
							12 (villas)		Villas	
7	Zhonghai Yujingxian villas	PuDong District	190,000	2012	1411	1.2	80	35%	High-rise	Shop/garden/gym
							15 (row houses)		Row houses	
							12 (villas)		Villas	
8	Zhonghai Ziyu Haoting	Putuo District	217,000	2014	1024	2.2	80	30%	High-rise	Shop/garden/gym
							15 (villas)		Villas	
9	Greenland Haiyuguanyuan	Jiading District	220,000	2011	1112	1.8	60	35%	High-rise	Gym/garden/shop
							15 (villas)		Villas	

Table 2.2 Quantitative and qualitative data of the case studies in Bogotá

	Name of the community	District	Area (m^2)	Year of construction	Number of households	Floor area ratio (F.A.R.)	Max. building height (m)	Green area ratio	Building type	Facilities
10	La Arborada de San José	Suba	13,000	N.A.	32	0.4	8	35%	Villas	Tennis/football pitch
11	Conjunto Residencial del Monte	Suba	35,530	N.A.	336	1.1	21	40%	Medium-rise	Playground/gym/common room
12	Tejares del Norte I	Suba	32,800	N.A.	394	1.04	16 (row house)	20%	Row house	Tennis
							10 (low-rise)		Low-rise	
13	Parque Central Colina 1	Suba	57,600	After 2010	864	4.8	63	30%	High-rise	Playground
14	Refugio de Gratamira	Suba	70,170	N.A.	40	0.70	10	20%	Villas	–
15	Hacienda San Sebastian	Suba	412,000	N.A.	139	0.49	7	65%	Villas	Tennis
16	Urbanización Maranta	Usaquén	138,200	After 1990	728	0.9	13 (row house)	20%	Villas	Multisport field/tennis/playground/BBQ
							10 (villa)		Row houses	
17	Conjunto Residencial Loira Real	Teusaquillo	17,800	2002	320	2.9	35	45%	High-rise	Multisport field/playground/gym/common room/shop
18	Conjunto Residencial Avenida Parque	Teusaquillo	41,694	2005	360	2.2	35	40%	High-rise	Multisport field/playground

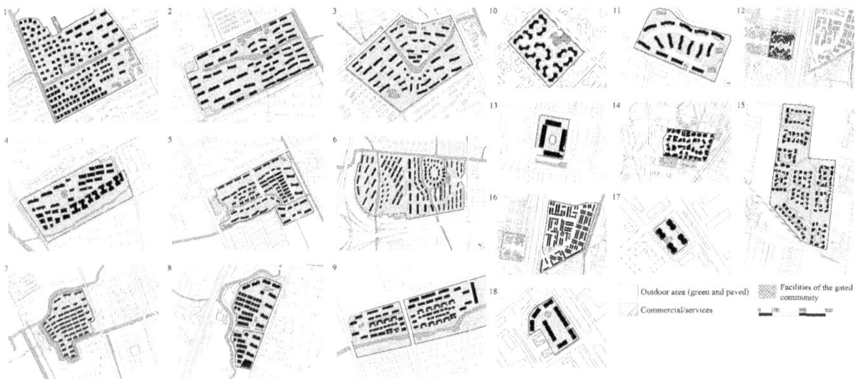

Fig. 2.3 Typo-morphological comparison between the case studies in Shanghai (1 to 9) and in Bogotá (10 to 18). Source: The Authors. 1 – Capital of New Hongqiao; 2 – Zhicheng Huayuan; 3 – Qingshui Yi Yuan; 4 – Baoli residential community (North phase); 5 – Beishangwan; 6 – Langting ShangjunHongjun/Langting ShangjunYuting/ Yiting Garden; 7 – Zhonghai Yujingxian Villas; 8 – Zhonghai Ziyuhaoting; 9 – Greenland Haiyuguanyuan; 10 – La Arborada de San José; 11 – Conjunto Residencial Del Monte; 12 – Tejares del Norte I; 13 – Parque Central Colina 1; 14 – Refugio de Gratamira; 15 – Hacienda San Sebastian; 16 – Urbanización Maranta; 17 – Conjunto Residencial Loira Real; 18 – Conjunto Residencial Avenida Parque

(Chelleri & Olazabal, 2012). This conception suggests that the position of urban resilience is at the center of all resilience factors and in correlation with other factors that have to be addressed in facing the pandemic (Cheshmehzangi, 2020). This is also associated with overarching conceptions, such as 'resilient urbanism' (Davoudi, 2014), which suggests the position of urban planning, urban design, and urban form (Crowe et al., 2016; Pickett et al., 2013; Sharifi, 2019; Singh, 2015). The arguments could then lead to the development of opportunities for urban transformations (Kabisch et al., 2018; Westley et al., 2011), which also touches on the central point of urban resilience policy development (Sanchez et al., 2018). The main argument is, therefore, related to how cities could prepare through better planning and design, in order to make them more resilient in facing pandemic events.

This study reflects on city resilience from one planning outlook, which is related to the morphological dimension of urban design. This particular outlook brings out an important factor that suggests how cities are developing or have developed to date and how this could lead to potential future urban design paradigms. The global example of gated community paradigm, however, is seen to be more contextualized to the functionality, spatiality, and typo-morphological features of the specific contexts. On the one hand, city resilience cannot just be simplified to the boundaries of urban form, but, on the other hand, it is possible to evaluate how a particular morphology could enhance the resilience of a city. The relationship between resilience and urban form (Sharifi, 2019) indicates how cities could be planned and designed better in order to be more resilient and more successful in preparing against an outbreak. Here, the study of gated communities from multiple contexts highlights their roles as prevention measures against a pandemic event. However, it is noted that gated communities are also criticized from other, different, standpoints. On the morphological side, a fragmented city made of parts disconnected with the rest of the urban fabric poses several problems in terms of urban space quality, urban space continuity, connections, etc. (Cheshmehzangi, 2018). Besides, a socially fragmented and divided city, with its inhabitants living inside 'bubbles', which denies interaction among different social classes (Blakely & Snyder, 1995; Janoschka & Borsdorf, 2004), can hardly be seen as an overall model for a resilient and sustainable urbanity.

Gated Communities and Prevention Measures in Shanghai and Bogotá: Commonalities, Differences, and Epidemic Resilience

In this section, we draw a comparison between the recurring functional, spatial, and typo-morphological features of the analyzed communities in Shanghai and Bogotá to highlight those elements that could have played an important role in containing the spread of the virus.

The first and more obvious feature of these compounds, both in China and Colombia, is that they are gated and accessible only by residents and authorized people. The access is granted through a series of pedestrian, vehicular, and mixed entrances surveilled by 24-h CCTV cameras and security personnel. This fact can be considered an ideal characteristic for the implementation of the pandemic prevention norms requested during a lockdown period. In Shanghai, where compounds are generally larger and provided with multiple accesses, circulation was diverted to the main entrance to allow greater control, with visitors and other people alien to the community rejected at the entrance gate by the security personnel, enabling immediate restriction on social activities and enhancing social distancing on a larger scale. In addition, at the entry points, residents' temperatures were regularly checked and recorded by security, and movements through checkpoints were also recorded. More importantly, the compound security had been enforced by the district government to monitor those under quarantine or those suspected of carrying the virus, not allowing their circulation outside their units instead. In Bogotá, private security had no responsibility nor legitimacy to carry out these controls and enforce such measures,[3] while single communities (and simple apartment buildings too) were left in confusion on how to deal with the pandemic and complaining to community managers for overreaching themselves (Tiempo, 2020).

At the same time, if we observe in more detail, it can be noticed that even the very physical element of a fence presents substantial differences between the Chinese and the Colombian contexts. In Shanghai, as well as in most of the enclosed

[3] In some buildings, security is still checking residents' temperatures but has no power to enforce any containment measure.

residential settlements realized around the country, the community's fence is usually interrupted by a two-to-three storey linear commercial podium facing the bounding arterial roads that defines the compounds' main urban fronts on at least one or two sides (Zhicheng Huayuan Community, case 2, features three commercial fronts). The shops are often connected to the interior space of the community, allowing the residents to directly purchase basic goods and daily groceries. This feature can be traced back to traditional Chinese urbanism, and it can be exemplified through the overlapping of two tendencies. On the one hand, the government enhanced and promoted a form of living within an enclosed compound that could satisfy the daily needs of its inhabitants while avoiding contact with the other blocks, especially during the early Tang Dynasty (Xu & Yang, 2008). On the other hand, during the mid-Tang to the Song era (ca. 800–1200), the urban settlements started to flourish and expand and "commercial premises made their first appearance in many residential wards. These premises then extended beyond the walled wards onto major thoroughfares and eventually replaced the isolated and highly regimented marketplaces" (Xie, 2020, p. 4). The presence of low-rise commercial podiums in contemporary communities reduces the contact among individuals coming from other compounds in a time of strict lockdown: the residents can rely on a varied choice of stores and services for their daily purchases without reaching congested malls and markets and thus reducing contact with other individuals who are potential virus carriers. However, in Bogotá, no commercial activities are usually embedded in gated communities. This may be primarily due to security reasons like avoiding unnecessary external access to the compound, but findings also support this in the planning regulations, which provide the transfer of land for basic commercial activities with local scope (Lozano Triviño, 2014, p. 108). Such conditions generally guarantee the availability of grocery and other stores and services at a walkable distance from the compound (see case 13 with a small commercial center at its external edge), but rarely within it (although case 17 features a commercial podium on the main boundary road). However, we can note that upper-class settlements (levels 5 and 6),[4] often based on individual villa typology, have no commerce within, while middle-class (levels 3 and 4) blocks that are more densely populated may include some basic activities. The theme of a commercial presence on gated communities' borders would be interesting to discuss further from different perspectives. In general, a commercial front guarantees not only a more urban appearance to fronts at street level but also an active street life, a basic condition for a safe urban environment as Jane Jacobs (1961) has already pointed out. Therefore, in cities like Bogotá, where gated communities are usually wholly surrounded by walls and fences, a walk along them, even in daytime, may appear scary and dangerous. In contrast, given the highly varied conditions of safety from street crime in Chinese cities, a walk along the edges of a gated community like Beishangwan or Greenland Haiyuguanyuan (cases 5 and 9) in Shanghai feels like quite a different

[4] The gated communities surveyed here are classified as levels 4 and 5, with one level 6 to allow for further considerations.

experience, not least because of the presence of commercial activities. In addition, the commerce within the compound increases the resilience of the system in a double-sided fashion: not only do the residents find basic goods easily available, but also commercial activities can maintain the majority of their clients during the lockdown, making their business sustainable even in difficult periods.

A second relevant feature of gated communities is the provision of a private, dedicated outdoor space accessible to residents. It connects all the buildings within the estate, and its quality changes according to various factors. In Shanghai, upper middle-class communities like those analyzed in this chapter generally enjoy rich and well-designed green spaces (Pow, 2009; Wu et al., 2014). They include sophisticated gardens with various species of plants, water features, such as ponds, cascades, canals, and fountains (all nine cases have at least one side defined by a canal, and in most of them the water strongly characterizes the landscape), pergolas, pavilions, and playgrounds, connected by paved walking paths, small plazas, and courtyards. Even if it is still not for sure whether this outdoor infrastructure has a proven ecological value (Cheshmehzangi, 2018), the advantage of compounds equipped with a large and varied green space is unquestionable. In fact, the residents could use such a large space for relaxation during the strict lockdown period, avoiding contact with people from 'outside' the community. Children could also spend some time enjoying outdoor activities. Quantitatively, data on our case studies suggest a similar provision of green area ratio (below 40%) in both contexts, although in Bogotá the variation among cases can be bigger, spanning from 20% to 65%. As for quality, the design of the outdoor space in Bogotá appears less sophisticated when compared to Chinese examples. In upper-class compounds (*Estratos* 5 and 6) like the Hacienda San Sebastián (case 15), common outdoor areas have no particular value, as every villa is provided with a generous individual garden. The quality of the outdoor area appears quite poor in the Maranta community (case 16), while the Del Monte estate (case 11), and another level 5 settlement of apartment buildings features a terraced system of paths and gardens, pleasant to the eye, but clearly resulting from leftover space after most of the plain surface facing the blocks has been used as a parking lot. However, it also enjoys a larger green area with sports equipment on one side. Furthermore, comparing more recent medium-rise compounds classified in socio-economic level 4 (cases 17 and 18) to older communities with row houses or villas of a higher level (case 16 is a level 5 settlement), we notice that the former ones enjoy a better outdoor space, characterized by a mix of hard and soft soil, piazzas and paths, playgrounds, and other equipment. This can be achieved thanks to the presence of underground parking lots freeing the ground level. However, this could also be a reason behind the generally low quality of the vegetation, as gardens appear almost devoid of large trees (cases 13, 17, and 18).[5]

Lastly, the presence of sports equipment within the compound is another important aspect that can be directly related to the quality of the outdoor and leisure facilities. Tennis courts, outdoor exercise machines, and club houses with indoor

[5] Another reason could be the relatively young age of the compounds and, consequently, their trees.

swimming pools and gyms integrated in the landscape design are very common features in the majority of the analyzed cases in Shanghai (see for example, cases 1, 2 and 6) and they are professionally managed by the estate management company. Bogotá also has some facilities generally available, although with differences. As previously stated, in upper-level settlements, like the Hacienda San Sebastián (case 15), the emphasis lies on the private dimensions of the outdoor area, with generous private gardens that leave little space for common areas; the only facility is a tennis court. Villas compounding La Arborada de San José (case 10) feature only a football pitch and a tennis court, as is the case with Maranta (case 16). In compounds with block typology, indoor gyms and a common room are diffused, as well as roof-top terraces for barbecues, available upon reservation for a daily fee. On the ground, basic sport areas (usually for basketball) may be available (cases 17 and 18), as well as playgrounds for children (cases 13, 17, and 18). Given Bogotá's climate, outdoor swimming pools are not provided. In the end, the availability of such facilities, together with a well-designed outdoor space, can allow residents to enjoy fresh air and a certain number of activities without leaving the estate. In China, for example, other than in the Hubei Province, outdoor spaces remained accessible during the February to March 2020 lockdown. In Colombia however, where selective lockdowns are still ongoing after re-opening and further closures, access to internal playgrounds, sport fields, and gardens have been explicitly prohibited in Bogotá (Cundinamarca, 2020). Nonetheless, in an uncertain future with possible soft, selective, or partial lockdowns, the opportunity for residents to enjoy (if legal) open air activities accessible to a more limited, thus controlled, number of people than in a public park or in a normal gym appears particularly important.

Results and Conclusions

At the time of writing, the total registered cases from the beginning of the outbreak in China are slightly above 90,000 and the transmission type classified as "cluster of cases," while in Colombia the total registered cases are well above 500,000, with a "community transmission" classification (World Health Organization, 2020). The reasons behind these figures can be related to a large variety of factors, such as the different institutional and economic arrangements, the promptness in implementing effective prevention measures, their strict observance by the population, and others that go far beyond the scope of this research. Nonetheless, it can be said that urban morphology and the way the two cities are structured and managed have also played a critical role in enhancing resilience against the pandemic outbreak.

Through this comparative study, it can be observed how the gated communities in Shanghai can be generally considered more resilient against acute shocks under the typo-morphological and functional perspective if compared with those in Bogotá. In other words, a 'city of islands' clearly outperforms other types of settlements when segregation becomes an unavoidable necessity; however, the inner qualities and the size of these 'islands' matter even more. In fact, even if some common elements can be found in both contexts, like the provision of green spaces for residents' use or the fact that they are enclosed and segregated from the rest of the city, Chinese compounds present a more effective balance between the satisfaction of people's daily necessities and the lessening of their mobility needs to avoid potential virus-spreading contact. The higher quality of designed outdoor spaces, the related amenities, and the presence of a series of basic services in the commercial podium ensure continuity of critical services even during a period of lockdown, while also providing the possibility for relaxation. This fact, coupled with the context-specific prevention measures implemented by the local institutions through the estate management, appears to be an effective tool in the containment of the disease outbreaks and can become an impactful adaptive urban planning example that enhances the city's resilience.

Acknowledgments Xuanrui Zhang and Qikai Li from the University of Nottingham Ningbo China, Department of Architecture and Built Environment, provided very helpful assistance with the illustrations and data elaboration.

References

100 Resilient Cities. (n.d.). *What is urban resilience?* http://www.100resilientcities.org/resources/. Accessed 20 May 2020.

Admiraal, H., & Cornaro, A. (2018). *Underground spaces unveiled: Planning and creating the cities of the future*. ICE Publishing.

Admiraal, H., & Cornaro, A. (2019). Future cities, resilient cities – The role of underground space in achieving urban resilience. *Underground Space* (in press).

Alexander, D. (2013). Resilience and disaster risk reduction: An etymological journey. *Natural Hazards and Earth System Sciences, 13*(11), 2707–2716.

Alterman, R. (1988). Adaptive planning. *Cognitive Science, 12*, 393–421.

Ban, K. (2012, May 23). The future we want. *The New York Times*. https://www.nytimes.com/2012/05/24/opinion/the-future-we-want.html

Barnes, D. S. (2006). *The great stink of Paris and the nineteenth-century struggle against filth and germs*. Johns Hopkins University Press.

Benchimol, J. L. (1990). *Pereira Passos, um Haussmann tropical: A renovação urbana da cidade do Rio de Janeiro no início do século XX*. Prefeitura da Cidade do Rio de Janeiro, Secretaria Municipal de Cultura, Turismo e Esportes.

Bigon, L. (2016). Bubonic plague, colonial ideologies, and urban planning policies: Dakar, Lagos, and Kumasi. *Planning Perspective, 31*(2), 205–226.

Blakely, E. J., & Snyder, M. G. (1995). *Fortress America: Gated Communities in the United States*. Brookings Institution Press/Lincoln Institute of Land Policy.

Borsdorf, A., Hidalgo, R., & Sánchez, R. (2007). A new model of urban development in Latin America: The gated communities and fenced cities in the metropolitan areas of Santiago de Chile and Valparaíso. *Cities, 24*(5), 365–378.

Breitung, W. (2013). Enclave urbanism in China: Attitudes towards gated communities in Guangzhou. *Urban Geography, 33*(2), 278–294.

Cabrera Laverde, O. D. (2013). Gated Communities en Latinoamérica. Los casos de Argentina, México, Colombia y Brasil. *Revista de Arquitectura, 15*, 44–53.

Caldeira, T. P. (2001). *City of walls. Crime, segregation, and citizenship in São Paulo*. University of California Press.

Chelleri, L., & Olazabal, M. (2012). *Multidisciplinary perspectives on urban resilience: A workshop report*. Basque Centre for Climate Change (BC3).
Chen, F., & Thwaites, K. (2013). *Chinese urban design. The typomorphological approach*. Routledge.
Chen, X. (Ed.). (2009). *Shanghai rising: State power and local transformations in a global megacity*. University of Minnesota Press.
Cheshmehzangi, A. (2018). The changing urban landscape of Chinese Cities: Positive and negative impacts of urban design controls on contemporary urban housing. *Sustainability, 10*(8), 2839.
Cheshmehzangi, A. (2020). *The city in need: Urban resilience and city management in disruptive disease outbreak events*. Springer.
Cheshmezangi, A., & Butters, C. (2016). Chinese urban residential blocks: Towards improved environmental and living qualities. *Urban Design International, 22*(3), 219–235.
Cookson Smith, P. (2011). *The urban design of concessions*. MCCM Creations.
Coy, M., & Pöhler, M. (2002). Gated communities in Latin American megacities: Case studies in Brazil and Argentina. *Environment and Planning B: Planning and Design, 29*(3), 355–370.
Crowe, P., Foley, K., & Collier, M. (2016). Operationalizing urban resilience through a framework for adaptive co-management and design: Five experiments in urban planning practice and policy. *Environmental Science and Policy, 62*, 112–119.
Cundinamarca. (2020, March 27). *Cerrarle el paso al COVID-19 en conjuntos cerrados depende de sus administradores y residentes*. http://www.cundinamarca.gov.co/Home/prensa2018/asnoticiasprensa/cerrarle+el+paso+al+covid+19+en+conjuntos+cerrados. Accessed 11 Aug 2020.
Davoudi, S. (2014). Climate change, securitisation of nature, and resilient urbanism. *Environment Planning C, 32*, 360–375.
Deng, X. (n.d.). Excerpts from talks given in Wuchang, Shenzhen, Zhuhai and Shanghai. *The selected works of Deng Xiaoping. Modern Day Contributions to Marxism-Leninism*. https://dengxiaopingworks.wordpress.com/2013/03/18/excerpts-from-talks-given-in-wuchang-shenzhen-zhuhai-and-shanghai/. Accessed 12 Aug 2020.
Engelmann, L., Henderson, J., & Lynteris, C. (2018). *The plague and the city in history*. Routledge.
Esherick, J. W. (1999). Modernity and nation in the Chinese city. In J. W. Esherick (Ed.), *Remaking the Chinese City: Modernity and national identity, 1900 to 1950* (pp. 1–16). University of Hawaii Press.
Frioux, S. (2013). *Les batailles de l'hygiène. Villes et environment de Pasteur aux Trente Glorieuses*. PUF.
Hajer, M., & Dassen, T. (2014). *Slimme Steden: de opgave voor de 21e-eeuwse stedenbouw in beeld*. Rotterdam: Nai010.
He, J. (2015). *Evaluation of plan implementation: Peri-urban development and the Shanghai master plan 1999–2020*. Delft University of Technology, Faculty of Architecture and the Built Environment, Department of Urbanism.
Hidalgo, R. (2004). De los pequeños condominios a la ciudad vallada: las urbanizaciones cerradas y la nueva geografía social en Santiago de Chile (1990–2000). *Eure, 30*(91), 29–52.
Jacobs, J. (1961). *The death and life of great American cities*. Random House.
Janoschka, M., & Borsdorf, A. (2004). *Condomínios fechados* and *barrios privados*: The rise of private residencial neighbourhoods in Latin America. In G. Glasze, C. Webster, & K. Frantz (Eds.), *Private neighbourhoods. Global and local perspectives* (pp. 92–108). Routledge.
Jiang, Y., & Waley, P. (2020). Who builds cities in China? How urban investment and development companies have transformed Shanghai. *International Journal of Urban and Regional Research, 44*(4), 636–651.
Kabisch, S., Koch, F., & Gawel, E. (Eds.). (2018). *Urban transformations: Sustainable urban development through resource efficiency, quality of life, and resilience*. Springer.
Kan, H. Y., Forsyth, A., & Rowe, P. (2017). Redesigning China's superblock neighborhoods: Policies, opportunities and challenges. *Journal of Urban Design, 22*(6), 757–777.
Lee, C. C. (2013). The city as a common framework. Rethinking the developmental city in China. In C. C. Lee (Ed.), *Common frameworks. Part 1: Xiamen* (pp. 10–28). Harvard University Graduate School of Design.

Lopez, R. (2012). *Building American public health*. Palgrave Macmillan.
Lozano Triviño, C. (2014). Los conjuntos cerrados en la conformación urbana de la ciudad contemporánea. La Colina como estudio de caso en Bogotá. *Universidad Nacional de Colombia*. Facultad de Artes.
Mendoza, F. R. (2015). Transformaciones urbanas vinculadas a barrios cerrados: evidencias para la discusión sobre fragmentación espacial en ciudades latinoamericanas. *Cuadernos de Geografía: Revista Colombiana de Geografía, 24*(1), 121–133.
Mendoza Jaramillo, A. (2016). Gestión urbanística de las urbanizaciones cerradas en Colombia: el caso de Chía. *Prospectiva. Revista de Trabajo Social e intervención social, 21*, 107–136.
Miao, P. (2003). Deserted streets in a jammed town: The gated community in Chinese cities and its solution. *Journal of Urban Design, 8*(1), 45–66.
Monson, K. (2008). String block vs superblock patterns of dispersal in China. *Architectural Design, 7*(1), 46–53.
Montoya Garay, J. W. (2018). *De la ciudad hidalga a la metrópoli globalizada: Una historiografía Urbana y regional de Bogotá*. Universidad Nacional de Colombia.
Pickett, S., Cadenasso, M., & McGrath, B. (Eds.). (2013). *Resilience in ecology and urban design: Linking theory and practice for sustainable cities*. Springer.
Pow, C. P. (2009). Neoliberalism and the aestheticization of new middle-class landscapes. *Antipode, 41*(2), 371–390.
Qian, J. (2014). Deciphering the prevalence of neighborhood enclosure amidst Post-1949 Chinese cities: A critical synthesis. *Journal of Planning Literature, 29*(1), 3–19.
Rowe, P. G., Forsyth, A., & Kan, H. Y. (2016). *China's urban communities: Concepts, contexts, and well-being*. Walter de Gruyter GmbH.
Saldarriaga Roa, A. (2000). *Bogotá siglo XX. Urbanismo, arquitectura y vida urbana*. Alcaldía Mayor de Bogotá, Departamento Administrativo de Planeación Distrital.
Sanchez, A., van der Heijden, J., & Osmond, P. (2018). The city politics of an urban age: Urban resilience, conceptualizations and policies. *Palgrave Communications, 4*(25), 1–12.
Shanghai Municipal People's Government. (2019). Total households, population, density of registered population and life expectancy (1978–2018). *Shanghai Statistical Yearbook*. http://tjj.sh.gov.cn/tjnj/nj19.htm?d1=2019tjnje/E0201.htm. Accessed 23 Aug 2020.
Sharifi, A. (2019). Urban form resilience: A meso-scale analysis. *Cities, 93*, 238–252.
Sims, S. (2020, May 3). How one of Brazil's largest favelas confronts coronavirus. *Bloomberg*. https://www.bloomberg.com/news/features/2020-05-03/how-one-of-brazil-s-largest-favelas-confronts-coronavirus
Singh, R. (2015). *Urban development challenges, risks and resilience in Asian mega cities*. Springer.
State Council. (1998). *A notification from the State Council on further deepening the reform of urban housing system and accelerating housing construction*. Beijing, China.
Swanson, M. (1977). The sanitation syndrome: Bubonic plague and urban native policy in the Cape Colony, 1900–1909. *Journal of African History, 18*(3), 387–410.
Tiempo, E. (2020, May 19). ¿Qué está permitido y qué no en una propiedad horizontal por pandemia? *El Tiempo*. https://www.eltiempo.com/bogota/coronavirus-en-bogota-que-esta-permitido-y-que-no-en-una-propiedad-horizontal-497364
Torres Tovar, C. (2007). Ciudad informal Colombiana. *Bitácora Urbano Territorial, 1*(11), 53–93.
Vogel, B., & Henstra, D. (2015). Studying local climate adaptation: A heuristic research framework for comparative policy analysis. *Global Environmental Change, 31*, 110–120.
Wainwright, O. (2020, April 7). How to build a hospital in nine days: Emergency architecture in a pandemic. *The Guardian*. https://www.theguardian.com/artanddesign/2020/apr/07/how-to-build-a-hospital-in-nine-days-emergency-architecture-in-a-pandemic-coronavirus-outbreak?CMP=Share_iOSApp_Other
Walcott, S. M., & Pannell, C. W. (2006). Metropolitan spatial dynamics: Shanghai. *Habitat International, 30*(2), 199–211.

Westley, F., Olsson, P., Folke, C., Homer-Dixon, T., Vredenburg, H., Loorbach, D., … Nilsson, M. (2011). Tipping toward sustainability: Emerging pathways of transformation. *Ambio: A Journal of the Human Environment, 40*(7), 762–780.

World Health Organization. (2020, August 27). *WHO coronavirus disease (COVID-19) dashboard*. https://covid19.who.int/table. Accessed 28 Aug 2020.

Wu, C., Wei, Y., & Wang, M. Y. (2014). Planned gated communities in urban China. Outdoor activities and designed leisure spaces. In M. Y. Wang, P. Kee, & J. Gao (Eds.), *Transforming Chinese cities* (pp. 188–210). Routledge.

Wu, F. (2003). Globalization, place promotion and urban development in Shanghai. *Journal of Urban Affairs, 25*(1), 55–78.

Wu, F. (2015). *Planning for growth. Urban and regional planning in China*. Routledge.

Wu, J., Wang, M., Li, W., Peng, J., & Huang, L. (2015). Impact of urban green space on residential housing prices: Case study in Shenzhen. *Journal of Urban Planning and Development, 141*(4), 05014023.

Xiao, Y., Lu, Y., Guo, Y., & Yuan, Y. (2017). Estimating the willingness to pay for green space services in Shanghai: Implications for social equity in urban China. *Urban Forestry & Urban Greening, 26*, 95–103.

Xie, J. (2020). *Chinese urbanism. Urban form and life in the Tang-Song dynasties*. World Scientific.

Xinhua. (2020, April 2). *New study shows transmission control measures greatly avert COVID-19 cases in China*. National Health Commission of the People's Republic of China. http://en.nhc.gov.cn/2020-04/02/c_78705.htm. Accessed 11 Aug 2020.

Xu, M., & Yang, Z. (2008). Theoretical debate on gated communities: Genesis, controversies, and the way forward. *Urban Design International, 13*(4), 213–226.

Xu, M., & Yang, Z. (2009). Design history of China's gated cities and neighborhoods: Prototype and evolution. *Urban Design International, 12*(2), 99–117.

Chapter 3
Cities' Health Dimension Post-pandemic: Brazil Urban Planning Aspects

Ana Maria Girotti Sperandio, Angela Alessandra Torezan Silingardi, Giovanna Gastaldo Cifoni, and Rafael de Souza Salomão

Introduction

The COVID-19 pandemic caused humanitarian challenges of major proportions, mostly related to the specific characteristics of today's cities, whether in the way they are configured socio-spatially, politically, or economically. Measures to control the advancement of the coronavirus involved changes in social dynamics within urban environments and required efforts never before undertaken by populations and governments worldwide.

In countries like Brazil, historical situations of national emergency caused by other pandemic events have not mobilized a comparable set of short-term adaptations and restrictions. Indicators of pandemic actions in this country pointed to social determinants of infections and deaths caused by COVID-19. A survey conducted by the United Health System (SUS) in partnership with the University of São Paulo pointed out that in high poverty areas, the relative risk of virus-related mortality was greater (Fioravanti, 2020).

This scenario highlighted the catalyst potential for health promotion and protection in urban planning, considering its capacity for spatial transformation and social determination, as well as revealing its relationship with the spread of diseases in structurally vulnerable urban regions not covered by social and economic public policies. Thus, doubts were raised regarding the theoretical and practical skills of planning conducted in this context, and the viability of urban planning in a future

A. M. G. Sperandio (✉)
Faculty of Civil Engineering and Architecture, University of Campinas, Campinas, SP, Brazil
e-mail: amgspera@fec.unicamp.brj

A. A. T. Silingardi
Architect and Urbanist, Safety Engineer, Campinas, SP, Brazil

G. G. Cifoni · R. de Souza Salomão
Architect and Urbanist, Campinas, SP, Brazil

© The Author(s), under exclusive license to Springer Nature Switzerland AG 2021

M. A. Montoya et al. (eds.), *COVID-19 and Cities*, The Urban Book Series,
https://doi.org/10.1007/978-3-030-84134-8_3

that will require profound changes in individual conceptions and collective provisions in the search for healthy cities.

COVID-19 is not the first disease to raise questions about changes in the ordering and planning of cities and the way in which public health policies are developed. In the second half of the nineteenth century and beginning of the twentieth century, hygienist transformations and reforms have been proposed in large cities in Europe, the USA, and Brazil, aiming to combat and control diseases such as malaria, cholera, and yellow fever (Guimarães, 2014). Thus, they became examples of how to relate urban planning and public health within a historical context. On the other hand, the Brazilian urbanization process during the twentieth century, combined with urban and sanitary legislation, triggered a series of interventions that ended up expelling the poorest people from the central areas of cities. These interventions are often motivated by an economic discourse about the need to promote improvements in circulation and urban infrastructure, allocating the central areas of cities to high-traffic road equipment and prioritizing the circulation of goods and services. With this movement, low-income housing projects are implemented in remote neighborhoods where the value of the land is lower and where the infrastructure, the provision of basic services, and public transport do not meet the demands of the population (Lefebvre, 2016).

Voluntary segregation, understood as a "natural" movement of the highest income population, also contributed to socioeconomic withdrawal between communities. These segregations are based on individuality, alienation, and removal from social crises and urban violence, for a life "between equals" inside gated condominiums and walled subdivisions (Lefebvre, 2016), and implemented on the edges of cities. People need to travel longer distances to reach work, study sites, shops, and services, demanding an effective public transport system or a road system that includes an increasing number of private vehicles, making it difficult to develop solutions for urban mobility. This socio-spatial and mobility situation triggered a series of problems common to urban centers, such as an increase in atmospheric pollution, time lost in displacements, and its consequences for the health of the population (Scifoni, 2016).

Understanding the processes of city formation and the natural history of diseases, combined with studies on the geography of health, may allow the insertion of new issues in urban planning. From this perspective, health goes beyond the scope of medical power and starts to occupy an important place in the political field (Guimarães, 2014). It is estimated that, after the COVID-19 pandemic, health promotion, disease prevention, urban planning, and mobility will have an important place in public policies in the search for healthy and resilient cities.

The situation imposed by the COVID-19 pandemic spurred studies and research in relation to urban planning, health promotion, and situations of vulnerability. This chapter presents initiatives to combat the pandemic that have contributed to the basic application of the concept of healthy cities in different scenarios around the world.

Revisiting Healthy Cities' Concepts and Premises

In a context in which urban planning must be a relevant instrument in decision-making focused on strategies that promote and protect health, healthy cities enable the creation of resilient communities and foment the development of collective potentialities and experimentation in equity.

The definition of healthy cities has been adapted from historical contexts. The World Health Organization (1998) defines healthy cities as those that allow the expansion of community resources through cooperation among people to carry out daily tasks, developing life to its maximum potential (WHO, 1998).

A frequent and current definition of healthy cities used by urban planning researchers was adopted in 2017 by author De Leeuw (2017), who states that:

> Healthy Cities, we feel, are quintessential vehicles to create a charming Anthropocene, an epoch in which community and creativity work together to shape institutions and governance arrangements that benefit equitable health and well-being for all in the new natural habitat of humanity: *urbs* and *civitas*, the city and its people. (De Leeuw, 2017, p. 19)

Adopted in this chapter, this definition aimed to connect people within city spaces and, beyond that, pointed out how questions related to life in a community can influence the population's health and well-being. Reinforcing this idea, Santana (2007) stated that the healthy city concept refers to a city as a community in which health social determinants interact with each other and influence the inhabitants' quality of life.

The inter-relations between community, academy, private institutions, and governance, as supporting actors in search for new urban planning solutions, are fundamental to developing healthy cities. Therefore, the intention to relate this concept to the rapid urban planning initiatives developed was to show that articulation and cooperation between the various sectors of society were essential in minimizing the impacts caused by the pandemic.

Methodological Tools

This study contemplated reviews of legal frameworks, international documents, guiding public policies, and records of experiences that denoted a new approach of urban planning focused on healthy and, therefore, resilient cities.

The relationship between city and health should be constantly addressed and continuously discussed by researchers, both at the national level and in international documents. For the development of this chapter, Brazilian legal frameworks were considered, such as Law 8080 (Brasil, 1990); the *National Health Promotion Policy* (Brasil, 2018); and Law 10,257 (Brasil, 2001). Regarding the international public policy guiding documents, the following ones were considered: *The Ottawa Charter* (1986) and the *Integrating Health in Urban and Territorial Planning Guide: A Sourcebook* (WHO & UN, 2020), which strengthen integration and the coalition for the construction of healthy cities with emergency public policies that address health and, consequently, life.

In the development of this chapter, initiatives for active mobility, the use of public spaces, and green areas were selected through news reports in the period between March and July 2020 in countries such as Italy, Colombia, the USA, Germany, and China. In these countries, such initiatives allowed the population to remain active during COVID-19. Social isolation stimulated active commuting, pop-up bike paths, and bicycle sharing systems. In addition, physical activity was encouraged through the opening of transit routes for the exclusive use of pedestrians and an improvement in green area distribution in cities.

Another theme selected was the urban community gardens. They are considered another way to face the critical periods in order to strengthen the notion of community through the articulation between the various social groups involved in health promotion. Some consolidated projects developed in Brazilian cities will be presented below.

The purpose of this chapter is to analyze and indicate actions and strategies that potentialized urban planning for a healthy city based on studies, virtual monitoring, and proposals for coping with the pandemic situation, and which also considered good living and the interaction between the city and its population. In addition, this chapter aims to present actions that stimulated the values and principles advocated by the legal frameworks studied, such as commitment, social participation, networking, social inclusion, happiness, and others. Such values and principles, when fully achieved, promote the resilience of communities and a strengthening of cities, not only in emergency situations but also on a permanent basis.

Selected Initiatives and Coping Strategies During the Pandemic that Reflected the Healthy City

In this section, some coping initiatives developed during the pandemic and other pre-existing actions in the cities are identified. Their results will be presented and some indication given as to how they can support urban planning for a healthy city, establishing the relationship between the social determinants of health and the principles and values of the *National Health Promotion Policy* (Brasil, 2018).

Active Mobility and the Well-being of the Population

In facing the pandemic, some cities stood out with their immediate actions related to mobility issues, allowing greater distancing between people during displacement.

Bogotá, Colombia, is known for its extensive network of cycle paths (about 550 km). During the pandemic, another 76 km of temporary bike lanes were created, partially using some major avenues, reducing the circulation of motor vehicles, and favoring active modes of transportation (Moloney, 2020). In an attempt to expand the cycle network, other cities have made parking spaces on the streets available for the circulation of bicycles.

In Berlin, Germany, bike lanes were enlarged using adhesive tape, thus creating pop-up bike lanes that allowed more social distance between cyclists during COVID-19. After the pilot test, it was observed that this measure provided greater safety for cyclists in relation to accidents and did not impair vehicle traffic because narrower lanes were used (Oltermann, 2020).

In general, wider lanes for automobiles allow them to travel faster and, consequently, the occurrence of occasional serious accidents. Narrower lanes imply greater care on the part of drivers, lower vehicle speeds and, therefore, streets are more favorable to cyclists and pedestrians (Speck, 2016). The pandemic accelerated the expansion of the cycle path system in several cities around the world and improved its acceptance by governments and populations, no longer seeing it as a high-risk facility (Moloney, 2020).

Another important point in encouraging active mobility was the shared bicycle system. Cities like New York and Beijing that already had this system in operation had an increase in the flow of users during the pandemic, which boosted a form of individual displacement and reduced the gathering of people on public transport (ITDP Brasil, 2020).

To encourage less polluting transport and greater social isolation during the pandemic, in Italy, on May 13, 2020, it was decreed that up to 500 euros would be provided for the purchase of bicycles, electric scooters, hoverboards, and Segways for cities with more than 50,000 inhabitants (Mobilize, 2020).

Studies have shown that higher rates of air pollution were related to higher rates of mortality from coronavirus, which indicates greater vulnerability of people exposed to pollution (Lisa Friedman, 2020). The reduced circulation of motorized vehicles during the pandemic also brought benefits, such as the reduction of noise and air pollution. It was pointed out, through satellite images, that this reduction can be favorable for the health of cities and, consequently, of urban populations (NASA, 2020), as shown in Fig. 3.1.

One action that could be preserved for the future is the practice of working from home, since the decreased movement of people commuting to work and limited vehicle traffic allows for a reduction in the emission of pollutants into the air, thus avoiding congestion and contributing to the physical and mental well-being of citizens. This type of working had already been used in some places but, after the pandemic, its more widespread application in large and medium-sized cities may contribute to the development of healthier cities.

It is imperative to reduce the circulation of motor vehicles, and for that, cities could invest in infrastructure and public policies for active transport, such as cycling and walking. To enhance this, wider, wooded, and accessible sidewalks should be considered, as well as lit paths and public roads with safe separation between cars

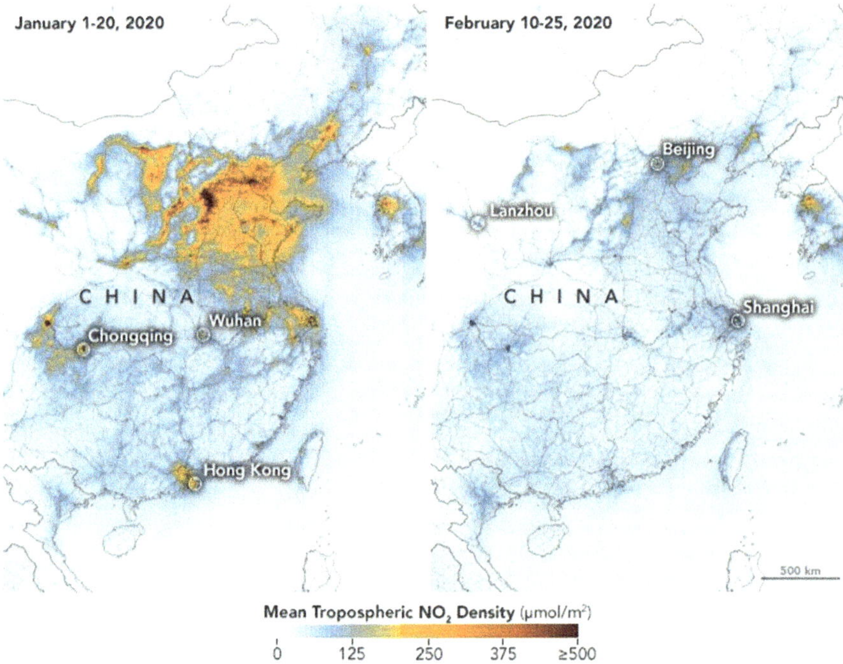

Fig. 3.1 Decreases in nitrogen dioxide (NO_2) over China. (Source: NASA & ESA, 2020)

and pedestrians. In a post-pandemic context, in which circulation is once again increasing, it is important to re-design spaces of social interaction and attractive elements along the way, such as fountains, squares, shops, and recreational activities. In tree-lined streets, conditions favorable to pedestrians are evident, but where these conditions do not exist, the environment proves to be inhospitable for passers-by (Duarte, 2000).

Sidewalks are part of the infrastructure of urban mobility; however, they are not administered by Brazilian municipalities as part of this system. Most Brazilian municipalities delegate the responsibility for the execution and maintenance of sidewalks to the owner of the adjacent property, with the public authority only in charge of carrying out inspections (Nunes et al., 2016). *Associação Brasileira de Normas Técnicas* (2015), the Brazilian Association of Technical Standards, through NBR 9050, establishes several criteria for sidewalks, such as dimensions, slopes, obstacles, urban furniture, accessibility, and safety standards, generally mandatory minimum conditions, but not necessarily the best conditions possible. The quality of the sidewalks reflects the stage of development of the city and reveals its concern with the mobility, security, and accessibility of its population. They are places of passage and also of social integration; therefore, the lack of adequate conditions on sidewalks causes not only a disincentive to active mobility (walking, cycling, etc.) but also a decrease in social connections and contact with public spaces and the city (Nunes et al., 2016).

Several elements can make a walk attractive and, in addition, the distances to be covered and the time spent on the route must be considered. According to a study prepared for the IPEA, the Institute of Applied Economic Research (Pereira et al., 2020), in the 20 largest cities in Brazil with low-income populations in vulnerable situations, it was estimated that there were more than 228,000 inhabitants living more than 30 minutes walking distance from a basic unit of public health care, and about 1.6 million people living more than 5 km away from a hospital with an intensive care unit. This study revealed weaknesses in the Brazilian urban mobility system in a pandemic scenario, as walking or using public transport with a sick or seriously ill person is neither feasible nor recommended when considering contagious diseases.

In addition, one cannot fail to consider that the viability of public transport, such as buses, subways, and trolleybuses, depends on the walking conditions of the city, as users must be able to cover the distance between the starting point and end point of their trip comfortably and safely (Speck, 2016).

Active transport contributes to the promotion of people's health in cities. In addition to allowing isolation and reducing the spread of diseases, it also emits less air pollution, thus preventing respiratory diseases. It is a way to get some exercise and provide autonomy, happiness, and well-being to people.

Green Areas, Public Spaces, and Their Equitable Distribution in the City

Green areas and parks were some of the first places allowed for use in some countries in the first period of reopening, as these spaces allowed contact with nature, helped in the treatment of the effects caused by isolation and, because they were wide and open, allowed larger distances between people. During the research, it was noted that another recurring situation in cities was the need to redefine the use of roads, turning them into free areas so that people could use them, get some exercise, and still maintain a safe distance from others.

In 2020, in Seattle, USA, there were more than 485 parks within the city and, according to Seattle Park and Recreation, 94% of the population lived within 10 minutes walking distance from any of them. This institution recommended that during the pandemic, people only go to green areas if they could walk there. If it were necessary to use a car to reach the destination it meant that it was distant and could contribute to the gathering of people. Other changes were the earlier closing time of parks, 8 pm rather than at 11:30 pm during normal periods, and the use of parks was only allowed for activities like walking, running, and cycling, and no longer for staying and having picnics. In neighborhoods without green areas, the mayor created the Stay Healthy Streets program, which determined the closure of streets for cars and made them available for pedestrians and cyclists, as well as for outdoor activities (Derrick, 2020).

In early May, as a proposal to minimize the effects of isolation, Domino Park in New York had circles of 2.5 meters in diameter painted on the grass to delimit spaces for groups of people, thus allowing the population to take advantage of the time spent in the park whilst keeping safe distancing (Harrouk, 2020). This strategy, of low cost and quick and simple execution, could easily be replicated in other cities. In San Francisco, USA, the Parks and Recreation Department based its actions on New York and established similar circles in Dolores Park and three other areas in different neighborhoods. These parks were at risk of closure due to the lack of respect of social exclusion rules by regulars and this was the option found to keep them open to the population. The circles also worked as a constant reminder of the atypical situation of the pandemic and the need for care and detachment (Keeling, 2020).

In Oakland, USA, the Oakland Slow Streets program, recently created, prioritized pedestrian and cyclist circulation by designating some streets (almost 10% of city roads) to be closed to high-speed traffic. This measure made it possible for people to get some exercise with the necessary distancing, converting the roads into a safe public space for them to use (Oakland, 2020). This program contributed to the shared use of open areas, promoted the physical and mental health of the population, and also favored equity in the city, as not all communities had a park close to their home.

The balanced distribution of public spaces and green areas in cities should be rethought so that more people have access to the benefits offered by them, such as leisure options, the possibility of outdoor exercise, social interaction, and improvement in air quality, benefiting the physical and mental health of all. A possible solution to this problem of unequal park distribution is the introduction of pocket parks, small green areas that can be distributed throughout the city, allowing equitable access to green areas by the population, in contrast to what commonly happens in cities, with the concentration of larger parks being in privileged areas (Lira, 2020). Another important issue is that of the routes and accesses to pedestrian and bicycle paths, which should be combined with parks and public spaces so as to promote walking in the city and encouraging people to visit places, since these routes favor movement and greater connection between spaces.

An interesting alternative to the development of new public spaces was the adaptation of streets and avenues for the intermittent use by pedestrians and cyclists at weekends, for example. This practice was consolidated in populous cities, such as New York, Santiago, and São Paulo (as in the case of Avenida Paulista and Elevado Costa e Silva) and constituted an alternative to make public spaces feasible in regions without land available for the implementation of new parks and equipment, providing the means for leisure, walking, exercise, etc. In addition, this alternative provided recreational areas for people who lived in densely populated regions far from squares and areas of shared use.

The transformation of these locations could offer a new consolidated look for certain areas of the cities due to the change in their use. A road once dominated by cars, buses, and other types of vehicles could become a place for pedestrians, even if only temporarily, providing a sense of belonging and autonomy, as well as breaking paradigms.

These initiatives require planning and communication between different sectors of society, involving public authorities, departments related to traffic flow, management of vehicles and pedestrians, commerce, and the local community, in order to make this transformation of practical use, meeting the demands imposed by each stakeholder, such as hours of operation, control, adaptation and containment of flows, actions for assembly and disassembly of equipment and furniture, places for storing equipment, and other measures (Frau & Neto, 2017; Garcia, 2014). In order to achieve this objective in Brazil, there are some difficulties to be overcome and many variables involved in addition to the usual bureaucracy of Brazilian public administration, but there are guidelines in this regard. The National Health Promotion Policy (Brasil, 2018) already dictates the creation of healthy environments and territories, the practice of physical activity, and the promotion of safe mobility as priorities for the promotion of health and determines those responsible for implementing these issues.

Considering the previously discussed alternatives that would result in a decrease in the flow of vehicles and, consequently, a decrease in the spaces designated for them on public roads, more adjustments in the use of these spaces within this scenario might be foreseen. In conjunction with the decrease in demand for street parking spaces, parklets could be used, which are proposals that have been tested and established in several cities around the world.

This set of proposals, involving the transformation of the consolidated urban space into an alternative form of appropriation and public use, did not require major urban interventions and resource mobilization, but actions aimed at effective public policies. It is also important to reaffirm that the proposals highlighted here were practiced in several cities around the world with a positive effect, both with regard to their practical and effective functioning, and in the results related to the search for healthy cities.

In view of the solutions presented here for the urban planning of a healthy city before and during COVID-19, it was noted that the promotion of public spaces and green areas in the urban environment contributed to the active life of the population, social inclusion, contact with the urban landscape, and consequently promoted health, happiness, autonomy, the feeling of belonging, and the strengthening of the notion of community in the population. In a post-COVID-19 transition scenario, these proposals could improve urban resilience and configure responses to the demands of the population in the search for spaces for public use and leisure areas, increasing the possibilities of necessary physical distancing without impeding the practice of physical activity.

Community Urban Gardens and Human Capital Development

Community urban gardens are successful examples of the application of a concept similar to that of small green areas, where smaller spaces distributed in greater number throughout the city can have positive effects for a greater number of people, offering healthy food, encouraging social interaction, and the appropriation of idle spaces, for example. The gardens were considered another way of coping with the pandemic. Three garden projects in the state of São Paulo (Brazil) will be presented: two in the countryside and one in the state capital. The projects implemented in the countryside, in the cities of Santa Bárbara d'Oeste and Conchal, were monitored by the *Laboratory of Urban Investigations* (LABINUR) linked to the Faculty of Civil Engineering, Architecture and Urbanism of the State University of Campinas (Unicamp), and the project in the state capital was monitored by the NGO *Cidades Sem Fome* (Cities Without Hunger).

In all cases, the gardens were set up on idle land with the collaboration of the community and local government with support from universities or non-governmental organizations. In São Paulo, the project initially intended to generate income by employing and training people living on the margins of the labor market. After implementation, it was noticed that the results exceeded the initial objectives, resulting in similar actions in the city (Belloni, 2018), validating and coinciding with what LABINUR observed in the experiences of Santa Bárbara d'Oeste and Conchal, where it was found that these actions went beyond the issue of food production (Sperandio & Bloes, 2020).

The *Cities Without Hunger* project, created in 2003, proposed the installation of community gardens on land within communities in the East Zone of São Paulo to provide work and food for the poor of the region, mostly the unemployed or retired and low-income families. Initially, the areas occupied were given by private organizations and public departments and, with the recognition of results, awards and dissemination in the media, individuals also began to assign unoccupied land to the NGO. Until 2018, the gardens followed a local marketing model that required daily dedication to work. With the increase in demand, it was possible to establish a second model, where the beneficiaries started to have formal work contracts and better salaries. In addition, new partnerships have emerged, with companies that have given land for planting or that have guaranteed the purchase of produce from the whole gardens (Belloni, 2018).

When implemented in 2003, these gardens had a positive impact on the surrounding community life by providing food and generating income for the families involved. In addition, by modifying the landscape of that area, they created a pleasant green space, shared with the population, making the place a reference point in the community, impacting the adjacent streets and alleys, and transforming the spaces of passage into spaces of contact and sharing. Involvement in the actions initially proposed, stimulated, and generated new collective practices, creating cooperation and networks, and strengthening the population as a community (Belloni, 2018).

Even though their initial purpose was not that of a green area intended exclusively for leisure, as with traditional squares, these gardens have become an option for meeting, talking, collaborating, and exchanging experiences. These characteristics of community space for social interaction could also be seen in the projects presented below.

In Santa Bárbara d'Oeste, the medicinal and unconventional plant garden project was developed in 2013 at the Municipal School of Elementary and Child Education Maria Augusta Canto Camargo Bilia (EMEFEI Maria Augusta Bilia) together with the College of Agriculture Luiz de Queiroz (ESALQ) at the University of São Paulo (USP) and with the support of the *Network of Potentially Healthy Municipalities* (RMPS). Installed on school grounds, it had about 50 species of vegetables that were cultivated by the students weekly (Fig. 3.2). There was a specific schedule, specially prepared for each school level, that involved knowledge of each plant, its origin, properties, cultivation, harvest, and preparation for consumption (Sperandio & Bloes, 2020).

According to the school principal (personal communication, June 10, 2020), the group expanded over the years and in 2020, in addition to the students, there was the involvement of school staff, parents, and community members who helped with the maintenance of the plantation and shared some of the produce for food and as medicine. A sanitary doctor who collaborated on the project (personal communication, June 10, 2020) emphasized that this was a way of creating awareness to the importance of social participation in simple and accessible actions that could be consolidated as public policies. According to her, this type of action, in addition to promoting a healthy diet, favored the sharing of theoretical and practical knowledge

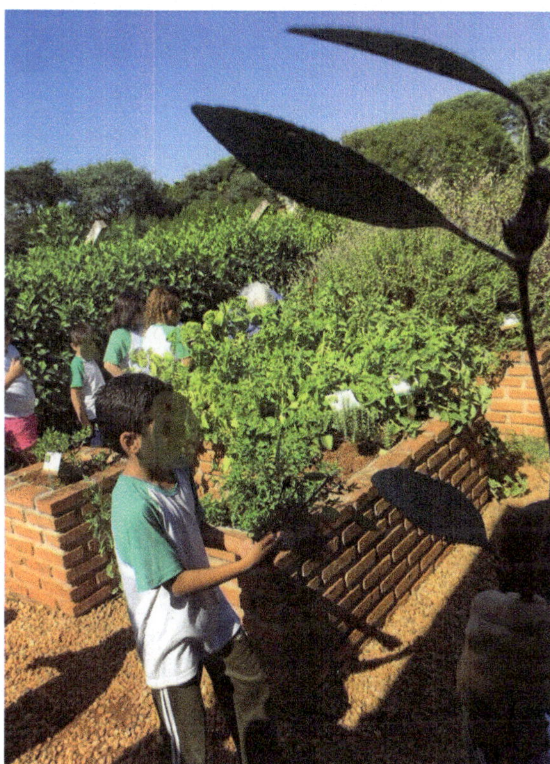

Fig. 3.2 Students taking care of the vegetable garden in Santa Bárbara d'Oeste. (Source: Sperandio, 2019)

and the dissemination of the community's culture, valuing the group and creating a sense of belonging and empowerment.

In Conchal, the community garden was implemented in 2010 with the support of LABINUR and RMPS, as well as involving the mobilization of the community and local government. That same year, Law 1.761 was created (Conchal, 2010), regulating public policies aimed at promoting health and the process of transforming the city of Conchal into a Healthy Municipality.

The area designated for the vegetable garden was idle land, used as a meeting point for drug addicts and a place for illegal waste disposal, which took advantage of the appearance of vectors and the insecurity of the nearby region. The community participated in the process of preparing the project through the development of light social technologies, as well as low cost and low complexity methodologies, which provided dialogue and interaction between people. In the initial stage, 20 beds were distributed among sixteen families (Fig. 3.3), changing that space and making it an instrument for health promotion and a first step toward a healthy city (Sperandio & Bloes, 2020).

According to the then coordinator of health promotion projects in Conchal (personal communication, July 22, 2020), the actions went through several issues, such as health, diet, education, and social promotion, when working with support for drug addicts and the resocialization of inmates. Furthermore, the community garden established effective management mechanisms that allowed work, production, and

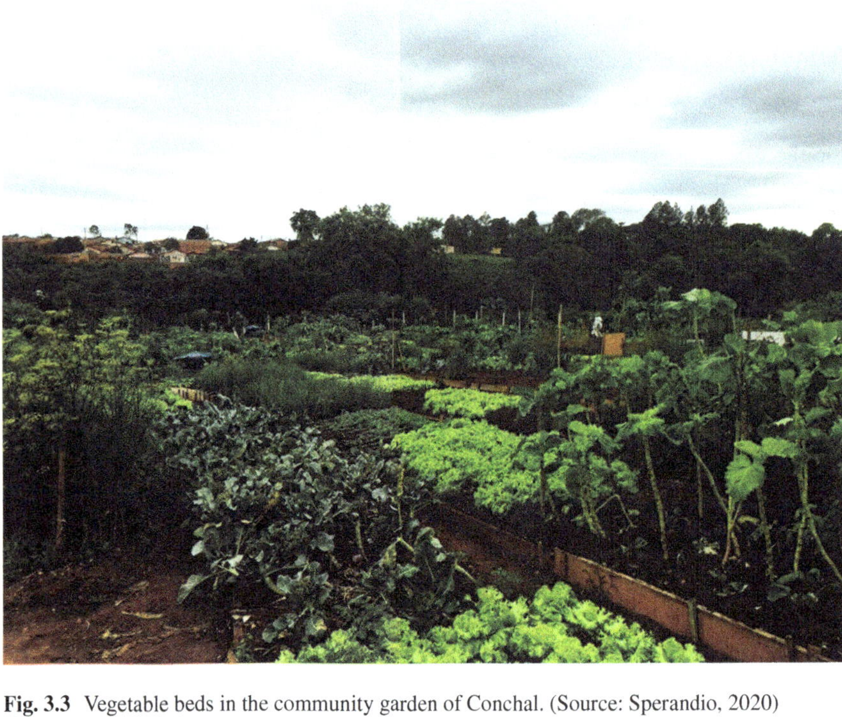

Fig. 3.3 Vegetable beds in the community garden of Conchal. (Source: Sperandio, 2020)

sales to continue, with adjustments, even during the pandemic. With the success of this first experience, other families joined the waiting list for new similar initiatives.

A garden of medicinal herbs, distributed with the guidance of professionals from the Family Health Unit in a neighboring area, was also set up on site. The nursing teams, doctors, and health agents became involved with this proposal, established by the National Policy of Integrative and Complementary Practices (PNPIC) in 2006, which was recently complemented with the addition of new topics (Brasil, 2015, 2018). The participation of professionals and community engagement was responsible for the success of this practice, causing other Family Health Units to seek information and support in order to replicate it.

In all the situations presented, it was found that the positive results exceeded the initial objectives and reverberated in similar actions being taken. These were connected to health promotion and urban planning in several aspects, such as healthy diet, income generation, respect for local culture, creation of a sense of belonging, encouragement in social interactions and autonomy, promotion of physical activity, encouragement in social dialogue, places of new training to face the pandemic, and the promotion of human resilience (Sperandio & Bloes, 2020), approaching to the Sustainable Development Goals (UN, 2015).

With the consolidation of positive results regarding new job opportunities, income generation, food, and social contact, it was noticed that the effective participation of the community, professionals, and entities increased. Their commitment was responsible for maintaining the activities and replicating this project in other parts of the city and nearby regions. The population's recognition of the vegetable garden as a positive practice that should be replicated motivated the group involved and made clear the effectiveness of this action (Globoplay, 2016).

Actions, such as community urban gardens, can be replicated, without major difficulties or impediments, in different regions of the cities because, when applying light technologies, they allow anyone, regardless of their education or income level, to have access to information and techniques for their realization, and few inputs are needed for its implementation. In addition, they rescue the social function of the city by occupying idle areas, contributing to the improvement of the urban environment, security, and appropriation of the city by the community.

It was noticed that the results obtained with urban gardens, both in the phase prior to the pandemic and during its establishment, met several demands of the population. The most obvious was the issue of healthy food production and its fair distribution to the community, but several others were also observed, such as job training, income generation, creation of a space for meeting and exchanging experiences, inclusion, contact and social participation, development of autonomy, creation of a sense of belonging and co-responsibility, strengthening community resilience, and happiness. All these factors contributed to the promotion of health and were essential for life in the community, so they should start to be considered as such and maintained even after the pandemic is over (Sperandio & Bloes, 2020).

Urban Planning for the Healthy City and Its Effects on People

Next, in a summarized form, words addressed during this chapter, arising from initiatives to confront the pandemic and from bibliographic reviews, will be presented. The set of these concepts point out strategies for network actions and directions for the development of a resilient and healthy city.

Figure 3.4 represents the healthy city as a central element, linked to urban planning issues (active mobility, public spaces, urban green areas, and community gardens). Around them are the results of these actions and the values generated by them.

Final Considerations

The process of urban readjustment in search of healthy cities can be made possible through the sum of successful and coordinated collective actions between local leaders, increasing the creation of coalitions between groups and communities, expanding governance networks capable of reverberating in cities and even on a global scale, overcoming social vulnerabilities, and promoting health beyond the limits of socio-spatial segregation, not only in crisis situations but also in usual circumstances, thus contributing to human and urban resilience.

It is essential to collect information and map the population and distances to health, education, commerce, and leisure services, and to encourage the involvement of governments, managers, professionals, specialists, health agents, and the population as a whole, for the definition, development, and implementation of

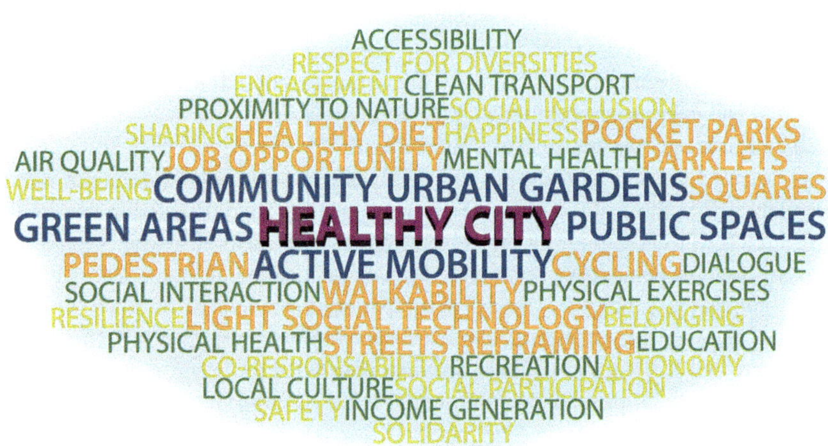

Fig. 3.4 Word Cloud with actions, concepts, and values related to the health city

strategies that make a city more accessible, walkable, resilient, and belonging to all its inhabitants.

All efforts made to face the pandemic cannot be abandoned at its end. Actions and strategies developed in several cities around the world should work as an example and starting point for solutions that are suitable for the particularities of each region and can only add to the urban planning process as a promoter of a healthy city. It is up to professionals, academia, and governments to take a major role in the community development processes in order to contribute to their strengthening, autonomy, and resilience in the face of new crises in the future.

References

Associação Brasileira de Normas Técnicas. (2015). *Norma brasileira ABNT NBR 9050: 2015 accessibility to buildings, equipment and the urban environment*. ABNT.

Belloni, L. (2018, November 18). Cidades sem Fome: A ONG que transforma terrenos abandonados em hortas orgânicas. *Huffpost*. https://www.huffpostbrasil.com/2018/11/18/cidades-sem-fome-a-ong-que-transforma-terrenos-abandonados-em-hortas-organicas_a_23591573/

Brasil. (1990). *Lei Orgânica da Saúde. Lei 8.080 de 19 de setembro de 1990*. Diário Oficial da União.

Brasil. (2001). *Estatuto da Cidade. Lei 10.257 de 10 de julho de 2001*. Diário Oficial da União.

Brasil. Ministério da Saúde. (2002). *As Cartas da promoção da Saúde, Carta de Ottawa 1986*. http://bvsms.saude.gov.br/bvs/publicacoes/cartas_promocao.pdf. Accessed 5 June 2021.

Brasil. Ministério da Saúde. (2015). *Política Nacional de Práticas Integrativas e Complementares no SUS: PNPIC*. Ministério da Saúde.

Brasil. Ministério da Saúde. (2018). *Política Nacional de Promoção da Saúde: PNPS*. Ministério da Saúde.

Conchal. (2010). *Lei 1.761 de 24 de setembro de 2010*. Prefeitura Municipal.

De Leeuw, E. (2017). Cities and health from the Neolithic to the Anthropocene. In E. De Leeuw & J. Simons (Eds.), *Healthy cities. The theory, policy, and practice of value-based urban planning* (pp. 3–30). Springer.

Derrick, A. (2020, May 7). Mayor Durkan urges residents to continue to stay home and announces stay healthy streets pilot will become permanent, bike projects will be expedited in 2020. *City of Seattle*. https://durkan.seattle.gov/2020/05/mayor-durkan-urges-residents-to-continue-to-stay-home-and-announces-stay-healthy-streets-pilot-will-become-permanent-bike-projects-will-be-expedited-in-2020/. Accessed 5 June 2021.

Duarte, D. H. S. (2000). *Padrões de ocupação do solo e microclimas urbanos na região de clima tropical continental*. [Unpublished doctoral dissertation]. Biblioteca Digital de Teses e Dissertações da Universidade de São Paulo. https://www.teses.usp.br/teses/disponiveis/16/16131/tde-18072006-182858/pt-br.php

Fioravanti, C. (2020, June 19). Novo índice detalha peso de variáveis socioeconômicas em doenças. *Pesquisa Fapesp*. https://revistapesquisa.fapesp.br/novo-indice-detalha-peso-de-variaveis-socioeconomicas-em-doencas/

Frau, F. M., & Neto, M. L. S. (2017, January). O destino do Elevado Costa e Silva, o Minhocão. *Vitruvius*. https://www.vitruvius.com.br/revistas/read/arquitextos/17.200/6394

Friedman, L. [Lisa]. (2020, April 7). New research links air pollution to higher coronavirus death rates. *The New York Times*. https://www.nytimes.com/2020/04/07/climate/air-pollution-coronavirus-covid.html

Garcia, R. (2014, June). Passagem para o sossego. *Apartes*. http://www.saopaulo.sp.leg.br/apartes-anteriores/revista-apartes/numero-8-junho-julho2014/passagem-para-o-sossego/

Globoplay. (2016, May 12). *Projeto transforma terreno com sujeira em horta para famílias de baixa renda em Conchal.* https://globoplay.globo.com/v/5019345/. Accessed 5 June 2021.

Guimarães, R. B. (2014). *Saúde: Fundamentos de Geografia humana [online].* Editora UNESP. https://doi.org/10.7476/9788568334386

Harrouk, C. (2020, May 27). Domino Park em Nova York introduz círculos no chão para garantir distanciamento. *Archdaily Brasil.* https://www.archdaily.com.br/br/940318/domino-park-em-nova-iorque-introduz-circulos-no-chao-para-garantir-distanciamento

ITDP Brasil. (2020, May 4). Mobilidade e pandemia: o que podemos esperar para o futuro da vida nas cidades? *Archdaily Brasil.* https://www.archdaily.com.br/br/938731/mobilidade-e-pandemia-o-que-podemos-esperar-para-o-futuro-da-vida-nas-cidades

Keeling, B. (2020, May 22) Mimicking Brooklyn, four SF parks adopt social distancing circles. *Curbed SF.* https://sf.curbed.com/2020/5/22/21266247/san-francisco-parks-social-distancing-circles-coronavirus

Lefebvre, H. (2016). *O direito à cidade*. Nebli.

Lira, P. (2020, May 6). Como retornar à vida em comunidade no mundo pós-pandemia? *ArchDaily Brasil.* https://www.archdaily.com.br/br/938922/como-retornar-a-vida-em-comunidade-no-mundo-pos-pandemia

Miana, A. C. (2010). *Adensamento e forma urbana: inserção de parâmetros ambientais no processo de projeto.* [Unpublished doctoral dissertation]. Biblioteca Digital de Teses e Dissertações da Universidade de São Paulo. https://www.teses.usp.br/teses/disponiveis/16/16132/tde-19012011-092832/publico/TESE_MIANA.pdf

Mobilize. (2020, May 18). Itália oferece 500 euros para pessoas comprarem bicicletas durante pandemia do coronavírus. *ArchDaily Brasil.* https://www.archdaily.com.br/br/939735/italia-oferece-500-euros-para-pessoas-comprarem-bicicletas-durante-pandemia-do-coronavirus

Moloney, A. (2020, May 28). Pedal on! Coronavirus lockdown spurs cycling momentum in South America. *Thomson Reuters Foundation.* https://news.trust.org/item/20200528151136-5to9y/?utm_campaign=new-land&utm_medium=newsletter&utm_source=topPicks&utm_content=link4&utm_contentItemId=20200528151136-5to9y

NASA. (2020, June 29). Airborne nitrogen dioxide plummets over China. *Earth Observatory.* https://earthobservatory.nasa.gov/images/146362/airborne-nitrogen-dioxide-plummets-over-china. Accessed 17 Aug 2020.

NASA, & ESA. (2020, February 25). *Decreases in nitrogen dioxide (NO_2) over China* [image]. https://commons.wikimedia.org/wiki/File:Nitrogen_dioxide_Density_Change_In_China_Due_To_Coronavirus.png. Accessed 17 Aug 2020.

Nunes, A. C. A. S., Oliveira, A., Callejas, A. G. H., Basile, R., Levy, R., & Cruz, S. S. (2016). Calçadas: o sistema de mobilidade urbana das cidades e a experiência do pedestre. In E. Almeida (Ed.), *Mobilidade urbana no Brasil* (pp. 253–264). Fundação Perseu Abramo.

Oakland. (2020, April 11). Oakland slow streets. *City of Oakland.* https://www.oaklandca.gov/projects/oakland-slow-streets. Accessed 17 Aug 2020.

Oltermann, P. (2020, April 13). Pop-up bike lanes help with coronavirus physical distancing in Germany. *The Guardian.* https://www.theguardian.com/world/2020/apr/13/pop-up-bike-lanes-help-with-coronavirus-social-distancing-in-germany?utm_medium=website&utm_source=archdaily.com.br

Pereira, R. H. M., Braga, C. K. V., Servo, L. M., Serra, B., Amaral, P., & Gouveia, N. (2020). *Mobilidade urbana e o acesso ao Sistema Único de Saúde para casos suspeitos e graves de covid-19 nas vinte maiores cidades do Brasil (Nota Técnica 14 Dirur).* Instituto de Pesquisa Econômica Aplicada – Ministério da Economía.

Santana, P. (2007). *A Cidade e a Saúde*. Almedina.

Scifoni, S. (2016). Urbanização brasileira e mobilidade urbana. In E. Almeida (Ed.), *Mobilidade urbana no Brasil* (pp. 23–32). Fundação Perseu Abramo.

Speck, J. (2016). *Cidade caminhável*. Perspectiva.

Sperandio, A. M. G. (2019). *Alunos cuidando da horta em Santa Bárbara d'Oeste* [image] (2019, March). LABINUR, Unicamp, Brazil.

Sperandio, A. M. G. (2020, March). *Canteiros de hortaliças na horta comunitária de Conchal* [image]. LABINUR, Unicamp, Brazil.

Sperandio, A. M. G., & Bloes, R. B. (2020). Community urban gardens: Social instrument for healthy and health-promoting cities. In W. Leal Filho, T. Wall, A. Azul, L. Brandli, & P. Özuyar (Eds.), *Good health and well-being. Encyclopedia of the UN sustainable development goals*. Springer. https://doi.org/10.1007/978-3-319-69627-0

UN. (2015). *Sustainable development goals*. https://sustainabledevelopment.un.org/post2015/transformingourworld. Accessed 17 Aug 2020.

UN-Habitat and World Health Organization. (2020). *Integrating health in urban and territorial planning: a sourcebook*. Geneva. Licence: CC BY-NC-SA3.0 IGO. https://www.who.int/publications/i/item/integrating-health-in-urban-and-territorial-planning. Accessed 17 Aug 2020.

World Health Organization. (1998). *Health promotion glossary*. Retrieved from https://www.who.int/healthpromotion/about/HPR%20Glossary%201998.pdf. Accessed 17 Aug 2020.

Chapter 4
Planning the Equitable Distribution of Services in Emerging Regions: Atizapán de Zaragoza, Mexico, and Yinchuan, China

Aleksandra Krstikj, Moises Gerardo Contreras Ruiz Esparza, Meng Wang, and Elsa A. Pérez-Paredes

Introduction

The last few decades revealed that infectious diseases caused by viruses, such as Ebola, MERS, and SARS, are increasingly becoming global and multidimensional phenomena (Alirol et al., 2011). For years, researchers have been warning that continuous expansion of the city's limits by an appropriation of natural areas and farmland for urban functions would probably lead to more frequent health contingencies (Lafferty, 2009). On the other hand, the inequitable distribution of services has been linked with increased vulnerability to infectious disease spread (Connolly et al., 2020). Thus, there is an urgent need for an assessment of the spatial equity of services in rapidly urbanizing regions that can be used as an indicator of resilience.

The specific context of the problem which gave rise to this study is the large-scale city lockdown, which was the primary response tool of many cities in an attempt to control the COVID-19 pandemic. Even though lockdowns and reduced mobility were criticized for being detrimental to mental health and other epidemic-related diseases of vulnerable groups (Belingheri et al., 2020; Füzéki et al., 2020;

A. Krstikj (✉)
School of Architecture, Art and Design, Tecnológico de Monterrey, Ciudad de Mexico, Mexico
e-mail: sandra.krstik@tec.mx

M. G. C. R. Esparza
Instituto de Ingeniería, Universidad Nacional Autónoma de México, Mexico City, Mexico

M. Wang
Department of Public Administration, Zhejiang University of Finance and Economics, Hangzhou, China

E. A. Pérez-Paredes
División de Ciencias Sociales, Licenciatura en Políticas y Proyectos Sociales, Universidad Abierta y a Distancia de México, Mexico City, Mexico

© The Author(s), under exclusive license to Springer Nature Switzerland AG 2021

M. A. Montoya et al. (eds.), *COVID-19 and Cities*, The Urban Book Series,
https://doi.org/10.1007/978-3-030-84134-8_4

Singh et al., 2020; Webb, 2020), in many cases it was the only available option to slow down the virus's spread (Melnick & Ioannidis, 2020). All six essential urban social functions—living, working, supplying, caring, learning, and enjoying (Moreno, 2019) —were significantly affected by the lockdowns. This study focused on the assessment of the spatial equity of parks for enjoyment, relaxation, socialization, and local stores for everyday supplies, to evaluate urban resilience in lockdowns from the aspect of walkable proximity. The walkable proximity was considered crucial in times of reduced mobility and especially relevant for vulnerable groups that depend on non-motorized transport. Thus, we hypothesized that spatial equity of services, such as parks and local stores, rather than density, plays a role in resilience to large-scale health crises since they are essential for enduring prolonged periods of reduced mobility. We aimed to develop a practical and easy-to-use tool for equity assessment that mathematically and spatially correlates proximity to services, marginalization, and population density. The tool also offers a possibility to quickly model new projective locations of services that can thus aid decision-making. An additional contribution of the study is the assessment of spatial equity in the two case studies: the municipality Atizapán de Zaragoza, part of the peripheral industrial belt of Mexico City metropolitan, and Yinchuan City, a second-tier city in Western China. The criterion for the selection of the case studies was that both are rapidly developing urban areas with high population densities that bring about significant sustainability implications.

This article has four sections: the first section introduces the problem context and research aim and reviews previous literature; the second section presents the methodological approach in the development of the tool for spatial equity assessment; the third section demonstrates the results of the tool's application in the spatial equity assessment of the two case studies; and the fourth section discusses the results obtained and their implication for decision-making oriented towards strengthening resilience to future lockdowns.

Literature Review

Resilience is a process, rather than a certain outcome, that includes the capacity for transformation or evolution when faced with a crisis (Davoudi et al., 2012; Vale & Campanella, 2005). In planning, urban resilience is defined by the potentiality of an urban form to return to "normal" through the concept of equilibrium to which planners always strive (Davoudi et al., 2012). Nevertheless, recent discourses on what is a normal state or a desired equilibrium (or if it exists at all) and how it can be maintained (or why) in an ever-changing world (Scheffer, 2009) highlights the question of whether planning is, in fact, obsolete if it does not integrate resilience and the community. Particularly in areas where spatial incoherencies of extended urbanization have been mounting risks for social disparities, for this and other types of disasters, planning must have a long-term vision that accounts for major shocks (sudden or more gradual) by providing adaptive models focused on resilience. Most of the international agendas for development and development bodies, such as the Sustainable Development Goals, the World Bank, and DFID, have explicitly focused on the same goals of inclusiveness, health, and resilience (Department for International Development [DFID], 2011: Jha & Stanton-Geddes, 2013; United Nations General Assembly [UNGA], 2015). In this context, a paradigm shift in planning is required that will focus on a supportive social context prior to a disaster as a key element to urban resilience (Plough et al., 2013). Since disasters occur in a socio-historical context of pre-existing health inequalities, vulnerability becomes a social construct where the most affected population in a pandemic will always be the people with chronic or mental illness, the marginalized, and the urban poor (Levac et al., 2012; Plough et al., 2013). Therefore, post-COVID-19 urban planning should explicitly incorporate spatial equity in the distribution of critical resources as a long-term preparedness strategy.

According to Frederickson (Frederickson, 2015), social equity in public administration deals with the fairness of organization, management, and delivery of public services, and is the third pillar in planning after efficiency and economy (Svara et al., 2005). The crucial difference between equality and equity lies in understanding the need for vulnerable groups to receive disproportionately more benefits (Folger et al., 1995; Talen & Anselin, 1998), also defined as "compensatory" equity (Crompton & Wicks, 1988). A study by Yuan et al. (2017) defined spatial equity using two characteristics: (1) horizontal equity, in which everyone receives the same public benefit following the concept of social equity; and (2) vertical equity, based on the different abilities and demands of various social groups, whereby socially vulnerable groups receive disproportionately more benefits (Yuan et al., 2017). Therefore, the term "vertical spatial equity" is related more to the spatial match of a facility's service level with the need and distribution of residents. The concept of equity in socio-spatial studies has been addressed in various ways and through indicators such as distribution, availability, access, and the quality of spaces, as well as power, governance, and decision-making (Borja, 2003; Jacobs & Appleyard, 1961; Jost & Kay, 2010; Harvey, 2010). Yet, research on how to evaluate spatial equity, especially on a neighborhood scale, is sparse and too complex for practical application in underdeveloped regions (Tsou et al., 2005). Any tool to measure resilience, such as the proposed spatial equity in this work, must be practical and easy to use by decision-makers to avoid a lag between research and practice that can undermine the implementation of resilience agendas (Clark-Ginsberg et al., 2020). Even though some studies argued that quantifying resilience often misses the point (Clark-Ginsberg et al., 2020), it can nevertheless provide significant support for informed decision-making and planning of services on the municipal or regional level that should be supplemented by qualitative research on the local level (cultural values, traditions, customs, etc.).

Urban services that have been identified as crucial for the community to sustain a prolonged period of lockdown or self-isolation are the neighborhood park and the local store. The public green space is essential for relaxation, recreation, and urban health in general (Maller et al., 2006; Sherer, 2006). Previous studies showed that people living close to parks enjoy mental and physical health benefits, stronger social ties, and a sense of security (Giles-Corti et al., 2005; Maller et al., 2006), which often increases property value (Crompton, 2001; Sherer, 2006). The Center for Disease Control and Prevention of the United States has identified mental health as one of the main concerns related to social distancing during the COVID-19 outbreak due to the high level of stress and anxiety caused by changes in daily life (Centers for Disease Control and Prevention [CDC], 2020). The National Recreation and Park Association of Mexico has established guidelines for municipal, state, and national authorities to keep parks, green areas, and public spaces open and accessible for as long as it is safe to do so (Ipas, 2020). On the other hand, the local store has become a significant part of people's routine supply of goods (BBC News, 2020). Even though local shopping might have started as a necessity due to the severely reduced mobility options, a recent YouGov poll by the trade body Co-operatives UK (undertaken on 4–5 June 2020), shows that 80% of consumers intend to continue their new habit once the crisis is over (Co-operatives UK, 2020). Thus, local stores can be understood as a significant factor in contributing to resilience during lockdowns, but also to the recovery phase since they create local jobs and reduce food waste.

The complexity of urban service planning is characterized by inequality (Boone et al., 2009), privatization (García, 2005; Weintraub, 1997), abandonment or lack of use (Secretaría de Bienestar [SEDESOL], 2020), inequitable geographical distribution in cities (Borja, 2003), internal insecurity (Campos-Vázquez & Cuilty, 2014), and the lack of fair decision-making processes by governments (Flores-Xolocotzi, 2012; Iracheta, 2012; Rabotnikof, 2003; Sassen, 2013; Schlosberg, 2004; UN-Habitat, 2015). For example, while the design of parks has often been studied in terms of their social, environmental, and economic value, the geographical park distribution across the urban landscape, in terms of equity, has received less attention (Talen, 2010). One of the biggest socio-spatial problems that have been recognized during the COVID-19 pandemic has been the lack of local parks for the public in walkable proximity to homes to meet various needs, such as physical and mental distraction activities that domestic spaces cannot provide (Canal Instituto de Investigaciones Sociales, 2020; Instituto de Investigaciones para el Desarrollo con Equidad [EQUIDE], 2020). Byrne and Wolch (2009) argue that the inequitable green space distribution is due to interlinked factors of park design, history of land development, evolving ideas about leisure and recreation, as well as histories of class and ethnic-racial inequality. It has been widely accepted that most Latin American cities lack sufficient public spaces and that existing public spaces are inadequately designed and their accessibility is limited by an unbalanced distribution throughout the urban area (Nyakairu et al., 2012; SEDESOL, 2020; United Nations Environment Programme [UNEP], 2010). For example, studies regarding the inequitable distributions of parks in Mexico City started appearing only a few years ago (Fernández-Álvarez, 2017). In the metropolitan periphery, where urban expansion is fastest and marginalization indices are usually higher, the problem of incomplete information systems is even more urgent.

Access to public services, especially in terms of walkable proximity, has been accepted as an integral component of a good urban form (Duany & Plater-Zyberk,

1991; Jacobs & Appleyard, 1961; Lynch, 1981) and sustainable urban planning (Cervero & Sullivan, 2012). The evaluation of access is particularly significant considering vulnerable populations who depend on non-motorized transport to reach urban services, e.g., the elderly, children, permanently or temporarily disabled, and the poor (Talen, 1998). Rigolon (2016) conducted an analytical literature review on inequity in access to urban parks which focused on three parameters of accessibility: proximity, acreage, and quality. He found that less work was done on proximity compared to the other two parameters, which resulted in a lack of unified methodology to evaluate this indicator. Moreover, the majority of research focused on developed countries, such as the US, the UK, and Canada, where information systems are more complete than in less developed regions. Geographical location and sampling of neighborhoods influenced the findings on proximity and reflected the divide between urban, suburban, and rural contexts, as well as the different patterns of park provisions in these contexts.

Method

First, georeferencing of centroids of public parks and stores is necessary. In some cases, the location of larger parks and commercial facilities are readily available from national or municipal open geodatabases. However, our research showed that for local neighborhood services that are open during the pandemic, the municipal office is always a better source of information. Nevertheless, the data from municipal offices in less developed countries could still be in a form of a non-georeferenced inventory datasheet. To georeference the location data, we used Google Geocoding API to automate the process of reading addresses from the inventory file and retrieving the corresponding geolocation with latitude and longitude. The locations were then transferred to QGIS 3.8.1. For local parks and stores, the approximation to a geometric center does not result in significant accessibility measurement error since their surface is relatively small.

Second, we analyzed the proximity of residential areas to parks and stores. In previous literature, the main place-based methodological approaches to measure proximity are *container, coverage, minimum distance, travel cost,* and *gravity* (Talen, 1998). The *container* measure, in Eq. (4.1), is a ratio Ci of the total sum of opportunities Sj for each area i (number of facilities) to population size P within the boundaries of area i:

$$Ci = \frac{\sum_{j=1}^{n} Sij}{Pi} \tag{4.1}$$

where n is the total number of facilities in area i. The *coverage* approach represents populations of interest as a centroid and delineates a critical distance around it to assess accessible services. These methods always run the risk of an aggregation error since the distance is over or underestimated as a result of using a centralized representation of administrative areas or populations. Additionally, the use of administrative units creates a boundary-supply error since it can be argued that people, especially those living at the boundary of administrative units, would rather walk to a closer service in another unit.

The *minimum-distance* approach in Eq. (4.2) measures the distance *D* from an origin *i* (e.g., neighborhoods) to a destination *j* (e.g., facility) as:

$$Di = \min_{i} \left\{ d_{ij} \right\} \tag{4.2}$$

The distance can be measured by the Euclidean straight line, Manhattan distance, or street network analysis. Mora-Garcia et al. (2018) and Comber et al. (2008) both argue that network analysis is better in measuring real distance since it accounts for actual access routes and barriers. However, most of the research has been done in developed countries where precise information on paths is readily available. Yet, many underdeveloped regions lack sufficient data for such analysis. For example, in Atizapán de Zaragoza, the wealthy live in gated estates that do have mapped roads but are inaccessible for people outside the estate. In other cases, gated estates do not allow road data to be collected, but people still use that road system. Moreover, many informal paths are not mapped but are constantly used. Thus, the Euclidean distance is still the most reliable approach in regions where data are unreliable.

The distance can also be estimated as a *travel cost* or a *gravity* measure that sums all facilities (weighted by size) divided by the frictional effect of distance. The aggregation and boundary-supply error are still limitations of these approaches if administrative units are used. The *radius* approach avoids these errors by using the service as an origin point to measure critical distance, or a buffer zone around it, and identify populations within the radius that have access.

All of the proximity assessment approaches described above measure distance, and distance is a constant. Nevertheless, the assessment of proximity is a two-dimensional districting problem, where the aim is to partition a territory into smaller units subject to some constraints, such as balancing, contiguity, and compactness (Novaes et al., 2009). Thus, the main challenge is to create a method for districting an area into continuous zones, where each zone obtained contains at least one service and is contiguous. The studies by Jia et al. (2014) and Abellanas & Palop (2008) use Voronoi diagrams to filter and cluster data on health center locations and census tract districting, respectively. In our study, we applied a Voronoi diagram to solve the problem of districting and measure proximity to parks and stores. A Voronoi diagram is a "fundamental structure in computational geometry that captures the notion of proximity in environments and provides a means of partitioning space into subregions to facilitate spatial data manipulation, modeling of spatial structures, pattern recognition, and locational optimization" (Okabe et al., 2009). Thus, an ordinary Voronoi diagram is a proximity region to a set of points, where *S* is a set of $n \geq 3$ point sites p, q, r, …in a Euclidean plane R^2. For points p = (p1, p2) and x = (x1, x2), the Euclidean distance is d (p, x) = $\sqrt{(p1\text{-}x1)^2} + \sqrt{(p2\text{-}x2)^2}$. For a straight-line segment pq that connects two points p, q ϵ S, the bisector is a perpendicular straight line through the midpoint of segment pq that separates the halfplane D (p, q) = {x | d (p, x) $\leq$ d (q, x)} closer to p from the halfplane D (q, p) closer to q. Finally, a Voronoi region VR (p, S) of a point *p* among a given set *S* of point sites, is the intersection of n-1 half-planes D (p, q), where q ranges over all the other sites in S, as in Eq. (4.3):

$$\mathrm{VR}(p,S) = \underset{\mathrm{q} \in S, \mathrm{q} \neq \mathrm{p}}{\cap} \mathrm{D}(\mathrm{p},\mathrm{q}) \tag{4.3}$$

In a Voronoi region created around point p, the Euclidean distances from all the points in that region to p are always shorter than the distance from those points to q, r, etc. The regions should be as compact and convex as possible and optimally take into account important geographical features. Novaes et al. (2009) and Feng and Murray (2018) developed advanced mathematical models that solve the problem of obstacles, such as rail lines, lakes, and rivers, and heterogeneity of space that the ordinary Voronoi tessellation cannot account for. Such solutions could be applied if sufficient resources were available because they would increase the precision of the proximity measurement.

The resultant Voronoi regions represent districts of residential areas closest to each specific park or store *(Vp)*. They allow us to identify residential districts that have walkable proximity to services on a pre-established threshold for walkability. In the US, the walkability limit has been defined as ½ mile (800 meters), a 10-min walk, or ¼ mile (400 meters), a 5-min walk (Boone et al., 2009; Rigolon, 2016). In Mexico, the distance ranges from 400 to 700 meters (Diario Oficial de la Federación [DOF], 2019; Subsecretaría de Desarrollo Urbano y Vivienda, 2013). In this study, we used the threshold of 800 meters to define walkable districts. The areas of such districts are less than 2 km^2. Next, we performed a spatial intersection of the identified Voronoi districts with neighborhoods of high and very high density *(Di)* and marginalization *(Mi)* to geolocalize the spatial inequity and identify critical areas. The critical neighborhoods are further classified with a green area proximity distress index (GAP) and commerce proximity distress index (CP) in categories of *medium, high, and very high*, depending on the combinations of *Di, Mi,* and *Vp,* according to the following criteria:

1. If Di = 3 or 4 and Mi = 3 or 4 and 2km^2 $\leq$ Vp $\leq$ 3 km^2, then distress index = medium.
2. If Di = 3 or 4 and Mi = 3 or 4 and 3km^2 $\leq$ Vp $\leq$ 4 km^2, then distress index = high.
3. If Di = 3 or 4 and Mi = 3 or 4 and Vp $\geq$ 4 km^2, then distress index = very high.

Finally, we designed an algorithm in Matlab to divide the perimeter of distressed neighborhoods by segments of 1 km that allowed us to tessellate them into triangles of walkable units based on the Delaunay triangulation. The centroids of the resultant triangles project approximate locations for future parks to balance the spatial equity between discriminated and affluent neighborhoods. This method for projective park planning, based on the Delaunay triangulation algorithm, is our original contribution to the ongoing debate and search for approaches to improve spatial equity of services, and can serve as a decision-support tool for resilience improvement strategies in preparedness planning.

Results

The Case Studies

Atizapán de Zaragoza is a peripheral municipality in the northwest Mexico City (CDMX) metropolitan area (Fig. 4.1, left), 23 km from Mexico City's center. The municipality has been undergoing metropolitan consolidation since the 1950s along the arterial road to Querétaro. By the 1970s, the municipality had 44,322 inhabitants and the urban growth had increased significantly, generating a lack of urban structure to ensure the efficient functioning of the area. By 2015, the municipality had a consolidated urban area of 91 km^2 and 489,937 inhabitants – 10 times more compared to the 1970s, with an average urban density of 5384 inh/km^2. The zone is largely a commuter municipality (Figueroa, 2014), where the lack of efficient public transport only emphasizes the need for services located in walkable proximity to housing. Atizapán is one of the municipalities worst affected by the pandemic in Mexico, with 4168 confirmed cases on April 11, 2021.

Yinchuan City is the capital of Ningxia Hui Minority Autonomous Region (Fig. 4.1, right). The administrative area of the city is 9025.38 km^2 and the total population is 2.16 million (2015). The population is housed in three urban districts (Xingqing, Jinfeng, and Xixia), two rural counties (Helan and Yongning), and one county-level satellite city (Lingwu). However, the continuous urban zone of the

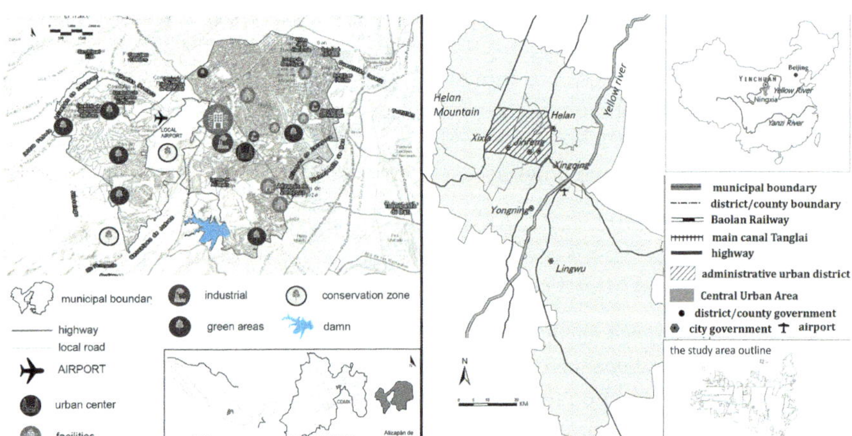

Fig. 4.1 Atizapán de Zaragoza, State of Mexico (left) and Yinchuan, Western China (right)

Central Urban Area (CUA) is 169.1 km^2 (2015), where half of Yinchuan's population is housed, resulting in a CUA's population density of 6387 inh/km2. The built-up urban area in Yinchuan tripled in the period between 2001 and 2015, which has posed a great strain on the sustainability of the development (Wang et al., 2017a). Recently, the city set the goal of becoming "smart" by improving urban services such as public transport, infrastructure, health centers, and garbage management, as well as housing (Bruni, 2019). The conditions with COVID-19 in Yinchuan have been significantly better than in Atizapán. The Ningxia region only had 75 cases (all recovered by May 2020) from which 39 were citizens of Yinchuan.

Materials

The material used for this research involved census records of population density and marginalization at the neighborhood level, as well as location data of public parks and stores. In the case of Mexico, the National Institute for Geography and Statistics (INEGI) and the National Population Commission (Conapo) provided us with extensive open databases of local-level socio-demographic characteristics. We clustered the data on population density in index values of D*i* 0 *(very low), 1 (low), 2 (medium), 3 (high) and 4 (very high)*, while marginalization was clustered in index values M*i* of 0 *(very low), 1 (low), 2 (medium), 3 (high), and 4 (very high)*. We obtained an inventory of urban public spaces from the updated Municipal Urban Development Plan (PMDU) of 2015, classified in local parks, squares, communal gardens, playgrounds, islands with sports use, and urban green areas (Pérez-Paredes, 2016). In China, we found data on population density and income level from the Special Issue of the Statistical Bulletin of Yinchuan (published on the 11th of January 2018).

Spatial Equity in Atizapán de Zaragoza

The marginalized neighborhoods in Atizapán occupy 26.8% of the urban area and are almost all located in the east zone (Table 4.1 and Fig. 4.2a). The marginalization coincides with high densities (Fig. 4.2b). We also obtained data on the location of senior citizens over 60 at the block level (Fig. 4.2c). The data revealed that neighborhoods with older populations are mainly located in the central and western zones and coincide with the more affluent ones.

The type of urban green space consists of large private golf and country clubs, undeveloped areas, and public local parks (Fig. 4.2d). The units of urban green space on which we focused in this study are consolidated local public parks (45) and communal gardens (18). The local parks comprise the highest percentage of public area and their surfaces range from 253 m^2 to 10,685 m^2, while the areas of communal gardens are from 446 m^2 to 5258 m^2.

Table 4.1 Marginalization Index Table—Atizapán de Zaragoza

Marginalization Index	No. of Hoods	West Location	Central location	East Location	Mean Area Km^2	% of Total Municipal Area
Very low	29	7	16	5	0.98	39
Low	27	1	17	9	0.55	20.25
Medium	24	0	9	15	0.42	13.95
High	36	3	2	31	0.37	18.27
Very high	17	0	1	16	0.36	8.53
Total	133 (53)	11 (3)	45 (3)	76 (47)		(26.8%)

Source: Elaborated by authors

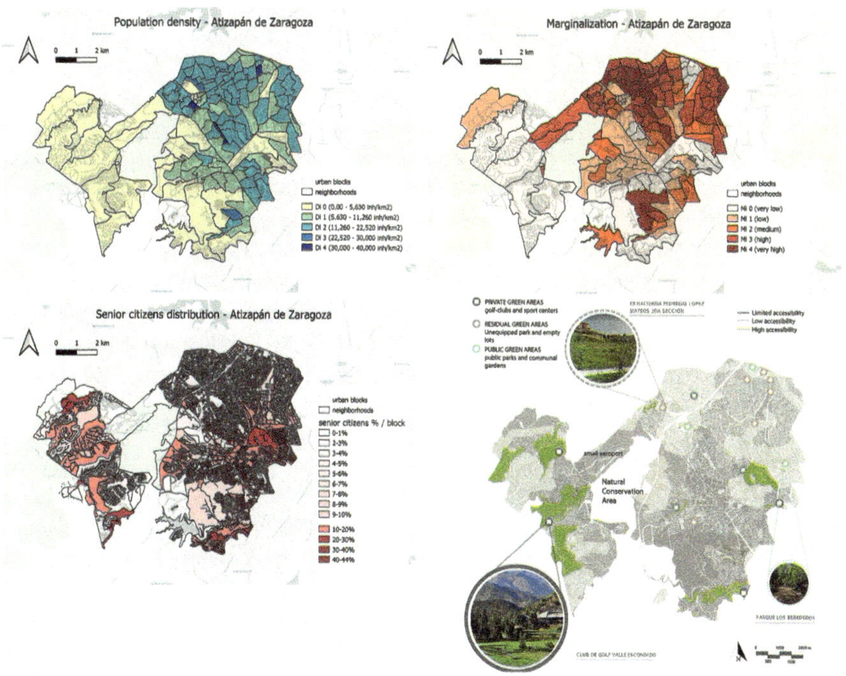

Fig. 4.2 Population density (**a**), marginalization (**b**), senior citizen distribution (**c**) and types of green areas (**d**) in Atizapán de Zaragoza

The resultant Voronoi districting (Fig. 4.3a) presents a significant mismatch between the distribution of parks and housing. The districts without walkable proximity together comprise 56.34% of Atizapán's area and are mostly located in the northeast (Table 4.2). There is one area of 10.07 km^2 (marked by *) in the northwest that is currently under development, so we did not consider it in future analyses. The districts with walkable proximity are located in the central and western parts where the majority of affluent and senior citizens live. The northeastern parts that have lower proximity to parks are settled by younger and highly marginalized populations. Thus, it seems that spatial equity of parks benefits the seniors but not the marginalized. The rethinking of local park distribution seems to be an urgent issue for the municipality.

The spatial intersection between districts without walkable proximity to parks and highly dense and marginalized neighborhoods found 29 with medium, 12 with high, and 10 with very high GAP distress indices, among which the most critical was Lomas de Tepalcapa, followed by Las Peñitas y Adolfo Lopez Mateos (Fig. 4.3c).

We performed a similar analysis for the distribution of stores (Fig. 4.3b). The Voronoi districts have a considerably denser number of stores, with central and northern zones having the best proximity. Nevertheless, the western zones that house a large part of the over 60 population seem quite destitute. Therefore, during

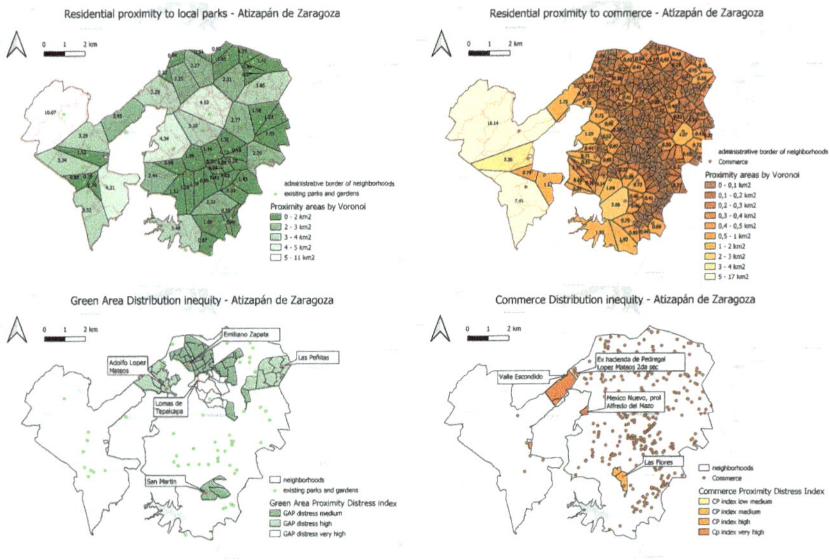

Fig. 4.3 Atizapán de Zaragoza: Residential proximity to local Parks (**a**) and commerce (**b**); Zones with high marginalization and low proximity to public green areas (**c**) and commerce (**d**)

a lockdown, this population will be exposed to higher risk considering the travel necessary to buy essential products. The spatial intersection of zones without proximity to shops and highly dense and marginalized zones was part of the reason for the urban area having a high CP distress index (Fig. 4.3d). Among these, the most concerning is Las Flores in the south, which is very highly marginalized and without proximity to stores.

In conclusion, the least vulnerable districts in lockdowns seem to only be the central ones, since the proximity of housing to both parks and stores is acceptable. On the other hand, the eastern districts are very vulnerable in terms of lack of proximity to parks, and the western districts were found to have a moderate risk due to a lack of stores. The most critical zones seem to be Lomas de Tepalcapa in the northeast and Las Flores in the south, with very high GAP and CP distress indices.

Spatial Equity in Yinchuan City

For Yinchuan, we found the population density at the neighborhood level (Fig. 4.4a). However, the data for the location of the Hui minority group (Fig. 4.4c) and income levels (Fig. 4.4d) were only available at the district level. Thus, the spatial intersection was performed only between large Voronoi districts and dense areas, while the income and minority distribution data were used only to clarify the context. We found that the eastern district of Xingqing, where the Old Town is located, has a

Table 4.2 Quantifying Voronoi proximity areas

Voronoi Proximity Areas	No. of Areas	No. of Parks	West Location	Central Location	East Location	Mean Area Km^2	% of Total Municipal Area
0–2%	40	39	4	24	12	0.61	33.59%
2–3%	***8***	***7***	***0***	***3***	***5***	***1.78***	***19.50%***
3–4%	***7***	***7***	***3***	***1***	***3***	***2.48***	***23.78%***
4–5%	***3***	***3***	***1***	***1***	***1***	***3.18***	***13.06%***
5–11%*	1	1	1	0	0	7.35	10.07%
Total	59 (***18***)	57 (***17***)	9 (***4***)	30 (***5***)	18 (***9***)		100% (***56.34%***)

(Italic bold letters emphasize values for Voronoi proximity areas beyond the walkability limit to parks)

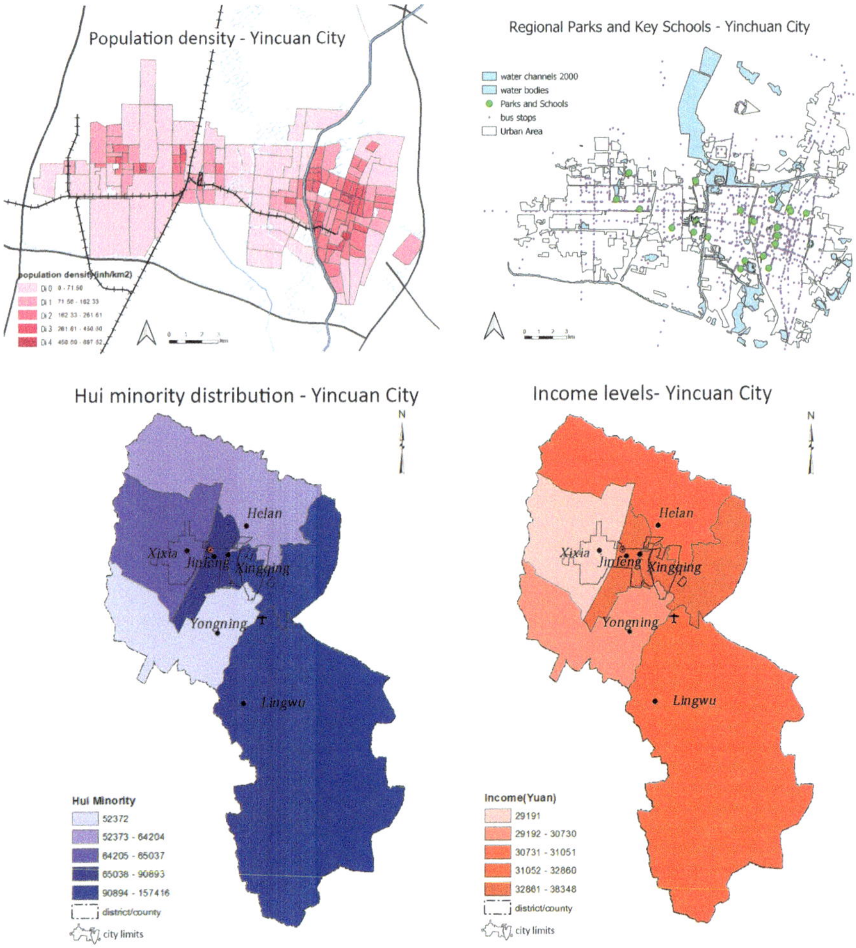

Fig. 4.4 Population density (**a**), location of regional parks and key schools (**b**), Hui minority group distribution (**c**), and income levels (**d**) in Yinchuan City

significantly larger population density than the rest of the city. The density is also significant in some of the western peripheral neighborhoods and a few communities of the central area around New Town. The east and central zones also have the highest incomes. The neighborhoods that seem to be characterized by high density and low-income levels are at the western periphery of the Xixia district.

In Yinchuan, we aimed to test the tool in a denser urban context with a good public transport network. The method was applied in the following way: the threshold for proximity area was raised to 5 km^2 and the researched units were larger urban district parks. Figure 4.4b presents the distribution of county parks, as well as key schools and bus stops.

The assessment of proximity was based on the centroids of 22 main parks and schools in Yinchuan (Fig. 4.5a). We found that the distribution of parks and schools matched the urban housing area much better than in the previously examined case. Even though the districts without proximity together comprise 63.42% of Yinchuan's area, those are predominantly special industrial zones at the southern outskirts of the city, with very little housing and low population density (Wang et al., 2017b). The two zones on the eastern border, however, house more residents than the southern zones, and, therefore, should be a priority in future planning. The few critical zones, identified with the intersection of high density and low park proximity, comprise less than 3% of the urban area and are located in the east, just outside Old Town, and in the western periphery (Fig. 4.5c). Attention should be paid to the small western zones since the income levels there are significantly lower as well. Thus, it seems that the spatial equity of the park and school distribution in Yinchuan performs favorably compared to Atizapán, even though the urban area is more densely populated. One significant reason could be the longer urban history of Yinchuan, which usually results in a more developed service network over time.

The analysis for the distribution of local stores (Fig. 4.5b) showed even more positive results than for green areas, with the zones of Old Town and the center of New Town having the best proximity. The districts without proximity (27.64%) are again the peripheral zones where the population density is insignificant. The high CP distress zones are less than 6% of the total urban area, with no zone exhibiting the characteristics of very high distress in this case. The high distress zones of the

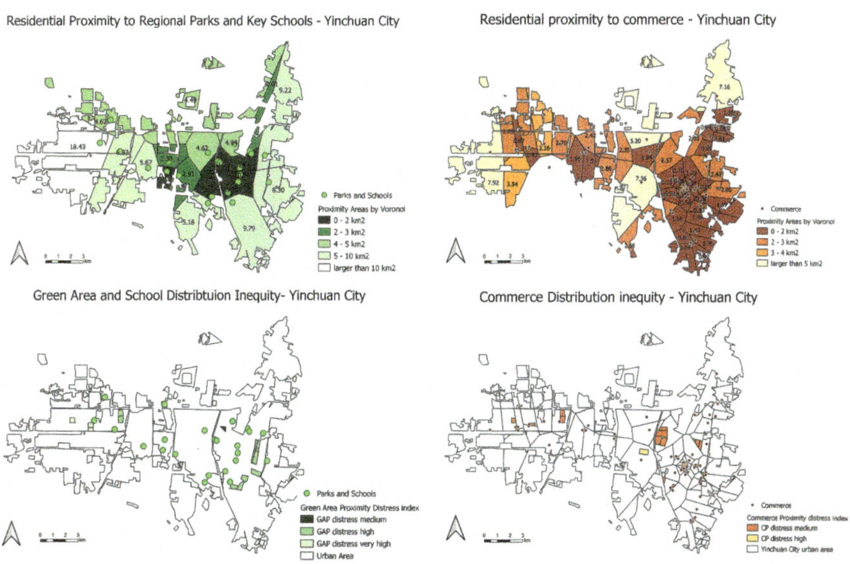

Fig. 4.5 Yinchuan: Residential proximity to regional parks and key schools (**a**), and commerce (**b**); Zones with high density and low proximity to regional parks and key schools (**c**), and commerce (**d**)

east zone have high-income levels, thus once again, the western peripheral zones seem to be more urgent for retrofitting.

We can conclude that even though Yinchuan has a significantly high population density, the distribution of services better matches the housing. Nonetheless, Yinchuan is facing other significant challenges in terms of sustainability, such as the low occupancy of the extensive peripheral special development zones and the unbalanced distribution of housing (Wang et al., 2017a, b).

Improving Equity in the Spatial Distribution of Parks

As a final step, we present the application of the Delaunay triangulation modeling in the case of Atizapán. First, we joined the discriminated areas in three polygons: AREAS 1, 2, and 3 (Fig. 4.6). We then divided the outline of each polygon into segments of 1 km along the perimeter. The code calculated the cumulative summation of the distance of all the vertices that define the outline of each polygon. Then, we calculated the ratio between that summation and 1 km, which gave us the *n* number of segments that can fit in the outline. With that variable and the cumulative summation of the distance, we found the pair of vertices where *n* segments should be located and calculated the coordinates of each vertex of the 1 km segment. In this way, we guarantee that at least one side of the triangles that will be generated by the Delaunay will be 1 km long. The centroids of the new triangles represent the approximate location of 45 future parks for the discriminated areas to achieve

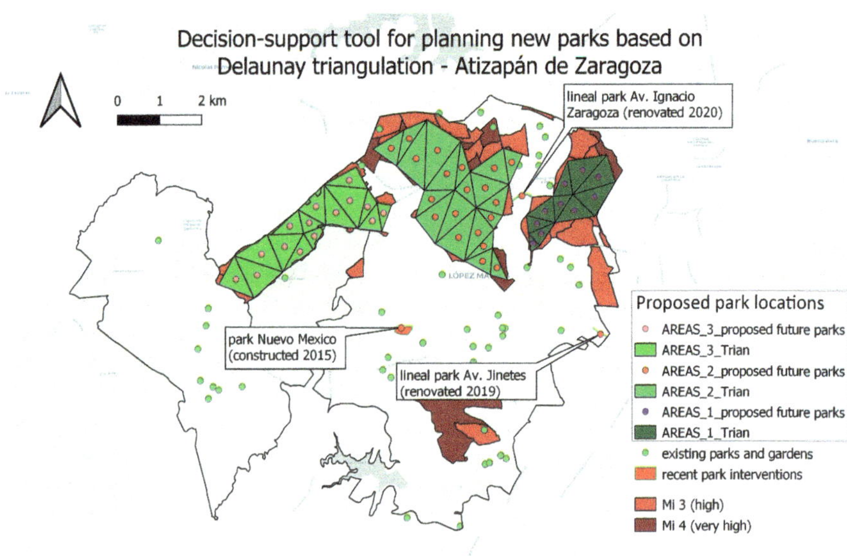

Fig. 4.6 Proposed new park locations to improve spatial equity based on Delaunay triangulation

similar spatial distribution as the most affluent neighborhoods. The locations of future parks are only indicative for planners to consider the possibility of redesigning underutilized open space in the vicinity, such as vacant lots, alleys, school sites, public or utility-owned property, unnecessarily wide streets, and abandoned riverbeds (Wolch et al., 2005). Part of the elongated Area 3 is currently a regional airport with very little housing. In case of future redevelopment, our work serves as a useful guide to consider equity before development. Finally, we also showed the location of three parks in Atizapán that have been recently developed and renovated. The current planning and investment in public parks miss the point of spatial equity since all three parks are located in zones with low to medium marginalization and density. The continuous resource allocation in low and medium marginalization/density zones can have a high cost for the community's inclusiveness and resilience.

Discussion

The assessment of spatial inequity as an indicator of resilience during lockdowns was proposed in this work. We acknowledge that resilience is a complex issue that cannot be measured only by spatial equity, nevertheless, equity is one of the crucial tools for resilience enhancement. In Atizapán de Zaragoza, where COVID-19 related stay-at-home orders have been in place for a year now, we noted a significant lack of walkable proximity to parks and stores in 56% of the housing area that is also highly marginalized. This prevents the formation of essential conditions for locals to comply with lockdown orders and increases the risk of outbreaks. The measurement in Atizapán confirms the findings by Fernandez-Álvarez (2017) on the 16 boroughs of Mexico City, that show park amenities inequitably distributed against marginalized populations. The results also support the conclusion by Segura (2014), that even though many large cities in emerging regions like San Paolo, Mexico City, and Buenos Aires, have managed to reduce income inequalities, the urban fragmentation and spatial discrimination of the growing metropolitan periphery persists. In Yinchuan, on the other hand, we found that the spatial equity of parks and stores matches the housing area much better, thus the planning is more aligned to form the conditions for urban resilience improvement.

Equity research is dominated by empirical studies of large cities from more developed regions (Rigolon, 2016). For example, in a study of spatial accessibility of playgrounds in Edmonton, Canada, Smoyer-Tomic et al. (2004) concluded that playgrounds are equitably distributed, with the highest social-need neighborhoods having the greatest accessibility. This type of study, although significant for the local context and in terms of methodology, does not provide insights for emerging regions with different socio-economic conditions. One of the few studies on small towns in South Africa by McConnachie and Shackleton (2010) found that newly built low-cost housing areas, occupied largely by poor black South Africans, have far worse green area provisions than the white low-density suburbs. In this context, our study is a valuable addition to the growing work focused on emerging regions, where investments that are not carefully planned would most likely benefit the wealthy rather than the deprived and aggravate the risk of social conflicts (Kabanoff, 1991).

The experiences during the crisis prompted a rethinking of the ways we consume urban public space and the importance of having accessible green spaces in "building back better" (Stockholm Environment Institute [SEI], 2020). Yet, during a health contingency, the distribution of other urban services, such as health centers, is undoubtedly crucial as well. However, our method is not constrained to the type of service and, in fact, can be used for various types of service spatial patterns. Thus, the value of the tool developed in this work is found in devising a more unified and practical approach for assessing spatial equity of various service patterns in different urban contexts. As a technology-based tool that measures spatial equity and identifies critical zones, it can inform decision-makers regarding priorities in resource allocation and contribute to more resilient outcomes in urban planning. For example, our model for future park distribution in Atizapán quickly revealed the approximate locations of future parks to strengthen resilience in the face of lockdowns and illustrated the priority missed in current planning. Particularly in developing regions faced with a lack of human and technological resources, an abundance of environmental justice issues, and pressure to contribute to national and international agendas for resilience and sustainability, this tool can provide evidence-based decision support and function as an interface between science and politics.

Finally, our study merely proposes a useful tool for improving equity in the distribution of services without analyzing public policies of local sustainable development. However, the issue of public policy, accountability, and governance is a crucial part of any effort to improve equity and resilience in the urban environment, since different strategies can have paradoxical results by excluding low-income communities and promoting gentrification (Checker, 2011; Dooling, 2009; Gould & Lewis, 2012; Krueger & Gibbs, 2007; Patrick, 2011). Therefore, the design of anti-gentrification policies aimed at rent control, affordable housing and housing trust funds, must be an integral part of any effort to improve the equity in future planning of services. Being 'just green enough', as Curran puts it (Curran & Hamilton, 2012), demands collaborations between local government and disparate community groups, and a readiness of local stakeholders to contest powerful real estate interests. In this context, our tool can be a starting point for involving urban planners, designers, and local stakeholders to develop strategies for urban service distribution that advance the quality of life and community resilience.

Acknowledgments We appreciate the information provided by public officials, consultants, and neighborhood leaders involved in the update of the Municipal Urban Development Plan (2015) of Atizapán de Zaragoza, in particular, Areli Figueroa Zuñiga, Marco Stout, and Alejandra Gudiño.

Funding This research received no external funding.

Conflicts of Interest The authors declare no conflict of interest.

References

Abellanas, M., & Palop, B. (2008, June). Urban data visualization with Voronoi diagrams. In *International conference on computational science and its applications* (pp. 126–136). Springer.

Alirol, E., Getaz, L., Stoll, B., Chappuis, F., & Loutan, L. (2011). Urbanisation and infectious diseases in a globalised world. *The Lancet Infectious Diseases, 11*(2), 131–141. https://doi.org/10.1016/S1473-3099(10)70223-1

BBC News. (2020, September 17). *People shopping more locally in lockdown, says Co-op*. https://www.bbc.com/news/business-54187672

Belingheri, M., Paladino, M. E., Piacenti, S., & Riva, M. A. (2020). Effects of COVID-19 lockdown on epidemic diseases of childhood. *Journal of Medical Virology, 93*(1), 153–154. https://doi.org/10.1002/jmv.26253

Boone, C. G., Buckley, G. L., Grove, J. M., & Sister, C. (2009). Parks and people: An environmental justice inquiry in Baltimore, Maryland. *Annals of the Association of American Geographers, 99*(4), 767–787.

Borja, J. (2003). *La Ciudad Conquistada* [The Conquered City]. Alianza Editorial.

Bruni, A. (2019, March 8). Unknown but intelligent: Yinchuan is a Smart City example from North-Central China. *Cifnews International New Cities*. https://en.cifnews.com/yinchuan-smart-city-example-china/

Byrne, J., & Wolch, J. (2009). Nature, race, and parks: Past research and future directions for geographic research. *Progress in Human Geography, 33*(6), 743–765.

Campos-Vázquez, R. M., & Cuilty, E. (2014). ¿Inversiones en espacios públicos genera capital social? Evidencia para México [Investments in public spaces generates social capital? Evidence for Mexico]. *Revista Bienestar Política Social, 9*, 129–162.

Canal Instituto de Investigaciones Sociales. (2020, May 22). *Condiciones de habitabilidad de las viviendas y el entorno urbano ante aislamiento por COVID*-19 [Conditions of habitability in houses and the urban environment against lockdown due to COVID-19] [video]. Universidad Nacional Autónoma de México. https://www.youtube.com/watch?v=jEGL93LmccA

Centers for Disease Control and Prevention. (2020, July 1). *Coping with Stress*. https://www.cdc.gov/coronavirus/2019-ncov/daily-life-coping/managing-stress-anxiety.html. Accessed 17 Aug 2020.

Cervero, R., & Sullivan, C. (2012). Green TODs. In T. Haas (Ed.), *Sustainable urbanism and beyond: Rethinking cities for the future* (pp. 126–132). Rizzoli.

Checker, M. (2011). Wiped out by the "Greenwave": Environmental gentrification and the paradoxical politics of urban sustainability. *City & Society, 23*(2), 210–229.

Clark-Ginsberg, A., McCaul, B., Bremaud, I., Cáceres, G., Mpanje, D., Patel, S., & Patel, R. (2020). Practitioner approaches to measuring community resilience: The analysis of the resilience of communities to disasters toolkit. *International Journal of Disaster Risk Reduction, 50*, 101714.

Comber, A., Brunsdon, C., & Green, E. (2008). Using a GIS-based network analysis to determine urban greenspace accessibility for different ethnic and religious groups. *Landscape and Urban Planning, 86*, 103–114.

Connolly, C., Keil, R., & Ali, S. H. (2020). Extended urbanisation and the spatialities of infectious disease: Demographic change, infrastructure and governance. *Urban Studies, 58*(2), 245–263. https://doi.org/10.1177/0042098020910873

Co-operatives UK. (2020, June 18). *Eight out of ten people will continue to shop locally more often* [Press release]. https://pressreleases.responsesource.com/news/99719/eight-out-of-ten-people-will-continue-to-shop-locally/

Crompton, J. L. (2001). The impact of parks on property values: A review of the empirical evidence. *Journal of Leisure Research, 33*(1), 1–31.

Crompton, J. L., & Wicks, B. E. (1988). Implementing a preferred equity model for the delivery of leisure services in the US context. *Leisure Studies, 7*(3), 287–403.

Curran, W., & Hamilton, T. (2012). Just green enough: Contesting environmental gentrification in Greenpoint, Brooklyn. *Local Environment, 17*(9), 1027–1042.

Davoudi, S., Shaw, K., Haider, L. J., Quinlan, A. E., Peterson, G. D., Wilkinson, C., Fünfgeld, H., McEvoy, D., Porter, L., & Davoudi, S. (2012). Applying the resilience perspective to planning: Critical thoughts from theory and practice, eds: Simin Davoudi and Libby Porter. *Planning Theory & Practice, 13*(2), 299–333. https://doi.org/10.1080/14649357.2012.677124

Department for International Development. (2011). *Saving lives, preventing suffering and building resilience: The UK Government's Humanitarian Policy*. https://assets.publishing.service.gov.uk/government/uploads/system/uploads/attachment_data/file/67468/The_20UK_20Government_s_20Humanitarian_20Policy_20-_20September_202011_20-_20Final.pdf

Diario Oficial de la Federación. (2019, February 28). REGLAS de Operación del Programa de Mejoramiento Urbano, para el ejercicio fiscal 2019. https://dof.gob.mx/nota_detalle.php?codigo=5551575&fecha=28/02/2019. Accessed 15 Nov 2019.

Dooling, S. (2009). Ecological gentrification: A research agenda exploring justice in the City. *International Journal of Urban and Regional Research, 33*(3), 621–639.

Duany, A., & Plater-Zyberk, E. (1991). *Towns and town-making principles*. Rizzoli.

Feng, X., & Murray, A. T. (2018). Allocation using a heterogeneous space Voronoi diagram. *Journal of Geographical Systems, 20*(3), 207–226.

Fernández-Álvarez, R. (2017). Inequitable distribution of green public space in the Mexico City: An environmental injustice case. *Economía, Sociedad y Territorio, XVII*(54), 399–428.

Figueroa, A. (2014). *Planificación y usos de suelo en el municipio de Atizapán de Zaragoza, estado de México, a partir del catastro y sus instrumentos de planeación urbana (1981–2012)* [Planning and ground uses in the city of Atizapan de Zaragoza, State of Mexico, base don cadastre and its instruments of urban Planning (1981–2012] [Master's tesis, Escuela Superior de Ingeniería y Arquitectura, Instituto Politécnico Nacional].

Flores-Xolocotzi, R. (2012). Incorporando desarrollo sustentable y gobernanza a la gestión de áreas urbanas [Incorporating sustainable development and gobernance to the management of urban areas]. *Revista Frontera Norte, 24*, 165–190.

Folger, R., Sheppard, B. H., & Buttram, R. T. (1995). Equity, equality, and need: Three faces of social justice. In B. B. Bunker & J. Z. Rubin (Eds.), *The Jossey-Bass management series and The Jossey-Bass conflict resolution series. Conflict, cooperation, and justice: Essays inspired by the work of Morton Deutsch* (pp. 261–289). Jossey-Bass/Wiley.

Frederickson, G. H. (2015). *Social equity and public administration: Origins, developments, and applications: Origins, developments, and applications*. Routledge.

Füzéki, E., Groneberg, D. A., & Banzer, W. (2020). Physical activity during COVID-19 induced lockdown: Recommendations. *Journal of Occupational Medicine and Toxicology, 15*, 25. https://doi.org/10.1186/s12995-020-00278-9

García, A. (2005). Miedo y privatización de los espacios públicos: ¿Hacer o deshacer la ciudad? [Fear and privatization of public spaces: Making or unmaking the city?]. In *La ciudad y el miedo* (pp. 209–221). Universidad de Girona.

Giles-Corti, B., Broomhall, M., Knuiman, M., Collins, C., Douglas, K., Ng, K., Lange, A., & Donovan, R. J. (2005). Increasing walking: How important is distance to, attractiveness, and size of public open space? *American Journal of Preventive Medicine, 28*, 169–176.

Gould, K., & Lewis, T. (2012). The environmental injustice of green gentrification: The case of Brooklyn prospect park. In *The world in Brooklyn: Gentrification, immigration, and ethnic politics in a global city* (pp. 113–146). Lexington Books.

Harvey, D. (2010). *The enigma of capital: And the crises of capitalism*. Profile Books.

Instituto de Investigaciones para el Desarrollo con Equidad [EQUIDE]. (2020). *Resultados de la encuesta de seguimiento de los efectos del COVID-19 en el bienestar de los hogares mexicanos. ENCOVID-19 junio y julio 2020* [Results of the follow-up survey of the effects of COVID-19 over the wellbeing in Mexican households. ENCOVID-19 June and July 2020]. https://equide.org/pobreza/https-equide-org-pobreza-impactos-del-covid-19-en-mexico. Accessed 10 Aug 2020.

Ipas, A. (2020, May 20). Coronavirus: 5 retos que transformaron a los parques [Coronavirus: 5 challenges that transformed parks]. *Asociación Nacional de Parques y Recreación de México*. https://anpr.org.mx/coronavirus-5-retos-que-transformaron-a-los-parques/. Accessed 10 July 2020.

Iracheta, A. (2012). Mejoremos las políticas públicas para hacer más eficiente la gestión urbana de las zonas metropolitanas del país [Let's improve public policies to make urban management more efficient in the metropolitan áreas of the country]. *Revista Economía, Sociedad y Territorio, 12*, 293–298.

Jacobs, A., & Appleyard, D. (1961). *The death and life of great American cities*. Vintage Books.

Jha, A. K., & Stanton-Geddes, Z. (Eds.) (2013). *Strong, safe, and resilient: Strategic policy guide for disaster risk management in East Asia and the Pacific. Directions in development: Environment and sustainable development.* The World Bank. https://documents1.worldbank.org/curated/en/230651468036883533/pdf/Strong-safe-and-resilient-s-strategic-policy-guide-for-disaster-risk-management-in-East-Asia-and-the-Pacific.pdf

Jia, T., Tao, H., Qin, K., Wang, Y., Liu, C., & Gao, Q. (2014). Selecting the optimal healthcare centers with a modified P-median model: A visual analytic perspective. *International Journal of Health Geographics, 13*(1), 1–15.

Jost, J. T., & Kay, A. C. (2010). Social justice: History, theory, and research. In S. T. Fiske, D. T. Gilbert, & G. Lindzey (Eds.), *Handbook of social psychology* (pp. 1122–1165). John Wiley & Sons.

Kabanoff, B. (1991). Equity, equality, power, and conflict. *Academy of Management Review, 16*(2), 416–441.

Krueger, R., & Gibbs, D. (Eds.). (2007). *The sustainable development paradox: Urban political economy in the United States and Europe*. Guilford Press.

Lafferty, K. D. (2009). The ecology of climate change and infectious diseases. *Ecology, 90*(4), 888–900. https://doi.org/10.1890/08-0079.1

Levac, J., Toal-Sullivan, D. O., & Sullivan, T. L. (2012). Household emergency preparedness: A literature review. *Journal of Community Health, 37*(3), 725–733.

Lynch, K. (1981). *A theory of Good City form*. MIT Press.

Maller, C. J., Townsend, M., Pryor, A., Brown, P., & St. Leger, L. (2006). Healthy nature healthy people: Contact with nature' as an upstream health promotion intervention for populations. *Health Promotion International, 21*(1), 45–54.

McConnachie, M. M., & Shackleton, C. M. (2010). Public green space inequality in small towns in South Africa. *Habitat International, 34*(2), 244–248.

Melnick, E. R., & Ioannidis, J. P. A. (2020). Should governments continue lockdown to slow the spread of covid-19? *BMJ, 369*, m1924. https://doi.org/10.1136/bmj.m1924

Mora-Garcia, R. T., Marti-Ciriquian, P., Perez-Sanchez, R., Cespedes-Lopez, M. F. (2018). *A comparative analysis of Manhattan, Euclidean and Network distances. Why are Network distances more useful to urban professionals?* 18th International Multidisciplinary Scientific Geo-Conference: SGEM. https://doi.org/10.5593/sgem2018/2.2.

Moreno, C. (2019, June 30). The 15 minutes-city: For a new chrono-urbanism! – Pr Carlos Moreno. Carlos Moreno*:* La Passion de L'Innovation. http://www.moreno-web.net/the-15-minutes-city-for-a-new-chrono-urbanism-pr-carlos-moreno/

Novaes, A. G., de Cursi, J. S., da Silva, A. C., & Souza, J. C. (2009). Solving continuous location–districting problems with Voronoi diagrams. *Computers & Operations Research, 36*(1), 40–59.

Nyakairu, J., Kuria, S., & Mbogori, S. (2012). *UN Habitat Annual Report (Nairobi)*. UN Habitat.

Okabe, A., Boots, B., Sugihara, K., & Chiu S. N. (2009). *Spatial tessellations: Concepts and applications of Voronoi diagrams* (Vol. 501 in probability and statistics). Wiley.

Patrick, D. J. (2011). *The politics of urban sustainability: Preservation, redevelopment and landscape on the high line* [Master's thesis, Budapest - Central European University].

Pérez-Paredes, E. A. (2016). Acciones y omisiones de las políticas públicas municipales dirigidas a los espacios públicos urbanos desde un enfoque socioambiental: Análisis de caso del municipio de Atizapán de Zaragoza, Estado de México [Actions and omissions of city pubic policies direct towards urban public spaces from a socioenvironmental approach: Case análisis of the city of Atizapan de Zaragoza, State of Mexico] [Doctoral dissertation, Centro Interdisciplinario de Estudios en Medio Ambiente y Desarrollo, Instituto Politécnico Nacional]. https://www.researchgate.net/profile/Elsa_Perez-Paredes

Plough, A., Fielding, J. E., Chandra, A., Williams, M., Eisenman, D., Wells, K. B., Law, G. Y., Fogleman, S., & Magaña, A. (2013). Building community disaster resilience: Perspectives from a large Urban County Department of Public Health. *American Journal of Public Health, 103*, 1190–1197. https://doi.org/10.2105/AJPH.2013.301268

Rabotnikof, N. (2003). Introducción para pensar lo público desde la ciudad [Introduction to think what's public from the city]. In P. Ramírez (coord.), *Espacio Público y reconstrucción de ciudadanía*. FLACSO; Librería Porrúa.

Rigolon, A. (2016). A complex landscape of inequity in access to urban parks: A literature review. *Landscape and Urban Planning, 153*, 160–169.

Sassen, S. (2013). Las ciudades como zona de frontera. La construcción de los sujetos urbanos [The cities as a frontier zone. The construction of the urban subjects]. *Revista Internacional de Arquitectura y Diseño, 14*, 140–146.

Scheffer, M. (2009). *Critical transitions in nature and society*. Princeton University Press.

Schlosberg, D. (2004). Reconceiving environmental justice: Global movements and political theories. *Environmental Politics, 13*(3), 517–540.

Secretaría de Desarrollo Social [SEDESOL]. (2020). Evaluación Complementaria de Percepción de Inseguridad, Satisfacción y Cohesión Social en Espacios Públicos [Complementary evaluation to the Annual Report regarding Perception of Insecurity, Satisfaction and Social Cohesion in Public Spaces]. http://www.normateca.sedesol.gob.mx/es/SEDESOL/Evaluacion_Complementaria_de_Percepcion_de_Inseguridad. Accessed 15 Nov 2019.

Segura, R. (2014). El espacio urbano y la (re)producción de desigualdades sociales. Desacoples entre distribución del ingreso y patrones de urbanización en ciudades latinoamericanas [The urban space and the (re)production of social inequality. Disconnections between income distribution and urbanization patterns in Latin American cities]. Universidad Nacional de San Martín.

Sherer, P. M. (2006). *The benefits of parks: Why America needs more City parks and open space*; Reprint of "Parks for People" (2003). San Francisco, CA, USA: The Trust for Public Land.

Singh, S., Roy, D., Sinha, K., Parveen, S., Sharma, G., & Joshi, G. (2020). Impact of COVID-19 and lockdown on mental health of children and adolescents: A narrative review with recommendations. *Psychiatry Research, 293*, 113429. https://doi.org/10.1016/j.psychres.2020.113429

Smoyer-Tomic, K. E., Hewko, J. N., & Hodgson, M. J. (2004). Spatial accessibility and equity of playgrounds in Edmonton, Canada. *The Canadian Geographer, 48*(3), 287–302.

Stockholm Environment Institute [SEI]. (2020, May 20). *Lockdown highlights the value of green space in cities*. https://www.sei.org/perspectives/covid19-value-of-green-space-in-cities/

Subsecretaría de Desarrollo Urbano y Vivienda, Dirección General de Rescate de Espacio Públicos. (2013). *Programa de Rescate de Espacios Públicos: Lineamientos Específicos para la Operación del Programa de Rescate de Espacios Públicos 2013* [Program to Rescue Public Spaces: Specific Guidelinesfor the Operation of the Program to Rescue Public Spaces 2013]. https://www.gob.mx/cms/uploads/attachment/file/5749/Lineamientos_PREP_2013_24-may-13_.pdf. Accessed 15 Nov 2019.

Svara, J. H., James, R., & Brunet, J. R. (2005). Social equity is a pillar of public administration. *Journal of Public Affairs Education, 11*(3), 253–258. https://doi.org/10.1080/15236803.2005.12001398

Talen, E. (1998). Visualizing fairness: Equity maps for planners. *Journal of the American Planning Association, 64*(1), 22–38.

Talen, E. (2010). The spatial logic of parks. *Journal of Urban Design, 15*(4), 473–491.

Talen, E., & Anselin, L. (1998). Assessing spatial equity: An evaluation of measures of accessibility to public playgrounds. *Environment and Planning A, 30*(4), 595–613.

Tsou, K. W., Hung, Y. T., & Chang, Y. L. (2005). An accessibility-based integrated measure of relative spatial equity in urban public facilities. *Cities, 22*(6), 424–435.

UN-Habitat. (2015). *Grupo de trabajo para Issue Paper 11: Espacio Público rumbo a la Conferencia de las Naciones Unidas sobre Vivienda y Desarrollo Urbano Sostenible—Hábitat III* [Work group for Issue Paper 11: Public Space towards the United Nations' Confereence about Housing and Sustainable Urban Development]. New York, NY, USA.

United Nations Envionment Programme [UNEP]. (2010). *Annual Report 2009: Seizing the Green Opportunity*. http://wedocs.unep.org/handle/20.500.11822/7824. Accessed 15 Nov 2019.

United Nations General Assembly. (2015). *Transforming our world: The 2030 agenda for sustainable development*. https://sdgs.un.org/2030agenda

Vale, L. J., & Campanella, T. J. (2005). *The Resilient City: How modern cities recover from disaster*. Oxford University Press.

Wang, M., Krstikj, A., & Koura, H. (2017a). Effects of urban planning on urban expansion control in Yinchuan City, Western China. *Habitat International, 64*, 85–97.

Wang, M., Krstikj, A., & Koura, H. (2017b). Study on the housing supply and public programs impacts on the housing development in Yinchuan city, Western China. *Journal of Architecture and Planning (Transactions of AIJ), 82*(732), 469–476.

Webb, L. (2020). COVID-19 lockdown: A perfect storm for older people's mental health. *Journal of Psychiatric and Mental Health Nursing, 28*(2), 300. https://doi.org/10.1111/jpm.12644

Weintraub, J. (1997). The theory and politics of the public/private distinction. In J. Weintraub & K. Kumae (Eds.), *Public and private in thought and practice: Perspectives on a grand dichotomy* (pp. 1–42). University of Chicago Press.

Wolch, J., Wilson, J. P., & Fehrenbach, J. (2005). Parks and park funding in Los Angeles: An equity-mapping analysis. *Urban Geography, 26*(1), 4–35.

Yuan, Y., Xu, J., & Wang, Z. (2017). Spatial equity measure on urban ecological space layout based on accessibility of socially vulnerable groups—A case study of Changting, China. *Sustainability, 9*, 1552. https://doi.org/10.3390/su9091552

Chapter 5
Appropriate Population Mobility Management in an Epidemic

Yuan Ren

In just a few months, COVID-19 spread to become a serious public health crisis on a national and global scale. The crisis highlights the complex challenges faced by high-density megacities amid rapid urbanization and the urgent need for enhanced urban governance capacity. This chapter discusses the relationship between population concentration and risk concentration in megacities, as well as the necessities and limits of population mobility management when facing the challenges of virus transmission, and illustrates how to execute effective and scientific population mobility management, including utilizing big data and new technologies for epidemic prevention and control. This chapter further argues that a good megacity's development should strengthen risk management, improve urban resilience, and enhance the efficacy of urban governance.

Risks and Challenges Posed by Population Concentration and Risk Concentration

Demographic Characteristics of Megacities and Related High-Risk Societies

Megacities are cities with a large size, high density, and high mobility population. They face complex risks and challenges, including the spread of infectious diseases. Megacities are highly prone to forming the centers of risk aggregation and are typical places of high-risk societies (Xiao, 2015). Obviously, here is a positive

Y. Ren (✉)
School of Social Development and Public Policy. Institute of Population Research, Fudan University, Shanghai, China
e-mail: yren@fudan.edu.cn

© The Author(s), under exclusive license to Springer Nature Switzerland AG 2021

M. A. Montoya et al. (eds.), *COVID-19 and Cities*, The Urban Book Series,
https://doi.org/10.1007/978-3-030-84134-8_5

correlation between population growth and virus spread. In cities with massive population concentrations, infectious diseases spread more rapidly and on a larger scale than in sparsely populated rural areas. The outbreak of COVID-19 is merely proof of the enormous risks inherent in high-density megacities and the vulnerability of big cities. For the prevention and management of highly infectious diseases such as COVID-19, there is no doubt that the public health management of megacities is under pressure.

Another issue is the mobility of the population. The high density of the population within megacities, with spatially connected and diversified urban life, brings a high degree of intra-city population mobility. The megacities are simultaneously characterized by intensive economic production, business and commerce, tourism and recreational services, and educational and cultural activities. These distinctive features of urban functioning expand the external population's mobility, making the megacity a hub for population movements in the urban system. Megacities also form the nodes of global urban connectivity, making it easy for health risks that have occurred in one single city, to expand into a global problem as populations move around the world. The high volume of population mobility in megacities has, to some extent, exacerbated the spread of the virus and brought about difficulties in controlling the virus, as well as posing real problems. The population mobility in high-density cities makes the internal reinforcement and external transmission of urban risks more obvious. It can significantly amplify the spread of infectious diseases. Hence, the large population size, high population density, and high population mobility in megacities result in risk complexification and risk concentration. Megacities need to address the considerable challenges of complex risks, including the challenge of managing infectious diseases. Megacities are inherently high-risk societies, and in high-risk societies any carelessness could lead to catastrophic events.

Population Concentration and Risk Concentration in Megacities

While we acknowledge that the huge population size, population density, and high population mobility of megacities put immense pressure on urban public health safety, we should also recognize that population size and population density are not the cause of pandemics like COVID-19. The concentration and mobility of urban populations are only external factors that become the conditions of and exacerbate the spread of infectious diseases. The pathology of urban development lies in the fast population growth and the disproportionate capacity development of urban management and services (Ren, 2015). In comparison to the urban population growth, the capacity of urban management and urban services are inadequate, which will result in various urban problems, for example, traffic jams, environmental deterioration, congested housing, etc. These factors also have a bearing on the spread of COVID-19. The spread of the epidemic should not be attributed to the large population size of megacities, it is fundamentally the result of the inefficient urban health services and the low efficiency of the disease prevention system. Therefore, to address the challenge of public health risks in megacities, it is in essence necessary to strengthen and refine urban governance by improving the capacity of urban management and services. That includes improving public health investment in staff and facilities, enhancing public health information and response mechanisms in a more efficient and integrated manner, etc.

Urban pathology is not the result of population concentration. On the contrary, objectively speaking, while urban population growth amplifies risk pressures, it creates positive ramifications for better risk resolution. The wealth effects of a population concentrated megacity improve the risk-response ability. The population concentration process also brings about knowledge spillover effects and economies of scale for public services. In addition, modern cities also possess normative and institutionalized management. All these factors have positive effects on risk management. Megacities have had significantly lower disease fatality rates, higher health security, better social protection, and a significantly better ability to deal with the pandemic compared to other areas. Megacities are also able to provide sufficient and better health services and can better support people's lives. It is true that there is a concentration of complex risks in megacities. As cities increase in size, the variety of risks to which megacities are exposed grows exponentially, however, the ability of megacities to cope with risks also grows exponentially. Throughout human history, the governance capacity of coping with risks during urbanization has always been faster than the speed of risk growth, thus bringing about prosperity in urbanization and continuous progress in humanity's wellbeing.

The COVID-19 pandemic seems to result in fearful impressions of large cities and disasters due to the public's misconception that population concentration has brought risk concentration. This inaccurate impression is unhelpful in forming an accurate and informed perception of China's urbanized development and associated risk management. Although megacities have dense and highly mobile populations which amplifies the risks and puts the residents under greater pressure, in the interrelationship between population concentration and risk concentration in megacities, urban problems are not simply attributable to an urban population. The simple correlation between population concentration and urban disaster is a very Malthusian view, which posits that urban population growth will always outpace urban development capacity. However, the history of the development of cities around the world shows that the capacity of urban management services is continuously improving and that cities are, in general, successful at promoting affluence and security, as well as achieving a better quality of life in the context of urban growth (Glaeser, 2011). It is precisely the competitive nature of urban development capacity and the high quality of urban management that have prompted the population to move into cities, which leads to population concentration. Similarly, it is precisely the improved capacity of urban management and services that have made it possible to address the challenges of modern society's complex risks. Directly attributing the spread of diseases to the population size would obscure the essence of the problem, ignore the reality that megacities provide more robust risk management and social protection, and would deviate from the urgent need to improve urban management services, modernize urban governance, and increase the capacity of cities in the process of urbanization.

Necessities and Limitations of Population Mobility Control

Although population concentration is not the cause of the spread of infectious diseases, high population density and high population mobility, as external conditions, objectively worsen the spread of the virus. Population mobility can exacerbate the spread of disease and increase the difficulty in disease control. Therefore, for epidemic control and prevention, the control of population mobility played a necessary role in curbing the spread of the epidemic, especially in the early stage of the outbreak. The slowing down of urban operations through population mobility controls can decelerate the spread of infectious viruses. Thus, the "city lockdowns" in Wuhan City and Hubei province during the epidemic, including the suspension of some public transport services, were temporary coping strategies given the rapid spread of the epidemic at that point in time. Considering the huge population mobility during the Spring Festival, we should regard the rigid control of population mobility as a proper and understandable response. Through measures such as implementing public opinion campaigns, encouraging the population to stay home and reducing outdoor activities, extending the Spring Break, and delaying the return to work, space was exchanged for time. The speed at which the virus spread was reduced due to the slowing down of spatial mobility, which won time to control the outbreak.

However, population mobility management is only a symptomatic approach to epidemic control and prevention and serves as an emergency response to the external conditions of disease transmission. The fundamental solution to coping with the epidemic includes the search for and identification of the source of infection and its total elimination, the acceleration of the development and use of testing reagents so that the control of population mobility can shift towards the control of viral mobility, and the strengthening of the development of vaccines and therapeutic drugs to treat the disease, etc. Through these methods, society could transfer to a kind of 'new normal', coexisting with the COVID-19 virus, as we now know that we will have to coexist with the virus and some of its mutations for a long time. With effective treatment methods and a scientific disease prevention system, it is possible that we can transform COVID-19 from an unknown infectious virus into a known and controllable one. Meanwhile, it is possible to change the emergent epidemic control and prevention system into routine disease management.

Facing the sudden impact of COVID-19, the implementation of population mobility control as an emergency epidemic control was a necessary response strategy as the rate of control and prevention of the epidemic did not keep pace with the spread of the virus. In some cases, we might hope that the implementation of these mandatory isolation and lockdown responses would be taken much earlier. However, we should still realize that slowing down urban mobility through lockdowns, social distancing, calling for less visiting between family and friends, and calling for people to stay at home and isolate themselves, are not a permanent cure to permanent disease responses.

We should also be aware that the act of controlling population mobility in megacities is incompatible with the very nature of megacity operations. There are also associated side effects of slowing or containing population mobility and urban operations, which can reduce the efficiency of a city's function and produce other problems, e.g., unemployment and economic slowdown, etc., which would then undermine other goals of megacity development.

Urban dysfunction due to population mobility control, and a slowdown in urban operations, can harm the city's, and national, economy. Due to short-term labor shortages, it will weaken production capacity. It affects upstream and downstream economic production through industry chains, significantly affecting life and social services that are heavily reliant on population size and people's consumption, particularly in these sectors: tourism, food and beverage, cultural and entertainment, as well as transportation. A decline in the efficiency of logistic network services could lead to a shortage of supplies, weakening supply, and leading to an increase in prices, thus hindering people's livelihoods. Inadequate material supplies can lead to planned arrangements and rationing, as we have seen online, for example, in some areas where vouchers for the purchase of masks have emerged, giving rise to associations with a return to the ticket economy. A slowdown in mobility is very detrimental to urban functioning in the long run, and its effects on epidemic control may not even be long-lasting. For example, in Wuhan, the lack of mobility in the city made it difficult for the city's inhabitants to provide services, and even medical supplies and logistics could not be provided in time.

Meanwhile, population mobility control and the freeze of urban operations are not conducive to effective social organization and social mobilization. If urban residents just stay at home, sleep and watch TV, lacking strong social organization and social participation, their social life is actually unhelpful to disease prevention and response. In the process of dealing with a major crisis such as the COVID-19 pandemic, it is necessary to mobilize social forces to participate in order to form social solidarity and initiate collective action against the pandemic. With active social charity activities, social organizations, and the intervention of social workforces, the capacity of urban epidemic control and prevention will be strengthened and meet the overall needs of urban residents in the process.

Thus, population mobility management, as a temporary, emergent approach for epidemic control and prevention, bears significant direct and indirect costs as a consequence, showing unsustainable outcomes. Mobility is to cities are as veins carrying lifeblood are to the body. Restricting the mobility of people and the mobility of urban operations will undermine the effective functioning of cities. While when facing the initial impact of the epidemic and dealing with the rapid increase of confirmed infectious cases it is necessary to reduce the spread of the epidemic through population mobility control, attention must be paid to the economic and social losses caused by the loss of urban mobility while implementing these measures.

Surely technology will offset the adverse effects of the loss of mobility to some extent. Considerable elements of economic and social activities can be conducted through online communications and telework. If there were some positive consequences to this great disaster caused by the pandemic, it is that the pandemic has been instrumental in accelerating the development of an information-based online economy or platform economy (Wan, 2020), and these developments will be helpful for future industrial restructuring and social changes. However, as mobility is still the essence of urban functioning, it is an obvious truism that weak population mobility and the slowdown of urban operations cannot support the effective functioning of either megacities or that of a vast country.

Implementing Scientific and Rational Population Mobility Management to Optimize Epidemic Prevention and Urban Functioning

Implementation of Dynamically Adjusted Population Mobility Management Based on Multi-leveled Risk Assessment

Regarding epidemic prevention, due to the lack of an adequate, reliable means of virus testing, as well as a lack of effective vaccines and medication, it is essential to adopt corresponding population mobility control for a highly contagious disease like COVID-19 to curb the spread of the epidemic. Precise population mobility management should, on the one hand, help to enhance the effectiveness of epidemic prevention, and on the other hand, strive to maintain economic and social development. Meanwhile, the practice of mobility restrictions should also take into account the limitations of public health provisions, including hospital beds and medical staff numbers. Instead of merely restricting the population mobility throughout the country on a "one-size-fits-all" basis, the scientific approach is to analyze the speed and trend of the virus spreading in order to assess the risks by levels, and then to make timely and dynamic adjustments of the population mobility management so as to optimize epidemic prevention and achieve targets of social and economic development.

China's epidemiological management has already acquired sufficient knowledge and experience. It needs to take into account the specific characteristics of the communicability and adverse health effects of COVID-19 to curate and implement scientific epidemic prevention schemes. In other words, public health and emergency management departments should conduct dynamic, graded alerts according to the extent and speed of the spread of the epidemic in different regions and adopt timely population mobility management strategies, including urban lockdowns and social distancing, etc. The strategies range from the cancellation of large public gatherings at lower alert levels to the cancellation of public events and public transport of a specific size at higher alert levels and to the reduction of outings and execution of community-based lockdowns at the highest alert levels. The social distancing standard should also adjust according to different risk levels. At the same time, there is a need to manage the population mobility between different regions in a multilevel manner, depending on the level of epidemic risks in different regions. Differential and multilevel population mobility management can also be implemented for different population groups based on factors such as the probability of individual infection and disease fatality rates among different groups. For example, with the increase in awareness of the viral fatality rate for the elderly population, it is necessary to encourage the elderly population, and those with underlying medical conditions, to strictly stay at home while implementing epidemic control and prevention measures. This suggests that scientifically refined population mobility management can indicate how these measures are conducted and improve their relevance and effectiveness.

Similarly, the gradual easing of mobility restrictions and the restoration of population mobility will be necessary after the COVID-19 pandemic has been brought under control. Epidemiological management in cities should also gradually retreat based on different risk levels. Cities should ease out of mobility restrictions as risk levels gradually fall in different areas, and with the risk of viral infection differing for different population groups. Urban development needs to strike the right balance between epidemic prevention and the gradual restoration of an economic and social order based on epidemic risk assessment. The key to the gradual restoration of population mobility, work, as well as economic and social activities in different regions, is to have accurate and dynamic information on the COVID-19 pandemic so that decision-makers can make accurate judgments. The gradual easing of restrictions on mobility through a multi-level assessment of epidemic risks will enable the national economy and social development to recover from the emergency period gradually, and steadily move towards a normalized state.

Therefore, population mobility management based on epidemic surveillance and multilevel risk assessment plays a fundamental role in epidemic prevention. In this regard, timely follow-ups and professional evaluations are needed to curate scientific and appropriate epidemic prevention and control measures. A scientific epidemic control scheme should constitute multilevel, dynamic, and streamlined measures to realize scientific and timely responses to the disease at the lowest cost, and to coordinate the relationship between epidemic control and the normal functioning of socio-economic development. This requires having an accurate and swift information system in place, as well as sound decision-making mechanisms integrated with scientific assessments, to enable the timely translation of scientific research into the guidelines for epidemic control and prevention.

Epidemic Control in Accordance with Rule of Law, and Avoidance of Social Discrimination in Implementing Population Mobility Management

Attention should be given to the potential moral hazards in population mobility management when it is used as a tool for epidemic prevention. There is a need to avoid the population mobility restrictions from morphing into geographical discrimination against special population groups in high-risk areas. We can see that during the control of the epidemic, some cities have barred people holding Hubei province identity cards from entering, even if those people could provide adequate proof of good health. That shows an exclusionary "beggar-thy-neighbor" mentality in view of self-protection. In some areas, local security staff have even forcibly disrupted the normal lives of urban-rural residents, violating the rights of people and infringing on their belongings. This shows the population mobility management has been exerted "excessively" and "improperly". The core purpose of mobility restrictions is to control the virus. If there are excessive mobility controls in place which convert the restrictions into a long-term population control policy, it would have deviated from the purpose, and this would result in the social exclusion of specific populations. This excessive mobility control is contrary to the legal basis of the free movement of people. The "beggar-thy-neighbor" mentality in the face of the great epidemic looming in the country speaks of the lack of a sense of brotherhood among fellow citizens and the lack of social ethics. This mentality is detrimental towards the building of a community of common destiny in the country.

We have, then, to carry out lawful administrative works and epidemic control measures within the framework of the Law on Prevention and Treatment of Infectious Diseases. There is a need to refine legal arrangements for emergency management and to identify the different levels of mobility control, the use of public and social resources, and restrictions on the freedom of movement of citizens at different levels of the State of Emergency. Such legal refinements include denoting what kind of population mobility is allowed and disallowed under different levels of urgency. Where necessary, it is imperative to implement programs for the control and punishment of population mobility in accordance with the legal mandate of the local People's Congress. For the public, we need to disseminate factually accurate epidemic prevention, disease transmission, and legal information, and encourage social solidarity, not social exclusion, in order to avoid the occurrence of discriminatory geographical labeling of groups.

Optimizing Risk management in High Density and High-Mobility Cities Using Big Data and Technological Innovations

The control and prevention efforts of the COVID-19 pandemic have shown unique characteristics compared to previous epidemic control management. Technological innovations using big data have played a significant role in epidemic prevention and public health management. Technological applications and big data usage can enhance outbreak control and emergency management capabilities tremendously, for example, people's mobile phones could provide data on people's dynamic spatial position so that the government and the communication company are technically able to trace people's commuting and to determine the risks of viral infection.

Through China's Baidu's big data, we can ascertain the direction and size of population movements, subsequently predicting the pressure on disease prevention in different regions. Big data technology can map the spatial variation of the population and conduct a simulation of the spread of the epidemic. In addition, it can capture the behavioral trajectory of the population through refined data analysis, calculate the resulting risk exposure opportunities, identify the population who came into close contact with infected personnel, and screen out the people at risk by calculating the probability of infection. With this technology, we can also identify the distribution and spread of the disease through demographic data, such as that consisting of confirmed, suspected, recovered, and deceased cases. These allow us to pinpoint the level of epidemic risk in different regions, identify outbreaks through incidence and infection rates, predict the spread of the disease, and adopt targeted responses, among other measures.

Technological innovation has given great superiority and effectiveness in epidemic prevention, emerging as salient support for modern public health management and playing a decisive role in staunching the pandemic. These tactics are well used in COVID-19 prevention practices in Singapore, South Korea, China, etc., and have contributed to the comparatively successful disease prevention achievements. These new techniques were inconceivable by traditional public health management standards. Without the support of technology, our response to this COVID-19 outbreak would have been more passive and faced more difficulties. Demographic data and related technological innovations for megacity health epidemic prevention and emergency management are beginning to manifest themselves, facilitating the realization of precision epidemic prevention driven by big data (Ma, 2020). It is foreseeable that big data will form an essential pillar for future public health management systems in megacities, providing more effective management and services, as well as more refined urban governance, through the provision of new data and analytical tools.

The application of big data technology to improve urban governance capacity and to provide more timely and refined management and services, once again demonstrates that megacities have a more substantial capacity for disease control and health services. One of the crucial measures to enhance the governance capacity of future megacities is the introduction of technological innovations, which will significantly boost the modernization of urban governance and achieve refined management. In this regard, some megacities in China have made substantial advancements. However, it is clear that, in practice, more progress is needed to truly apply the scientific and technological advancements to the modernization of urban governance.

Another concern arising from combining technological innovations in population data and urban epidemic control is the conflict between the privacy of personal details and the needs of public health management. Even for epidemic prevention purposes, overexposure of private information, whether released by the government or by business companies, is effectively a misuse and improper disclosure of personal information. The mobilization of big data information and privacy protection will increasingly become prominent issues in modern urban technology governance.

There is a need to strike a balance in public safety management between establishing efficient and targeted urban management and avoiding a breach of the legitimate rights of individuals (Ren et al., 2019). In addition, there is a need to delineate the legal obligations and responsibilities of individuals in the process of disease control and public health management. It is also important to determine the authoritative legal powers of the public sector in emergency management and its extent in urban management. It is through establishing the rule of law that efficiency can be achieved, propelling law-abiding, ethical urban management.

Hopefully, if we can thoroughly distinguish the infected and uninfected demographics, or can procure sufficient vaccines and effective medication, we can essentially win the fight against COVID-19 and bring life back to normal. However, due to a lack of adequate testing coverage and disease treatment methods so far, we have to rely on population mobility management to curb the outbreak. Meanwhile, scientific and rational population mobility management responses also serve as one component of the overall public health system facing the challenges of epidemic diseases and pandemics. We should optimize population mobility management to better balance urban operation, social-economic development, and epidemic control and prevention. If there were some lessons we learned on population mobility management during the COVID-19 pandemic, they might include adopting dynamic adjustments based on timely multi-level risks assessment, standardizing mobility management according to the rule of law, and better utilizing big data and technological innovations to implement accurate tracing, tracking and epidemic prevention. Based on scientific improvement and innovations, effective and professional rules-based public health responses are important to strengthen urban resilience.

Historically, human development has constantly coexisted with viruses and infectious diseases. The virus is daunting but its existence is inevitable and can never be eradicated. It is through the repeated battles we have had with the outbreak of diseases that human society has developed and evolved, medicine has advanced, and the capacity of urban public health management and services has improved. In the process of urbanization, active preparedness to strengthen infectious disease control and prevention systems are vital to improving urban resilience. Strengthening public health systems and capacity building is still very much reliant on the refinement of management. Megacities, including Shanghai, have accumulated considerable experience in actively addressing various risk challenges. The rapid development of science and technology also provides more effective tools to enhance megacities' management capacity and risk response.

One quintessential tip in life is that a child's cold could be considered as an "exercise" for improving the baby's immune system. Likewise, for megacities, public health events and epidemic outbreaks could also be regarded as an "exercise" to improve the city and the country's immune system for public health. We need to remain hyper-vigilant about the challenges that megacities face, as megacities are high-risk societies, while also having confidence in modern urban governance. To some extent, the enormous cost of disasters could be regarded as an inevitable trade-off for improving urban resilience for sustainable development. The numerous problems within the public health management system exposed in this COVID-19 pandemic further illustrate the need to improve the health management system and urban governance system. When tackling the pandemic, the varied responses, practices, and mechanisms adopted by different countries and megacities are invaluable lessons for us to work on for improving our health management systems and urban governance systems in the future. Important objectives that need to be accomplished in the rapid urbanization process in China include strengthening urban resilience, improving the capacity of urban governance, and modernizing the governance of megacities.

Acknowledgments Support for the research was provided by Shanghai Municipal Education Commission Grant (No. E00026).

References

Glaeser, E. (2011). *Triumph of the city: How our greatest invention makes us richer, smarter, greener, healthier, and happier*. New York: Penguin Press.

Ma, L. (2020, February 4). Big data driven precise epidemic prevention: What can be done and how to do better? *Six Tone*. https://tech.sina.com.cn/roll/2020-02-04/doc-iimxxste8824735.shtml

Ren, Y. (2015). Reflection of Mega-City population synthetic control. *Nanjing Social Science, 1*, 83–90.

Ren, Y. et al. (2019). *Development and application of population big data and Megacity social governance research*. Science and Technology Commission of Shanghai Municipal Soft Science Research Report.

Wan, J. (2020, February 3). How the epidemic affects the economy. *Sina.com*. http://finance.sina.com.cn/review/jcgc/2020-02-03/doc-iimxxste8480829.shtml

Xiao, Y. (2015). Risk generation mechanisms and their operating logics in Megacities. *Exploration and Free Views, 3*, 16–18.

Chapter 6
Diversification of Urbanism in the Process of City Region Transformation

Hisako Koura

Introduction

Since its outbreak in Wuhan at the beginning of 2020, COVID-19 (coronavirus) has spread globally and has brought about a socioeconomic crisis, as well as a crisis of the public health system in many countries. The short but intensive experience of coping with COVID-19 during the first 6 months of the emergency response implies several planning issues for future urban transformation.

First, teleworking, as an alternative to commuting, was requested and has actually become accepted as one of the new working styles. The diversification of working styles has already affected residential preference, with more of the population transferring outside of Tokyo after the first 6 months of the crisis than those moving in. Second, density control, to reduce the risk of infection, demands a new planning concept for the reorganization of the intensive layout of urban functions, including enough open space, as a requisite aspect of a "walkable city." The third is the mobility issue, which goes hand-in-hand with commuting on a local scale and inbound movement on a regional and global scale, as a consequence related to social and economic conditions.

The three issues mentioned above, working style, density control, and mobility, are becoming considerable aspects in the planning field and inspire us to seek an alternative approach that can function within the existing urban and rural transformation due to the uneven conditions of land use and distribution of the local population. In Japan, we now confront the necessity of smart shrinkage in many urban and rural areas studded with abundant vacant housing and land (Ministry of Land, Infrastructure, Transport, and Tourism of Japan [MLIT], 2017b, 2018).

H. Koura (✉)
Graduate School of Arts and Design, Kobe Design University, Kobe, Japan
e-mail: koura-h@kobe-du.ac.jp

© The Author(s), under exclusive license to Springer Nature Switzerland AG 2021

M. A. Montoya et al. (eds.), *COVID-19 and Cities*, The Urban Book Series,
https://doi.org/10.1007/978-3-030-84134-8_6

Considerable Signs of Change

Working Style Diversification

During the COVID-19 emergency in April and May 2020 in Japan, people were requested to self-isolate. Many had to choose between closing offices, factories, shops, restaurants, and other facilities, or developing an individual teleworking system. Some were forced on turning to a remote office working style and telecommuting, utilizing more sophisticated online systems to continue their business. Schools also struggled to continue the educational process under various limitations.

These struggles reveal the gap in the potentiality of business continuity, depending on the type of business and industry, their targeted market, and most of all, on IT literacy and ICT infrastructure conditions. Moreover, employment conditions were affected by the business continuity. Though working style alternatives in this period relied significantly on IT literacy and the infrastructure of companies and institutions, younger generations have become aware of the fact that alternative working styles allow them to migrate to the countryside or other places with internet connection availability, while the business remains in the urban center. At the moment, the number of those individuals who can choose a job unrestrained by the physical location is not large, but it is certainly increasing during the current crisis. Nevertheless, it has already been observed that some move out to the countryside while retaining their business in the city office. This new situation allows individuals to engage simultaneously as part-time workers in agriculture, creating a small local income on the side. Some firms have permitted employees to engage in side-work, which is not normally allowed.

The diversification of working styles opens up the constraint of residential choice, which in turn functions as a positive factor to promote relocation and migration for a more balanced local renovation and urban transformation on a regional scale.

Autonomous Neighborhoods

The importance of the daily market is another factor that has been recognized during the self-isolation period. The neighborhood food market and commodity shops were busy even during the emergency period since they support our daily life. On the other hand, many shops and restaurants targeting visitors and inbound tourists, even those located in the immediate surroundings of the daily market, have been having serious problems keeping their business operational. The decrease of daily commuting and reduced mobility of visitors opened a severe gap between the urban center and suburbia. During this emergency period, the density of ordinary life in suburbia is unusually high, whilst the urban center is left empty.

The proportion of the world's urban population in the 1950s used to only be 30%. In 2018, the portion was estimated at 55% and is expected to increase to 68% by 2050, according to the United Nations [UN] projections (UN, 2018). In the EU and the US, the urban population rate reaches a staggering 80%. In Japan, over 59% of the population lives in the three major metropolitan areas. The Japanese metropolitan areas, where people commute to the center to work, might appear monotonous, but they are more akin to a mosaic of unique local cohesion grounded in land-use, landscape, geography, local history, culture, and social and economic features.

In Japan, each mosaic that composes the metropolitan region is highly networked to the center, thus only during the self-isolation and reduced mobility period have people realized the locality of their neighborhood. Even though people in urban areas have been using delivery services and online shopping more than usual to avoid unnecessary contact and infection, while the drive-through shopping style has been developing in the countryside, we experienced the vital necessity of a daily market to sustain our ordinary life. We also realized the large number of essential workers who make our lifestyle possible.

Even though businesses, services, and communications continued the online network functions with relative ease, the efficiency of the daily market and essential work that demands real contact is delivered from within the local cohesion, which implies that a reorganization process is required to improve the urban units and their networking. This process develops autonomous neighborhoods generated only in the real sphere of daily existence, where individual comfortable places are embedded. Such neighborhoods will work as a planning unit in local coherence.

Optimization of Urban Spatial Values

Social distancing is a required condition to support coexistence with COVID-19 while it continues to rage. The capacity of facilities is limited to under half or one-third of the normal usage, and adequate ventilation is required. Thus, sufficient parks and green open spaces in the living environment have become highly valued. While cafés and restaurants deal with this issue by providing open-air tables, museums, halls, and events are having a hard time implementing their programs.

It is still not clear whether social distancing will affect urban density, facility design, and layouts in future planning. However, it is quite certain that streets, community places, shop fronts, cafés, gardens, and even vacant land will be local resources for public space, which will activate social living under any circumstances and improve urban resilience during any crisis. During the last 10 years, both placemaking movements and tactical urbanism renovated abandoned and/or underutilized space into live public space through voluntary local initiatives. These movements seek optimized social density, which is coincidentally happening with the reevaluation of spatial value in today's crisis.

Besides this, creating various public spaces promoted by autonomous and voluntary approaches, future social associations of urban life, and farming at the fringe, as well as rural living in the countryside, will generate local collaborations and thus enhance resilience. Therefore, at the regional scale, urban transformation with appropriate consideration towards the natural and social environment will be demanded, which might lead to relevant spatial coherence.

Implication for Changes

The COVID-19 crisis is, in a sense, an opportunity to open up another potentiality for planning, such as urban-rural re-structuring and networking, which have been long discussed but never put into practice. The MLIT (Ministry of Land, Infrastructure, Transport, and Tourism of Japan) conducted an interview survey of experts on urban planning, mobility, landscape, disaster prevention, and medical care, the result of which highlighted five planning issues as crucial for consideration in future planning.

The five indicated discussion issues comprise: (1) A future urban policy on business function in the center, multi-functions in local and suburban living, and the association and sharing of roles under unbalanced density; (2) A transportation policy to cope with the reduction in commuting density and the development of modal options in local mobility; (3) An open space policy in high-density urban centers and a reappraisal of greenery relaxation values in the context of green infrastructure developments; (4) The development with efficient utilization of distal services, internet, and advanced information technologies; and (5) Preparedness for complex disaster emergencies.

The signs of change that are discussed above, such as working style diversification, autonomous neighborhoods, and the optimization of urban spatial values, are shared as general understandings in the MLIT interview survey report (MLIT, 2020). These signs that emerged in the crisis have the potential to promote the "Compact Plus Network" policy (MLIT, 2014) of MLIT, which demands advancing the urban transformation in both metropolitan and local cities with the relocation of urban functions and living density in order to realize a more efficient structure to cope with the shrinkage of populations and local businesses. At the same time, we have learned that there is an appropriate density and accumulation of functions to achieve high efficiency of services and social care. In both cases, COVID-19 revealed latent planning issues, while the experiences of alternative working and living styles, and the confrontation with business continuity, accelerated the changes for urban transformation.

Urban Transformation

Growth and Shrinkage

The present City Planning Act of Japan, enacted in 1968 (Japanese Ministry of Justice, 2009), aimed to control excessive urban expansion without infrastructure developments during the period of rapid growth. The Act established the zoning system of the Area Division into an Urbanization Promotion Area and the Urbanization Control Area in the City Planning Area (MLIT, 2007). With the expectation of future growth, the Urbanization Promotion Area was considered a crucial tool by the authorities to manage and control the development. Nevertheless, urban density did not reach the planning index outside of the three major metropolitan areas of Japan. On the contrary, motorization and weak planning tools against development in the agricultural zones at the urban fringe promoted urban sprawl.

The national population of Japan has declined since its peak in 2008 (Statistics Bureau of Japan, 2016). Even though this shrinking phenomenon differs from place to place, depending on social and economic conditions, we are confronted with an urgent necessity of developing a new planning tool to cope with shrinking and to manage the inevitable urban transformation, for which purpose the City Planning Act of 1968 is obsolete. In an attempt to revitalize urban centers and relocate daily urban functions to form compact and walkable local neighborhoods, including disaster prevention, the present legal framework is enforced through a special measures law, although it has a limited legal period.

Urban transformation whilst the population is shrinking, is very much associated with the issue discussed above concerning the reorganization of living and working styles. This issue can be looked at through the concept of the commuting working style, brought about by modernization, industrialization, and waged earnings as a general lifestyle that resulted in the centralization of urban functions, and the development of suburbia. However, in the present context, with a lack of the appropriate planning tools to lead much needed urban transformation, the alternative working style might function as a trigger to promote migration and awaken an interest in such a daily life and enhance local resilience according to the general concept of "Compact Plus Network."

Polycentric Urban Region: Kansai

Kansai is a polycentric urban region with Kyoto, Osaka, and Kobe as major cities. The region nearly equals the area covered by the Osaka metropolitan area, but each of the three cities occupies a unique position. Kyoto is the old capital that nowadays attracts global tourism. Kobe has been struggling to evolve its urban functions due to the loss of its global position as a major port, and Osaka intends to be a global business center. The Kansai region appears as one agglomeration composed of various types of local cohesion.

The Kansai agglomeration was rapidly growing during the 1960s. The expansion had already settled down by the 1980s, even though housing developments and land use conversions have continued since then. The five-year census indicates the DID (Densely Inhabited District), which is an urbanized district with 4000 or more inhabitants per square kilometer that forms an aggregate with adjacent districts of similar population density in a municipality of more than 5000 people. A recent assessment of the Kansai region's DIDs (Fig. 6.1) (Geospatial Information Authority of Japan, n.d.) showed that urban expansion has been limited by geographical conditions, which is a typical feature of the area. The urbanization after the economic growth of the 1960s has never been well controlled. A comparison between the built-up area of 1976 and 2016, expressed with the Fringe Index,[1] presents evidence of the continuous expansion in the region brought on by developments at the urban periphery (Fig. 6.2). On the other hand, the area of DIDs has been rather stable

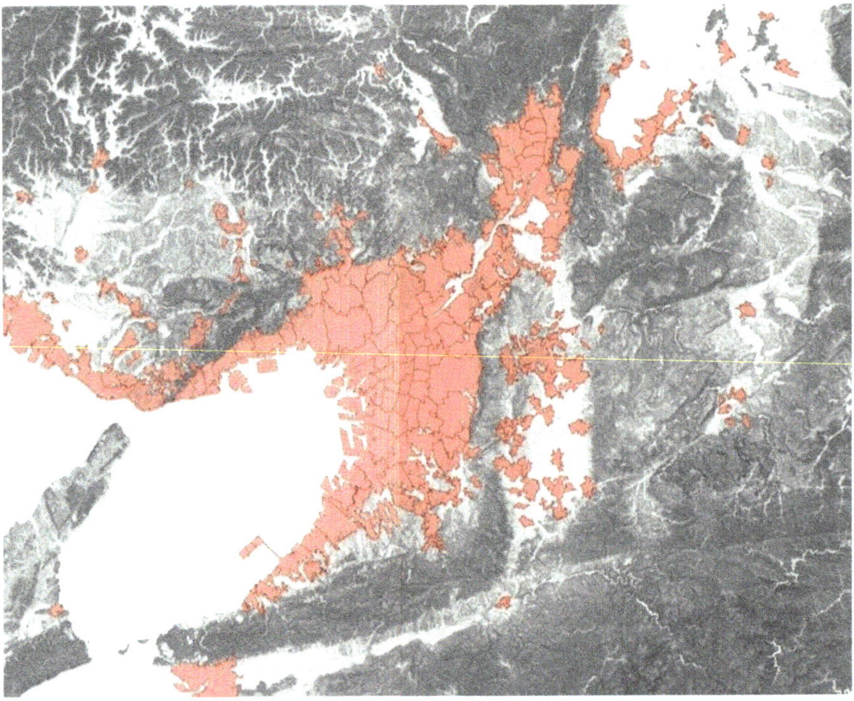

Fig. 6.1 DID of Kansai Region in 2015

[1] Fringe index: Fringe Index indicated by the range of 1-0 is calculated by the land-use data of 100m mesh provided by MLIT. It is the average numberof land-use index of 100m mesh in the radius of a 1km area. The land use Index is calculated by "0" for the mesh of built-up land and "1" for the mesh of forestry and farming land. In the figure, white is "1," dark grey is "0."

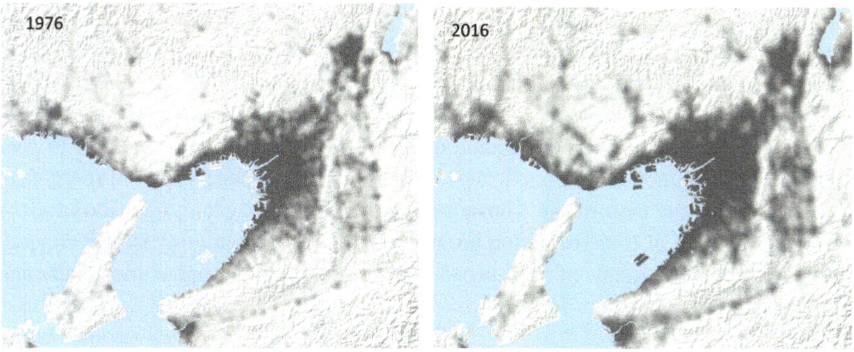

Fig. 6.2 Urban fringe land use of 1976 (left) and urban fringe land use of 2016 (right)

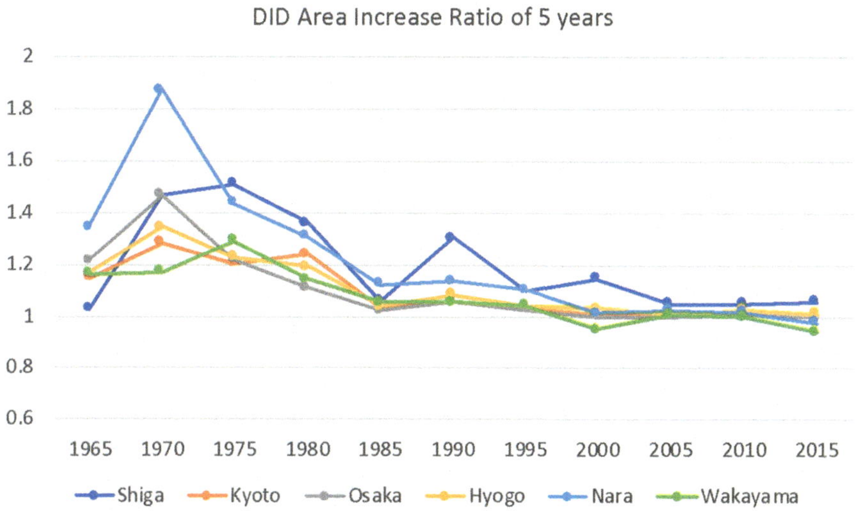

Fig. 6.3 DID area increase ratio of five years (prefectures in Kansai Region)

(Fig. 6.3)[2] during the last 20 years. In fact, the population of the area has decreased since 2005 (Union of Kansai Governments, 2021), which means that the inhabitants have been scattered across the newly developed area, decreasing the density.

The Kansai region is now entering a shrinking phase. Thus, priority issues related to the city region transformation should be the revitalization of the urban center and the reorganization of the suburban land use to sustain efficient public services under a tight budget. Smart measures for shutting downtowns and villages are becoming a realistic discussion. In this shrinking phase, the Kansai region has some advantages due to its polycentric feature and wide range of unique local cohesions generated by history and geography, which provide various alternatives for life in the future.

---

[2] The difference of DID area is calculated based on the Census data.

This unique local cohesion undoubtedly works as an advantage, yet, at the same time, its autonomy makes coordinating collaborative efforts difficult. Due to the recent decentralization of the planning authority, municipalities have the responsibility for planning decisions. The "Compact Plus Network" policy sets up a legal framework for this through the Location Optimization Plan (2014)[3] in order to concentrate urban function and residential land use in the planned area and reorganize urban form. In the case of the Kansai region, collaborative planning efforts for the regional concept of transformation are urgently needed. Such efforts must concentrate on the developments of rural-urban relations, including urban compactness and a networked structure.

Potential of Smart Sustainability Management in Kobe

Kobe, one of the three major cities in the Kansai region, is a port town developed in the modern age that has been gradually losing its position as a global center as a port. The future establishment of a diverse business field and the revitalization of the urban center are significant urban issues for the city. The investment in medical technology and its related innovative services is one attempt in the process of restructuring the port yard with infill development. Recently, the city's government has concentrated on the city center's redevelopment to create a more legible mobility hub, with livable public spaces. At the same time, there is a need to cope with the smart shrinking in the new towns filled with housing complexes and the countryside behind the Rokko mountains.

Owing to Kobe's geographical position, urbanization is limited to a narrow strip between the inland sea and the Rokko mountains. Thus, new towns and housing developments were located behind the mountains, where they coexisted with farmland and the natural environment. However, the ratio of senior citizens in those housing complexes is getting higher, while at the same time the number of vacant houses that cannot be inherited by the next generation is growing. This situation has prompted a discussion about restructuring, including the shrinkage of housing.

On the other hand, it has been observed that migration to the countryside by citizens who take advantage of its proximity to the city center for work, has already taken place. These citizens have the opportunity to be simultaneously engaged in a new farming business while doing teleworking, so doubling their income by combining farming with another type of revenue. This movement is often accompanied by some social conflicts between the new migrants and old inhabitants, which could be solved by mutual efforts to understand the lifestyles of others and their involvement in the community.

---

[3]The Plan is framed in the Urban Renaissance Special Measures Law (2002) that is legally requested to be reviewed and revised within 10 years. The Plan was set up in the amendment of this Special Measures Law of 2014 (https://www.mlit.go.jp/en/toshi/city_plan/compactcity_network.html).

The migrants' lifestyle is compatible with the alternative working style related to the COVID-19 crisis. Such migration is expected to increase in the process of Kansai's regional transformation and could provide a base for the concept of a compact city and network, with a balanced and efficient distribution of population and functions creating the diversity of rural-urban relations. The younger generation is becoming aware that the closeness of the urban center has the potential to support life in the countryside and commuting to work. On the other hand, the large consumption market supports the challenges of new agricultural businesses. This consciousness, experienced through the recent COVID-19 crisis, will affect the movement of migration.

Urban Transformation Evolved with COVID-19 Experience

Transformation Scheme for Smart Shrinkage

In the legal framework of Japan, the Location Optimization Plan (2014) was implemented for location control of residential development and urban functions to promote urban transformation towards a compact and networked region. 399 municipalities have already decided their own plans in order to obtain the necessary subsidy provided by MLIT for the implementation of the local projects. The plan's aim of transformation with strict land-use control should clearly be about sustainable development. However, it is extremely difficult to decide on a plan when considering the right of occupation and land ownership. Thus, the plan is often a result of compromise rather than an ambitious restructuring concept. Nevertheless, the implications of the three significant processes discussed above, prompted by the COVID-19 crisis, are expected to give impulse to a more favorable practice for local restructuring.

According to the White Paper of MLIT (MLIT, 2017a), 1/4 of the citizens in their 20s are interested in migrating to rural areas to start farming or other small businesses and practice slow living. Such a tendency might have been promoted by recent experiences. Meanwhile, whilst we stayed at home trying to find a convenient daily lifestyle, we came to pay more attention to the value of living in an environment found in a walkable neighborhood, with several alternatives for working styles and mobility. Living locally will be the basic unit of local cohesion and this concept is compatible with both the urban and rural domains.

The legal actions needed to support the coexistence of urban-rural living and farming have already started. The "Countryside Residential Zone" was set up as a new category of land-use zoning in 2017. The re-evaluation of the urban farmland, in the context of the urban planning framework, was initiated with the approval of other management bodies besides farmers. These actions prepared the way for the promotion of urban farmland revitalization as a valuable green open space as well as the residential potential of the countryside. Yet, even though the planning framework is set up, it is still not easy to encourage the advancement of urban alterations.

Migration becomes more of a selectable alternative. The experiences of teleworking and the enhanced consciousness of a local daily life environment will lead people to prefer to live in a lower density area. The fluidity of relocation movements is a favorable sign for the advancement of transformation with the reorganization of urban functions, where the local neighborhood is a comfortable and unique unit. The transformation of the city's regions should, in fact, be an interactive process between a regional framework and local initiatives with strategic management of developments for a sustainable region with local identification. In this way, local diversity will improve regional resilience.

Urban Resilience

Resilient cities are defined in the OECD (Organization for Economic Co-operation and Development) report of 2017 (OECD, 2016) as cities that have the ability to absorb, recover and prepare for future shocks and stresses to ensure sustainable development, well-being, and inclusive growth. Having an adaptive, robust, redundant, flexible, resourceful, inclusive, and integrated urban system is an essential feature of resilience. The transformation for smart shrinkage demanded in Japan is expected to improve resilience in both rural and urban domains.

From the viewpoint of promoting urban transformation, the experiences in coping with the COVID-19 crisis have significant implications. Among them: (1) A teleworking and/or remote office working style that might change office locations and residential preferences; (2) An increased interest in the neighborhood unit, with a daily market and other shared places that arc essential for living; and (3) An intimate natural environment and daily use of open space that is recognized for enhancing both mental and physical conditions of life. These are all significant factors for the future of urban planning. All of them are related to the evolution of urban transformation involving the rural domain, and at the same time, might work as a driving force in reorganizing urban centers to an appropriate accumulation of functions and density.

We should make the most of the opportunities brought about by the changes which have emerged since the crisis, such as working style diversification, concerns about autonomous neighborhoods, and the optimization of urban spatial values. Each of these advances local diversity, autonomy, and redundancy, to build up the capacity to enhance urban resilience. Cities are perceiving the recovery process from the crisis as a good opportunity for transformation towards more sustainable and resilient societies.

The following statement by Kristiaan Borret[4] is also meaningful when we proceed towards the planning of urban transformation: "Slow urbanism takes the time to do things properly. It proceeds from the local context, incorporates time and variation in a natural way, and considers change during the process, not as a problem but welcomes it. In the end, slow urbanism produces a more organic, more authentic, and therefore more culturally sustainable city." Even though transformation is an urgent planning issue, its inclusive process should be a priority.

References

Geospatial Information Authority of Japan. (2021, June). *GSI Maps (Electronic Land Web)*. http://maps.gsi.go.jp/#10/34.727505/135.596695/&base=std&ls=std%7Cdid2015&blend=0&disp=11&vs=c1j0h0k0l0u0t0z0r0s0m0f0&d=m. Accessed July 2020.

Japanese Ministry of Justice. (2009, June). *Japanese City Planning Act enacted June 15, 1968 (English translation)*. http://www.japaneselawtranslation.go.jp/law/detail/?id=1923&vm=&re=. Accessed June 2020.

Ministry on Land, Infrastructure, Transport, and Tourism of Japan [MLIT]. (2007). *Urban Land Use Planning System in Japan*. https://www.google.com/search?q=Urban+Land+Use+Planning+System+in+Japan&client=firefox-b-d&ei=x6XGYMCBH4WosgXQup6ADw&oq=Urban+Land+Use+Planning+System+in+Japan&gs_lcp=Cgdnd3Mtd2l6EAMyBAgAEBM6BwgAEEcQsANQzLQWWMy0FmCKvBZoAXACeACAAagBiAG1ApIBAzA-uMpgBAKABAqABAaoBB2d3cy13aXrIAQfAAQE&sclient=gws-wiz&ved=0ahUKEwi-Agd748ZXxAhUFlKwKHVCdB_AQ4dUDCA0&uact=5#. Accessed Aug 2020.

MLIT. (2014). *Grand Design of National Spatial Development towards 2050, Japan*. https://www.google.com/url?sa=t&rct=j&q=&esrc=s&source=web&cd=&ved=2ahUKEwj-i%2D%2DY8JXxAhVEIKwKHc4xCIYQFjAAegQIAhAD&url=https%3A%2F%2Fwww.mlit.go.jp%2Fcommon%2F001088248.pdf&usg=AOvVaw18ZPQV0haEaIVsH2Sz6JdR. Accessed Aug 2020.

MLIT. (2017a). *2017 White Paper on Land, Infrastructure, Transport and Tourism*. https://www.mlit.go.jp/hakusyo/mlit/h29/hakusho/h30/pdfindex.html. Accessed Aug 2020.

MLIT. (2017b). *Report of the Urban Planning Committee*. https://www.mlit.go.jp/common/001197384.pdf. Accessed Aug 2020.

MLIT (2018). *Report on Case Studies of Special Measures for the Vacant Land Issue*. https://www.mlit.go.jp/common/001258292.pdf. Accessed July 2020.

MLIT. (2020). *Town Development Triggered by the New Corona Crisis (translated by the author from the original Japanese title: 新型コロナ危機を契機としたまちづくり)*. https://www.mlit.go.jp/toshi/machi/covid-19.html. Accessed Mar 2021.

Organization for Economic Co-operation and Development. (2016). *Resilient Cities – Policy Highlights*. https://www.mlit.go.jp/common/001136418.pdf. Accessed June 2020.

[4] Kristiaan Borret was bouwmeester of the City of Antwerp From 2006 to 2014. Since 2017, he is the Supervisor of Oostenburg for the City of Amsterdam (Netherlands). The statement quoted in the chapter is taken from the proceedings of the International Conference "POLYCENTRIC CITY REGIONS IN TRANSFORMATION" in 2015.

Statistics Bureau of Japan. (2016). *Statistics Today No.115: 2015 Census, Short Review of Population Decline*. https://www.stat.go.jp/info/today/115.html. Accessed Aug 2020.
Union of Kansai Governments. (2021). *Kansai Data*. https://www.kouiki-kansai.jp/koikirengo/koikirengo/kansaidata/index.html. Accessed Mar 2021.
United Nations. (2018). *Revision of World Urbanization Prospects*. Department of Economic and Social Affairs. https://esa.un.org/unpd/wup/. Accessed Mar 2021.

Part II
Responses

Chapter 7
"The Great Equalizer"? The Long-Term Effects of the COVID-19 Pandemic on Poverty, Inequality, and the 2030 Agenda in Latin America

Ana Luíza Matos de Oliveira and Ana Paula Emídio

Introduction

As the COVID-19 pandemic erupted, some argued that it would have an equalizing effect, as all were seen as equally vulnerable to this disease. However, as the pandemic transitioned to the global south, especially to Latin America (LA), inequalities have been highlighted. The poorer and the non-white population in LA are suffering the most from the virus and COVID-19 has taken an obvious toll, both in health and in socioeconomic terms, on those who were already vulnerable all around the region. It also widens various gaps and inequalities in the long run, in this already very unequal part of the world.

There is no conventional or easy way of dealing with the COVID-19 crisis, especially when considering it is not simply a complex temporary reality. Cities might have to deal with the virus for a long time, and the impacts of the virus in the short term might influence trajectories for a longer period of time. Our objective in this chapter is to discuss the long-term effects of the COVID-19 pandemic on poverty, inequality, and sustainable development in LA, with a special focus on cities. This is a difficult task as the COVID-19 crisis is still unfolding. However, this debate needs addressing, as the pandemic will pose further challenges to public policy to which academics and policy makers need to adjust. In the long term, what are the expected impacts of the COVID-19 pandemic on poverty and inequality in LA? Could this be an opportunity for the region to reflect on a social policy reform to truly assist the vulnerable and reduce inequalities?

A. L. M. de Oliveira (✉)
FLACSO, São Paulo, Brazil

A. P. Emídio
Universidade Federal de Minas Gerais, Belo Horizonte, Brazil

© The Author(s), under exclusive license to Springer Nature Switzerland AG 2021
M. A. Montoya et al. (eds.), *COVID-19 and Cities*, The Urban Book Series,
https://doi.org/10.1007/978-3-030-84134-8_7

The chapter begins with a section on the Social Development Goals (SDGs) for LA before the pandemic, especially those connected to inequality and poverty. The third section discusses preliminary data on how the pandemic of COVID-19 impacted LA in the short term, followed by the fourth section on its long-term social impacts on LA. Focus will be given in this section to poverty and inequality. Finally, the fifth section discusses the challenges faced by the region to reach 2030 targets amid the new scenario.

The 2030 Agenda and the Indicators for Latin America Before the Pandemic

In 2015, the international community adopted the 2030 Agenda (with goals to be reached by 2030), which consists of 17 Sustainable Development Goals (SDGs) and 169 targets which detail these goals. The 2030 Agenda is a global effort to seek sustainable development and builds on years of work from the international community and the expertise of the eight Millennium Development Goals for the year 2015 (United Nations [UN], 2015).

The 17 SDGs are: (1) No Poverty; (2) Zero Hunger; (3) Good Health and Well-being; (4) Quality Education; (5) Gender Equality; (6) Clean Water and Sanitation; (7) Affordable and Clean Energy; (8) Decent Work and Economic Growth; (9) Industry, Innovation, and Infrastructure; (10) Reduced Inequality; (11) Sustainable Cities and Communities; (12) Responsible Consumption and Production; (13) Climate Action; (14) Life Below Water; (15) Life on Land; (16) Peace and Justice Strong Institutions; and (17) Partnerships to achieve the Goal. This framework was built considering poverty and inequality as transversal and multidimensional issues (Oliveira, 2019) present in all targets, although both issues have specific goals, SDG 1 for poverty and SDG 10 for inequality. However, the United Nations Conference on Trade and Development [UNCTAD] (2020b) argues that the inclusion of inequality in the 2030 Agenda was quite broad and that "none of the 10 targets actually address economic, income or wealth inequality directly" (UNCTAD, 2020b, 141–2). SDG 11 is also of relevance to our analysis.

LA had an active role in pushing for this agenda in the UN. However, just before the pandemic, Latin America and the Caribbean (LAC) were not on a good track. The Economic Commission for Latin America and the Caribbean [ECLAC] (2020b) shows that more than 70% of the SDGs targets analyzed (which were 72) for the region show that a public policy intervention is required to reach the SDGs by 2030. The evaluation was carried out in May 2020 with data prior to the pandemic.[1] Of the 72 targets analyzed: only 4 had been met (relating to SDGs 3 and 14); 15 could be reached following the trend at the time (relating to SGDs 1, 3, 4, 6, 7, 8, 9, 15, and

[1] A complete assessment of SDGs for each country in LA is available at https://agenda2030lac.org/estadisticas/datos-indicadores.html

17); 8 could be reached only with public policy intervention (relating to SDGs 1, 2, 4, 5, 8, and 15); 13 could be reached only with a high degree of public policy intervention (relating to SDGs 1, 2, 3, 4, 5, 8, and 11); 27 were stagnant (relating to SDGs 1, 2, 3, 4, 5, 6, 7, 8, 9, 10, 12, 14, 16, and 17); and 5 were in reversal (relating to SDGs 2, 9, 13, 15, and 17) (see categories in Fig. 7.1).

Regarding specific SDGs of interest for this chapter (1, 10, and 11), according to ECLAC (2020b): of the 4 targets met in LA, none relate to SDG 1, 10, and 11; of the 15 targets which could be reached following the trend at the time, 2 relate to SDG 1 (extreme poverty by international standards and total poverty by international standards); of the 8 targets which could be reached only with public policy intervention, 1 relates to SDG 1 (working poor in extreme poverty by international standards); of the 13 targets which could be reached only with a high degree of public policy intervention, 2 relate to SDG 1 (extreme regional poverty and working poor in extreme poverty by regional standards) and 1 relates to SDG 11 (the proportion of urban population living in marginal neighborhoods, informal settlements, or inadequate housing); of the 27 stagnant targets, 2 relate to SDG 1 (coverage of social protection programs and public expenditure in education) and 1 relates to SDG 10 (inequality by the participation of wages in GDP); and of the 5 targets in reverse, none relate to SDG 1, 10, or 11.

In June 2020, the SDG Index 2019 for LAC (Centro de los Objetivos de Desarrollo Sostenible para América Latina y el Caribe [CODS], 2020) was released, also with data prior to COVID-19. In this report, SDG 11 stands out as the second highest average score in the subregion (equivalent to 81.8), having advanced 1.1% in

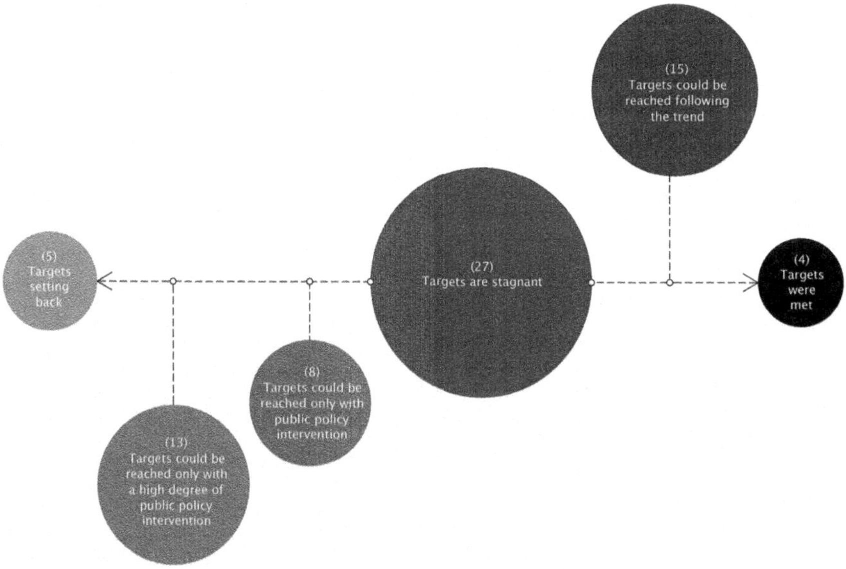

Fig. 7.1 ECLAC's assessment of the 2030 Agenda targets in Latin America prior to COVID-19. (Source: Authors' own elaboration from ECLAC 2020b)

comparison to the same score assessed in 2015 (80.91). However, 12 countries in the region (Argentina, Bolivia, Brazil, Colombia, Costa Rica, Guatemala, Guyana, Honduras, Jamaica, Nicaragua, Peru, and Uruguay) experienced only a moderate advancement toward the goal, still being below what is necessary to achieve it. None of the countries analyzed showed a setback in their evolution, but five countries (Dominican Republic, Haiti, Suriname, Trinidad & Tobago, and Venezuela) were still stagnant regarding this SDG and only seven (Belize, Chile, Ecuador, El Salvador, Mexico, Panama, and Paraguay) met the required progress to achieve the targets defined by SDG 11 in 2030. However, nine countries (Barbados, Cuba, Saint Lucia, Bahamas, Saint Vincent & the Grenadines, Granada, Antigua & Barbuda, Dominica, and Saint Kitts & Nevis) did not have the minimum 80% of the indicators required to be included in the analysis.

Therefore, LAC were in a dire situation regarding the 2030 Agenda, even before the pandemic. The CODS (2020) argues that, following the historic trend, the SDG goals will not be achieved in LA even in the next 50 years. ECLAC (2020b) also argues that the comprehensiveness of the 2030 Agenda was already at risk: "The world that existed when the 2030 Agenda was approved in 2015, today seems far away" (ECLAC, 2020b, p. 53, own translation). COVID-19 reinforces, then, the need for urgent action to guarantee the SDG's resilience to handle the most extreme and intense disruptions caused by the pandemic. There are many unforeseen needs being triggered that limit the chances of citizens' surviving, which brings the vulnerability of the targets set to light. Reframing the resilience of those referred targets will be mandatory to prevent the increase of the lags in the achievement of the goals and the setback of those in which the region was on the right track.

How the COVID-19 Pandemic Impacted Latin America

Prior to the outbreak of the pandemic, ECLAC (2020a) estimated that the LAC's Gross Domestic Product (GDP) would grow by a maximum of 1.3% in 2020. When COVID-19 hit, estimates for growth became much more pessimistic. ECLAC (2020b) first projected the region's GDP to decline by 5.3% in 2020, and then, ECLAC (2020d) revised estimates to 9.1% in 2020, consolidating a new "lost decade." The reduction in economic activity would lead the GDP per capita in LAC to the same level observed in 2010 (ECLAC, 2020d).

The disturbance in economic activity in 2020 in LA occurred first as a reflection of the pandemic abroad (especially in China and Europe), and then with the disruption of economic activity in the region itself due to the arrival of the virus. The region is expected to grow at a slower pace than the global north, increasing the gap between these realities (ECLAC, 2020c; International Monetary Fund [IMF], 2020).

According to ECLAC (2020d), the value of regional exports could have fallen 23% in 2020. Another issue is remittances; in the main economies which generate remittances for LA, such as the USA and Europe, unemployment has risen. In Haiti, for instance, remittances represent 33% of the GDP. In El Salvador and Honduras,

20%. Tourism also fell by 44% in the first 4 months of 2020, hitting Central America and the Caribbean (ECLAC, 2020d; Haywood, 2020).

The services sector, which is very prominent in LA, was strongly hit. The informal sector, which comprises 53.1% of the total workforce in LAC (International Labor Office [ILO], 2018a), was also very affected, leaving those in this sector with lower schooling levels and income stranded. Social protection programs have not been able to maintain the constant income of workers, especially those in the informal sector. This dynamic has an obvious impact in the short term, but it impacts workers' trajectories in the long run too. How workers are able to overcome this period matters.

ECLAC (2020c) estimates that 2.7 million companies will go bankrupt due to the crisis, with a greater impact on small and medium businesses. Furthermore, ECLAC (2020d) estimates unemployment rates to be around 13.5% by the end of 2020 in LA, 5.4 p.p. over the value of 2019. Thus, the number of unemployed would reach 44.1 million people, 18 million more than in 2019. For those working, working from home was not a possibility for everyone due to differences in economic sectors/occupations or due to poor Internet access (ECLAC, 2020a, e; Instituto de Estudos para o Desenvolvimento Industrial [IEDI], 2020; ILO, 2020b).

Urban populations in LA (the most urbanized region on the planet) were particularly hit by the virus. About 81% of the population in LAC live in urban areas (UN, 2019), facing various vulnerabilities regarding work, housing, sanitation, and health. As countries all around the region struggled with the challenge of social distancing, the pandemic exposed the underfinancing of social infrastructure in urban areas, as well as the interrelations between poverty, informality, and inequality (Corburn et al., 2020). Those living in the outskirts of large cities faced the impossibility of social distancing due to overcrowded housing conditions, while the lack of sanitation made it difficult to maintain the hygiene standards necessary to fight the spread of the virus. The flaws in the availability and access to accurate information about the use of masks and other forms of prevention as well as the official discourse on hydroxychloroquine as an alleged cure for COVID-19 in the case of Brazil (Palmeira et al., 2020), plus, the high dependence on the informal sector, made incomes highly volatile in this time of crisis. All over LA, preexisting urban inequalities and vulnerabilities have shaped the spread of COVID-19. In São Paulo, neighborhoods where public transportation trips originated during the pandemic (meaning, those which kept traveling to work by public transportation) presented a higher number of hospital admissions with COVID-19 (Stern, 2020); the risks of dying from COVID-19 in the city being 50% higher in areas of lower socioeconomic status (Toledo, 2020). In Mexico City, the weight of population density fueled transmissions, while in Bogotá, the economic divide between the Northeast of the city (a poorer area) and the rest reflects itself in the spread of the disease. In Buenos Aires, the divide between the North and the more vulnerable South shaped contagion and the attention each area received from authorities (Galindo & Arroyo, 2020). Meanwhile, in Santiago, tense protests and lootings of those starving in the poorest areas occurred (Clarín, 2020). Therefore, it is evident that the most vulnerable were largely hit. For example, indicators suggest that seven out of ten people who died from the coronavirus in Mexico were people with primary education and no formal work (Hernández, 2020). At the same time, Brazil is "rejuvenating" the profile of the deceased by COVID-19 (Azevedo, 2020).

The Sustainable Development Report 2020 (Sachs et al., 2020), which includes the COVID-19 crisis, classifies the pandemic as having a "mixed or moderately negative short-term impact" on SDG 11 due to the reduction in pollution levels observed in urban areas all over the world since the start of lockdown. However, this perception can be considered widely optimistic as stimuli to economic recovery are not necessarily considering the climate emergency (UN, 2020). In fact, SDG 11 will be one of the most affected goals right away as over 90% of the reported COVID-19 cases worldwide are in urban areas (UN, 2020) and LAC will need to recalibrate urban planning and urban development, infrastructure, and services, so as not to allow SDG 11 to become irreparably out of reach in the long run. Notwithstanding, the complex conditions of urbanization all over LA make it challenging to offer territorial responses to the pandemic. Simplified readings of the cities, a disregard for their heterogeneity, and the lack of accurate data compromise the need for a deep and multidisciplinary strategy on promoting assertive ways to mitigate the negative urban impacts of the pandemic (Rolnik et al., 2020). Only the adequate handling of data and information is capable of articulating urban resilience in a quantifiable, evidence-based, and accessible way. From this, it will be possible to predict and better enable urban communities to survive and thrive despite the multiple shocks and stresses caused by the pandemic (Rockefeller Foundation, 2013).

Filling data gaps on COVID-19 issues will then be critical, not only to more deeply understand and manage the effects of the crisis, but also to design both short- and long-term solutions to each urban context.

Long-Term Social Impacts of the Pandemic in Latin America: Poverty and Inequality in the Urban Context

Long-term impacts of the pandemic are to be expected and create challenges for social policy in the region. ECLAC (2020b) argues that COVID-19 is pushing the SDGs beyond reach. The UNCTAD (2020a) argues that poverty, inequality, the climate crisis, unsustainable production, and other pressing challenges require even more urgent action in developing countries due to COVID-19. Meanwhile, the International Labour Organization (ILO) and United Nations Children's Fund (UNICEF) argue that the pandemic will increase poverty and inequality in LA, risking the fulfillment of many indicators of the 2030 Agenda for sustainable development (ILO, 2020b; ILO & UNICEF, 2020).

Poverty and extreme poverty have been on the rise in the region since 2015 (ECLAC, 2020b). Estimations at the beginning of the year showed that poverty in LA was to increase in 2020 to up to 35.8% and extreme poverty to up to 14.2% (ECLAC, 2020b), making it almost impossible to reach the 2030 Agenda target of reducing extreme poverty to 3% of the population by 2030. If the region's GDP grew 5% from 2021 to 2030 and the Gini Index fell by 1.5% a year, extreme poverty rates in the region would reach 5.7%. Therefore, it would take a very impressive effort to reach almost double the target. However, new estimations paint a grimmer picture: according to ECLAC (2020d), the number of people in poverty in the region could grow from 185.5 million to 230.9 million in 2020 (from 30.2% of the population in 2019 to 37.3% in 2020); and extreme poverty could increase from 67.7 million in 2019 to 96.2 million in 2020 (from 11.0% of the population in 2019 to 15.5% in 2020). According to these estimations, the highest increase in poverty is projected to happen in Argentina, Brazil, Ecuador, Mexico, and Peru, while the highest increase in extreme poverty is concentrated in Brazil, Colombia, Ecuador, El Salvador, and Nicaragua. These new projections add to the difficulties in reaching the SDGs.

According to Food and Agriculture Organization of the United Nations [FAO], International Fund for Agricultural Development [IFAD], UNICEF, World Food Programme [WFP], and World Health Organization [WHO] (2020), the number of undernourished people in LAC was already growing before COVID-19 (from 38.8 million in 2015 to 47.7 million in 2017), putting the region in a worse shape than it was when it agreed to the 2030 Agenda in 2015. However, projections from these institutions show an increase to 66.9 million undernourished people in the region by 2030, a projection which does not take into account the impacts of the COVID-19 crisis. In LA, warning signs come from Venezuela (considered an extreme hunger hotspot) and Brazil (considered an emerging hotspot) (Oxfam, 2020a).

Gender and racial inequalities are also stressed under COVID-19. The sexual division of labor structurally places women as responsible for domestic work and has significant implications for the place of women in the labor market. It is one of the factors pushing women into part-time jobs, informality, and hindering promotions (Gibb & Oliveira, 2015). With the disruption of the social apparatus for social reproduction, such as schools, daycare centers, etc., and with the increase in domestic work during the pandemic, households were forced into a new configuration. Women, who already have the burden of being responsible for domestic/care work, might suffer from an extra overload during the pandemic, widening gender gaps and having long-term effects on the place of women in the labor market. Another gender-related issue regarding the pandemic, which has long-lasting effects, is the increase in domestic violence under social distancing or lockdown (Oliveira et al., 2020).

Racial inequalities might also increase as black and indigenous individuals suffer from more social and economic vulnerability than the white population in LA (Alloatti & Oliveira, 2021). Due to intersectionality[2] (Hirata, 2014), the situation of black and indigenous women is even more dire. Migrants, people with disabilities,

[2] The effects of intersectionality (understood as the multiple interacting influences of social location, identity, and historical oppression) in inequalities and health are not a new phenomenon to science (Kapilashrami et al., 2015). These pose challenges for researchers as different axes of inequality cannot be analyzed in isolation from one another, but a structural approach must be pursued. To understand health inequalities, Gkiouleka et al. (2018) suggest an integrative analytical framework that accounts for the complexity of the intertwined influence of both individual social positioning and institutional stratification on health. According to the authors, intersectionality provides a strong analytical tool for an integrated understanding of health inequalities by addressing the multiple layers of privilege and disadvantage, such as race, migration/ethnicity, and gender/sexuality.

the elderly, the homeless, people in rural areas, among others, are more vulnerable. Disarray in the labor market and in education can also have a generational impact, scarring the trajectories of children and youth, and increasing inequalities. The United Nations Educational, Scientific and Cultural Organization (UNESCO) and ECLAC (2020) argue that access to technology in LA is scarce and unequal, yet it is even more important now in order to access education during the pandemic. In this sense, if no measures are taken, educational inequalities might increase, influencing students' trajectories in the long term (ECLAC, 2020e). ECLAC (2020a) also adds that around 85 million children in LA receive at least one meal a day in school. Schools also allow for parents to work. If they are not opened, mothers might be particularly overburdened due to the sexual division of labor. Furthermore, as families are pushed into poverty and schools are closed, more children might be forced into child labor (ILO & UNICEF, 2020), scarring their trajectories for life. Girls are particularly at risk.

Another issue is the youth entering the labor market, which will be an even harder situation (ILO, 2020a; Zerega et al., 2020). Youth is a group which, structurally, faces greater vulnerability, lower wages, and higher unemployment. According to ILO and UNICEF (2020), 328 million young workers (or 77% of youth worldwide) were in informal work, while for older workers, this rate is 60%. During the COVID-19 crisis, ILO and UNICEF (2020) estimate that 17.1% of workers aged 18–29 have stopped working (the "generation lockdown"). For young workers in low-income countries, this rate is 19.1%.

As a result of the various processes brought by the pandemic, ECLAC (2020d) estimates that the Gini Index might grow between 5% and 5.9% in Brazil, Chile, El Salvador, and Mexico, and over 6.0% in Argentina, Ecuador, and Peru. The Gini Index is estimated to increase between 1% and 8% in the 17 countries analyzed. Therefore, inequality is one of the defining traits of the region and is set to worsen. In this period of crisis, those with savings, support, and social capital are in a better position to move forward.

The various preexisting vulnerabilities for specific groups interact during the pandemic, combining health and socioeconomic conditions, so creating and enhancing various inequalities (Fig. 7.2). From an intersectional perspective, in the case of COVID-19, due to environmental racism, which exposes the indigenous and black population to pollution and a lack of sanitation (Behre, 2020), preexisting conditions were generated, making this population more vulnerable to the disease (or to a more serious form of it) and affecting choices regarding exposure to the virus and obtaining income. This intersection of vulnerabilities is likely to have a long-term impact. Another example of an intersection of vulnerabilities is how a precarious access to social rights, such as education, derived from an unequal system based on the region's colonial heritage, can generate a reality in which some children had access to Internet and remote schooling during the pandemic, while others faced an interruption in the formal learning process.

The pandemic has highlighted an ongoing and deep crisis in the city models predominant in LAC that are now proven to not only be unable to preserve and

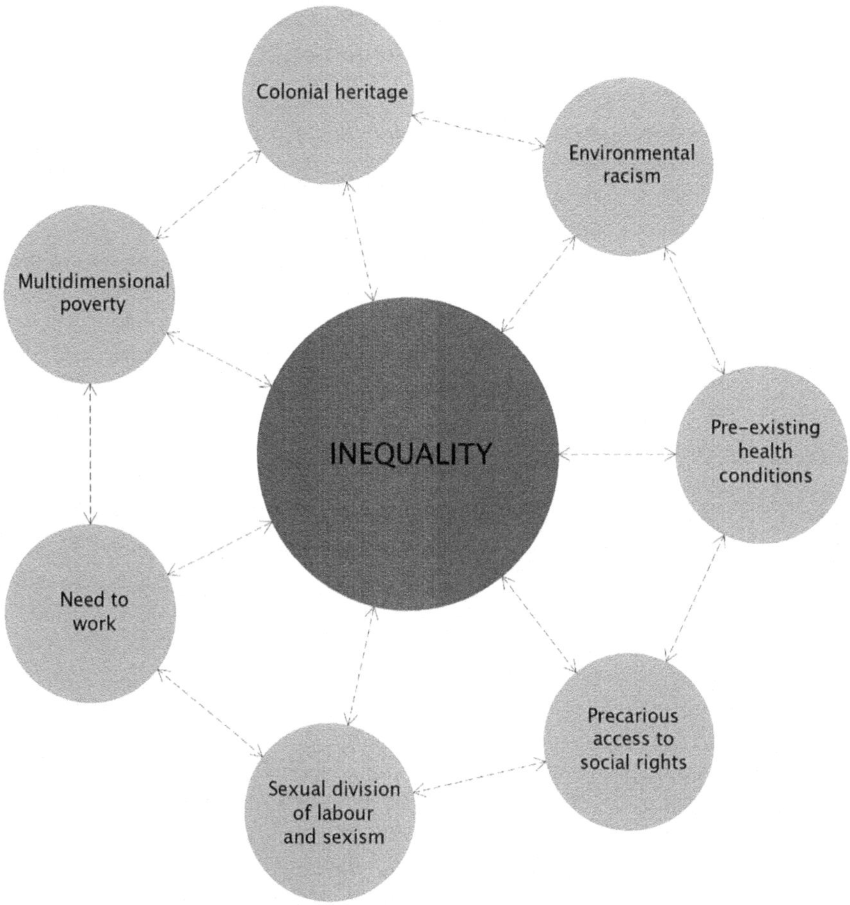

Fig. 7.2 The intersections of vulnerabilities and the negative long-term social impacts of the COVID-19 pandemic in Latin America. (Source: Authors' own elaboration)

protect life during a health emergency, but also systematically expose people to the toxicity of disorderly growth and the idea of profit at any cost (Escola da Cidade, 2020). Neoliberal urban policies have consistently generated segregated and fragmented cities in the region (Carrión & Dammert-Guardia, 2019), perpetuating social and spatial inequalities previously settled. In Latin American cities, basic urban public policies, such as housing, mobility, and sanitation, were turned into profitable goods (Maricato, 2015). This generates conflicts and sparks tensions that can no longer be overlooked, and makes it particularly challenging for LA to plan cities in ways that prioritize the needs of the majority of the population rather than the economy and the elite's petty interests.

Challenges Faced by the Region to Reach 2030 Targets Amid the New Situation: Avoiding a "K" Shaped Recovery

COVID-19 has raised the issue of the need to protect the most vulnerable. The crisis challenges the limitations of social protection programs, and the pandemic may set back many efforts in fighting vulnerability and fulfilling the 2030 Agenda. In our cities, it has become clear that inequalities in income, gender, and race, as well as poverty, are connected to a higher vulnerability to COVID-19 due to poor sanitation, housing, working conditions, and, for some, preexisting health conditions. In such a scenario, for poorer households and smaller enterprises in Latin America, with lower savings, it is more difficult to obtain credit.[3] Even the mayor of São Paulo, Bruno Covas, who does not usually raise issues of inequality, argued in an interview that COVID-19 has highlighted inequalities due to the virus being more lethal in the poorer outskirts of the metropolis (UOL, 2020).

One proposal which stands out in public debate now is to have a basic or universal income. This has been an issue for quite some time as productivity and automation threaten to lead to structural unemployment. Even before the pandemic, these societal changes led the ILO (2018b) to estimate that the unemployment rates in LA would rise from 12% in 2020 to 16% in 2030, 20% in 2040, and 25% in 2050. In this sense, progressive taxes were already needed to finance a basic or universal income. With the pandemic, this is an even more pressing issue.

In theory, the implementation of this measure is possible, as from 2018 to 2019, the number of millionaires in LA grew by 2.7% (Capgemini Research Institute, 2020), and during the pandemic, the wealth of billionaires also grew (Oxfam, 2020b). However, it has always been challenging in LA, a region known for the concentration of wealth and power, to increase progressive taxation.

Programs such as providing a basic or universal income can have an impact on state revenues in the short term as they possess a high multiplier effect: Neri et al. (2013) estimate, for the *Programa Bolsa Família* (a cash transfer program) in Brazil, a multiplier effect of 1.78. A basic income could have a similar positive impact on revenues and might avoid a recovery in a "K" shape, in which the richer get richer and the poorer get poorer. Additionally, in the long term, investing in the most vulnerable can have an impact on well-being, but, above all, investing in a stronger safety net for the most vulnerable, and not leaving aside the need to implement a comprehensive welfare system,[4] is a question of rights and social justice.

[3] Studies for the USA argue that high-income households have increased savings during the pandemic as expenditures for this group have dropped 17% compared to 4% for low-income households (Galiley, 2020). We are not yet aware of such studies for LA.

[4] Even before the pandemic, there was a growing need for public intervention to guarantee the 2030 Agenda. The pandemic increases the need for social expenditure in the future, not only in the present moment. For example, as ECLAC and OPS (2020) argue, during the pandemic, treatments for many chronic diseases were interrupted. Furthermore, some people infected by COVID-19 were left with side effects, which will have a future toll on health care systems, especially the public ones (Salehi et al., 2020).

In the case of Brazil, as the federal government's systematic denial of the seriousness of the COVID-19 crisis and its negative impacts unravels, it is clear that local-level initiatives can play a major role in economic revival. A good example of how basic income programs can offer an efficient response during prolonged times of emergency lies in Maricá, a municipality in the state of Rio de Janeiro, southeast of Brazil. With a consolidated basic income program since 2013, Maricá is arguably the most well-equipped city in Brazil, if not in LA, to manage the side effects of the pandemic, having experienced an increase of 15% in its tax collection during the months of April and May of 2020, while in the rest of the State, tax collection decreased by 30% (Betim, 2020). This was only possible thanks to the systematic payment of the so-called Basic Citizenship Income, a unique policy structured alongside the Community Bank and a currency called Mumbuca (Mumbuca 1 = Brazilian Real (R$) 1.00[5]), which can only be used within the city's limits, dynamizing the local economy and helping to create a thriving market (Ferreira & Katz, 2020). Back in 2019, the program reached its most ambitious height by paying the equivalent of R$130.00 to each of the city's 42,000 lowest-income residents. With a remarkably fast response, and contrary to the denial of Brazil's president, in March 2020, the city managed to quickly adapt its system to provide R$ 300.00/month to the poorest and the economically vulnerable (unemployed and informal workers) between the months of April and September (Silva et al., 2020).

Nonetheless, strategies to tackle the long-term effects of the pandemic must consider the environmental emergency. The dependence of our economic model on the depredation of the environment is not sustainable and can cause other pandemics. The Amazon, for example, hosts 3,200 types of coronaviruses and, as deforestation grows, they could be transmitted to humans (Pontes, 2020). On the other hand, Carrington (2020) argues that the cost of preventing a possible new pandemic due to the destruction of wildlife would be equal to 2% of the COVID-19 economic damage. In this sense, economic development toward a "better GDP," one that is not so predatory on the environment, is a question of survival.

Another set of strategies of interest refer to new urban planning actions to adjust cities to the reality of a pandemic. As cities work on adapting their urban designs and predefined zoning, the need for quality public spaces becomes clearer, as well as rethinking the location of urban services to provide safe and healthy access to essential facilities (Organisation for Economic Co-operation and Development [OECD], 2020). It is also possible to predict a trend in creating more hybrid spaces by diluting preestablished uses for zoning and establishing new building parameters, such as density capacity, natural ventilation norms, and flexible constructions, to ensure any kind of activity. LA's mainstream urban development model, which privileges cars and individual transportation, has a major challenge: if the need for social distancing continues, more pedestrianized spaces should be encouraged (Constable, 2020).

[5] As of August 20th, 2020, USD 1 equals R$ 5.61.

Even though creating more green spaces and promoting innovative guidelines for building designs are effective and, therefore, an essential approach, this does not necessarily represent an effort to make LA more inclusive; its cities can be very hostile for the most vulnerable. Urban planning in LA systematically considers the "formal city" (taken as "planned and civilized") first, leaving the "informal city" (taken as "erratic and marginalized"), where the marginalized are, stranded. This establishes a barrier to fully comprehend urban matters in LA and to formulate effective strategies to act on its territorial inequalities (Angotti, 2015). The access to quality spaces, both public and private, is still held by a privileged minority, which is likely to remain that way if the capital's influence keeps being the one and only force adjusting the new parameters of what living a safe life means in a pandemic and controlling who can afford to do so. It is mandatory that structural social thinking follows the new urban planning, so the attempts to mitigate the negative impacts of the pandemic in the cities do not become just another profitable product with the potential to worsen what was already problematic.

On a brighter note, good policies are being applied in influential Latin American cities, bringing to light some promising approaches to long-term planning that will not only enhance the resilience of its urban systems to recover from adversity, but also respond to it in a more considered way. The city of Medellín, in Colombia, is planning ahead by expanding its bike lanes by almost 50% and doubling the number of public transport lines in the next 3 years, while committing to electrifying all public transport by the end of the decade (World Economic Forum [WEF], 2020). Bogota is also working to promote a more sustainable city model, having added 35 km of lanes for cyclists during the quarantine and now planning, among other measures, to promote urban and peri-urban agriculture to make the city more livable and eco-friendly in the years to come (Medina, 2020). Mexico City, the second most crowded city in Latin America, is also setting the bar high by announcing an economic recovery plan that aims to cover urban infrastructure and social housing and is expected to develop 13 urban corridors through housing projects in areas with already good transport connections (Infobae, 2020).

The pandemic proved once more that the complexity of urban systems that perpetuate social inequalities goes far beyond specific individual and isolated elements. For there to be effective resilience strategies, such as the ones previously presented, that aim to guarantee truly viable solutions, it is necessary for them to be collaborative and integrated. When applied to the long-term situation, the pandemic is likely to deflagrate, so resilience actions should be seen as an evolutionary process in which it is possible to understand cities and communities, not as isolated study objects or neutral containers, but rather as complex and interconnected socio-spatial systems (Davoudi et al., 2012). Each city, alongside their respective entities, must address its own adjustments, ensuring more resilience through integrated flows and better optimization of its preexisting resources.

Final Remarks

Even though it might be comforting, or even necessary, to evolve resilience in order to handle the unpredictability regarding all the aspects of the COVID-19 pandemic, it is very important that we keep in sight that preserving what we had (Davoudi et al., 2012) might be pointless, since we are not talking about a temporary situation; the disruptions we are experiencing are most likely to remain as the norm.

The COVID-19 pandemic is no "equalizer." It is not only affecting economic variables per se, but also life trajectories. As Florida (2020) argues, the full impact of COVID-19 on our geography and our cities remains to be seen. However, it appears that the virus may reinforce some key faults in our existing economic and geographic divides.

The pandemic appeared in a context of vulnerability and inequality in LA, and amplifies social, economic, and sanitary vulnerabilities. It is a baseline change for sectors in LA. In the long term, inequalities might increase due to: poorer children who had no means to pursue distance learning, or might even have had to drop out of school in order to work; youth entering a labor market scarred by the lack of jobs due to the increase in domestic labor; and domestic violence which might increase gender inequalities in the long term; as well as many other forms of increase in racial, regional, and social inequalities.

Even before the pandemic, there was a growing need for public intervention to guarantee the 2030 Agenda. Now, new public policies will have to be designed to accommodate the new reality. Therefore, once the pandemic is under control, resuming a fiscal approach which does not consider the reality brought by the pandemic could worsen its negative long-lasting social impacts.

References

Alloatti, M., & Oliveira, A. (2021). Deepening and widening the gap: The impacts of Covid-19 pandemic on gender and racial inequalities in the labor market, domestic work and domestic violence in Brazil. Manuscript under preparation.

Angotti, T. (2015). América Latina urbana: violência, enclaves e luta pela terra [Urban Latin America: Violence, enclaves and the struggle for land]. *Margem esquerda – ensaios marxistas, 24*, 37–44.

Azevedo, A. L. (2020). O Brasil pode rejuvenescer a Covid-19 [Brazil can rejuvenate Covid-19]. *Jornal O Globo*. http://www.ensp.fiocruz.br/portal-ensp/informe/site/arquivos/anexos/d5382480b4c86924ea23a199865745c0ad0ef3c2.PDF. Accessed Nov 2020

Behre, A. A. (2020, July 9). The climate-change community desperately needs to address historic inequities. *Time*. https://time.com/5864693/climate-change-racism/. Accessed Nov 2020.

Betim, F. (2020, July 19). Maricá, no Rio, preserva empregos e negócios na pandemia e coloca a renda básica no centro do debate [Maricá, in Rio, preserves jobs and businesses in the pandemic and places basic income at the center of the debate]. *El País*. https://brasil.elpais.com/sociedade/2020-07-19/marica-no-rio-preserva-empregos-e-negocios-na-pandemia-e-coloca-a-renda-basica-no-centro-do-debate.html. Accessed Nov 2020.

Capgemini Research Institute. (2020). *World Wealth Report 2020*. https://worldwealthreport.com/wp-content/uploads/sites/7/2020/07/World-Wealth-Report-WWR-2020_Final_web.pdf. Accessed May 2021.

Carrington, D. (2020) Cost of preventing the next pandemic 'equal to just 2% of Covid-19 economic damage'. *The Guardian*. https://www.theguardian.com/world/2020/jul/23/preventing-next-pandemic-fraction-cost-covid-19-economic-fallout. Accessed Nov 2020.

Carrión, F., & Dammert-Guardia, M. (2019). *Derecho a la Ciudad: una evocación de las transformaciones urbanas en América Latina* [Right to the city: An evocation of urban transformations in Latin America]. IFEA, CLACSO, FLACSO.

Centro de los Objetivos de Desarrollo Sostenible para América Latina y el Caribe. (2020). *Índice ODS 2019 para América Latina y el Caribe* [2019 ODS Index for Latin America and the Caribbean]. https://cods.uniandes.edu.co/wp-content/uploads/2020/06/%C3%8Dndice-ODS-2019-para-Am%C3%A9rica-Latina-y-el-Caribe-2.pdf. Accessed Aug 2020.

Constable, H. (2020, April 26). How do you build a city for a pandemic? *BBC*.

Corburn, J., Vlahov, D., Mberu, B., Riley, L., Caiaffa, W. T., Rashid, S. F., Ko, A., Patel, S., Jukur, S., Martínez-Herrera, E., Jayasinghe, S., Agarwal, S., Nguendo-Yongsi, B., Weru, J., Ouma, S., Edmundo, K., Oni, T., & Ayad, H. (2020). Slum health: arresting COVID-19 and improving well-being in urban informal settlements. *Journal of Urban Health, 97*(3), 348–357.

Davoudi, S., Shaw, K., Haider, L. J., Quinlan, A. E., Peterson, G. D., Wilkinson, C., Fünfgeld, H., Mcevoy, D., Porter, L., & Davoudi, S. (2012). Resilience: A bridging concept or a dead end? "Reframing" resilience: Challenges for planning theory and practice interacting traps: Resilience assessment of a pasture management system in northern Afghanistan urban resilience: What does it mean in planning practice? Resilience as a useful concept for climate change adaptation? The politics of resilience for planning: A cautionary note. *Planning Theory & Practice, 13*(2), 299–333. https://doi.org/10.1080/14649357.2012.677124

Clarín. (2020, May 19). *Coronavirus en Chile: se disparan los casos y estalla la furia en los barrios más pobres* [Coronavirus in Chile: Rise in cases and the fury outburst in the poorest neighborhoods]. https://www.clarin.com/mundo/coronavirus-chile-disparan-casos-estalla-furia-barrios-pobres_0_ujm0mMuQp.html. Accessed Nov 2020.

Economic Commission for Latin America and the Caribbean [ECLAC]. (2020a). *América Latina y el Caribe ante la pandemia del COVID-19: Efectos económicos y sociales: Informe Especial Covid-19 N1* [Latin America and the Caribbean against the COVID-19 pandemic. Economic and social effects: Special report Covid-19 N1]. https://repositorio.cepal.org/bitstream/handle/11362/45337/4/S2000264_es.pdf. Accessed Nov 2020.

ECLAC. (2020b). *La Agenda 2030 para el Desarrollo Sostenible en el nuevo contexto mundial y regional: Escenarios y proyecciones en la presente crisis* [2030 agenda for sustainable development in the new global and regional context: Situations and projections in the current crisis]. https://repositorio.cepal.org/bitstream/handle/11362/45336/6/S2000208_es.pdf. Accessed Jan 2021.

ECLAC. (2020c). *Panorama Fiscal de América Latina y el Caribe 2020* [Fiscal outlook of Latin America and the Caribbean 2020]. https://repositorio.cepal.org/bitstream/handle/11362/45730/3/S2000154_es.pdf. Accessed Jan 2021.

ECLAC. (2020d). *Enfrentar los efectos cada vez mayores del COVID-19 para una reactivación con igualdad: nuevas proyecciones. Informe Especial Covid No 5* [Facing the progressively bigger effects of COVID-19 for a reactivation with equality: New projections. Special report Covid N. 5]. https://www.cepal.org/es/publicaciones/45782-enfrentar-efectos-cada-vez-mayores-covid-19-reactivacion-igualdad-nuevas. Accessed Aug 2020.

ECLAC. (2020e). *Universalizing access to digital technologies to address the consequences of COVID-19*. Special report No 7. https://repositorio.cepal.org/bitstream/handle/11362/45939/5/S2000549_en.pdf. Accessed Sept 2020.

ECLAC, & Organización Panamericana de la Salud [OPS]. (2020). *Salud y economía: una convergencia necesaria para enfrentar el COVID-19 y retomar la senda hacia el desarrollo sostenible en América Latina y el Caribe* [Health and economy: A necessary convergence to fase

COVID-19 and resume the path towards sustainable development in Latin America and the Caribbean]. https://repositorio.cepal.org/bitstream/handle/11362/45840/4/S2000462_es.pdf. Accessed Aug 2020.

Escola da Cidade. (2020, May 13). *Utopias e distopias urbanas em tempos de pandemia*. [Video file]. https://www.youtube.com/watch?v=31sXhys8qe8&t=. Accessed Aug 2020.

Ferreira, L., & Katz, P. (2020, April 9). What a solidarity economy looks like. *Boston Review*. https://bostonreview.net/class-inequality/paul-katz-leandro-ferreria-brazil-basic-income-marica. Accessed Aug 2020.

Food and Agriculture Organization of the United Nations [FAO], International Fund for Agricultural Development [IFAD], UNICEF, World Food Programme [WFP], & World Health Organization [WHO]. (2020). *The state of food security and nutrition in the world 2020. Transforming food systems for affordable healthy diets*. FAO. http://www.fao.org/documents/card/en/c/ca9692en. Accessed Feb 2021

Florida, R. (2020, April 3). *The geography of coronavirus*. City Lab. https://www.bloomberg.com/news/articles/2020-04-03/what-we-know-about-density-and-covid-19-s-spread. Accessed Aug 2020.

Galiley, A. (2020, July 31). *The pandemic has resulted in record savings, but only for some*. Next Advisor. https://time.com/nextadvisor/banking/savings/us-saving-rate-soaring/?utm_source=newsletter&utm_medium=email&utm_campaign=the-brief&utm_content=20200803&et_rid=70754059. Accessed Sept 2020.

Galindo, J., & Arroyo, L. (2020) Os mapas da pandemia revelam as desigualdades na América Latina. *El País*. https://brasil.elpais.com/internacional/2020-08-04/os-mapas-da-pandemia-revelam-as-desigualdades-na-america-latina.html. Accessed Sept 2020.

Gibb, L., & Oliveira, A. (2015). A desigualdade na distribuição do trabalho total no Brasil: a quem favorece? *Revista Pesquisa & Debate, 26*(2 (48)), 87–104.

Gkiouleka, A., Huijts, T., Beckfield, J., & Bambra, C. (2018). Understanding the micro and macro politics of health: Inequalities, intersectionality & institutions – A research agenda. *Social Science & Medicine, 200*, 92–98. https://doi.org/10.1016/j.socscimed.2018.01.025

Haywood, K. M. (2020). A post-COVID future: Tourism community re-imagined and enabled. *Tourism Geographies, 22*(3), 599–609.

Hernández, H. (2020). *Mortalidad por covid-19 en México. Notas preliminares para un perfil sociodemográfico*. Notas de coyuntura del Crim No. 36 [Mortality due to Covid-19 in Mexico. Preliminary notes for a sociodemographic profile. Crim Coyunture Notes No. 36]. CRIM-UNAM. https://web.crim.unam.mx/sites/default/files/2020-06/crim_036_hector-hernandez_mortalidad-por-covid-19_0.pdf. Accessed Aug 2020.

Hirata, H. (2014). Gênero, classe e raça: Interseccionalidade e consubstancialidade das relações sociais [Gender, class and race: Intersectionality and consubstantiality of social relations]. *Tempo Social, 26*(1), 61–73.

Instituto de Estudos para o Desenvolvimento Industrial [IEDI]. (2020). *Entraves à digitalização na América Latina e o combate da Covid-19*. Carta IEDI 1041 [Barriers to digitization in Latin America and the fight against Covid-19. Barriers to digitization in Latin America and the fight against Covid-19]. https://www.iedi.org.br/cartas/carta_iedi_n_1014.html. Accessed 17 July 2020.

International Labor Office [ILO]. (2018a). *Women and men in the informal economy: A statistical picture* (3rd ed.). Geneva: ILO. https://www.ilo.org/wcmsp5/groups/public/%2D%2D-dgreports/%2D%2D-dcomm/documents/publication/wcms_626831.pdf

ILO. (2018b). *The future of work: A literature review*. https://www.ilo.org/wcmsp5/groups/public/%2D%2D-dgreports/%2D%2D-inst/documents/publication/wcms_625866.pdf. Accessed July 2020.

ILO. (2020a). *Covid-19 and child labour: A time of crisis, a time to act*. https://www.ilo.org/wcmsp5/groups/public/%2D%2D-ed_norm/%2D%2D-ipec/documents/publication/wcms_747421.pdf. Accessed Aug 2020.

ILO. (2020b). *Working from home: Estimating the worldwide potential: Policy brief.* https://www.ilo.org/wcmsp5/groups/public/%2D%2D-ed_protect/%2D%2D-protrav/%2D%2D-travail/documents/briefingnote/wcms_743447.pdf. Accessed July 2020.

ILO, & United Nations Children's Fund [UNICEF]. (2020, May). *ILO monitor: COVID-19 and the world of work.* Fourth edition updated estimates and analysis. https://www.ilo.org/wcmsp5/groups/public/%2D%2D-dgreports/%2D%2D-dcomm/documents/briefingnote/wcms_745963.pdf. Accessed July 2020.

International Monetary Fund [IMF]. (2020). *World economic outlook update, June 2020.* https://www.imf.org/en/Publications/WEO/Issues/2020/06/24/WEOUpdateJune2020. Accessed July 2020.

Infobae. (2020, June 24). *Coronavirus en la Ciudad de México: gobierno planea generar 987,183 empleos tras crisis por COVID-19* [Coronavirus in Mexico City: Government plans generating 987,183 jobs after the COVID-19 Crisis]. https://www.infobae.com/america/mexico/2020/06/24/coronavirus-en-la-ciudad-de-mexico-gobierno-planea-generar-987183-empleos-tras-crisis-por-covid-19/. Accessed Aug 2020.

Kapilashrami, A., Hill, S., & Meer, N. (2015). What can health inequalities researchers learn from an intersectionality perspective? Understanding social dynamics with an inter-categorical approach? *Social Theory & Health, 13*, 288–307.

Maricato, E. (2015). *Para entender a crise urbana* [To understand the urban crisis]. Expressão Popular.

Medina, E. (2020). *Así cambió el Plan de Desarrollo de Bogotá por el coronavirus (COVID-19)* [Bogota's development plan changed like this due to coronavirus (COVID-19)]. https://bogota.gov.co/mi-ciudad/administracion-distrital/asi-cambio-el-plan-de-desarrollo-de-bogota-por-el-coronavirus. Accessed Nov 2020.

Neri, M. C., Vaz, F. M., & Ferreira de Souza, P. H. G. (2013). *Efeitos macroeconômicos do programa bolsa família: uma análise comparativa das transferências sociais* [Macroeconomic effects of the Bolsa Família program: a comparative analysis of social transfers]. https://www.ipea.gov.br/portal/images/stories/PDFs/131015_bolsa_familia_cap11.pdf. Accessed July 2020.

Organisation for Economic Co-operation and Development [OECD]. (2020, July 23). *Cities policies responses.* https://read.oecd-ilibrary.org/view/?ref=126_126769-yen45847kf&title=Coronavirus-COVID-19-Cities-Policy-Responses. Accessed Aug 2020.

Oliveira, A. (2019). Desigualdade no início do século XXI: o Brasil na contramão mundial? *Argumentum (Vitória), 11*, 171–168.

Oliveira, A., Fares, L., Silva, G., & Nassif-Pires, L. (2020, March 29). *Home quarantine: Confinement with the abuser?* Multiplier Effect. http://multiplier-effect.org/home-quarantine-confinement-with-the-abuser/. Accessed May 2020.

Oxfam. (2020a). *The hunger virus: how Covid-19 is fuelling hunger in a hungry world.* https://oxfamilibrary.openrepository.com/bitstream/handle/10546/621023/mb-the-hunger-virus-090720-en.pdf. Accessed Aug 2020.

Oxfam. (2020b). *Quem paga a conta? Taxar a riqueza para enfrentar a crise da Covid-19 na América Latina e Caribe* [Who pays the bill? Taxing wealth to tackle the Covid-19 crisis in Latin America and the Caribbean]. https://rdstation-static.s3.amazonaws.com/cms/files/115321/1595622094Nota_informativa_da_Oxfam_Quem_Paga_a_Conta.pdf. Accessed Aug 2020.

Palmeira, V., Costa, L., Perez, L., Ribeiro, V., Lanza, K., & Silva, A. (2020). Do we have enough evidence to use chloroquine/hydroxychloroquine as a public health panacea for COVID-19? *Clinics, 75*, e1928.

Pontes, N. (2020, April 15). *O elo entre desmatamento e epidemias investigado pela ciencia* [The link between deforestation and epidemics investigated by science]. Deutsche Welle. https://www.dw.com/pt-br/o-elo-entre-desmatamento-e-epidemias-investigado-pela-ci%C3%AAncia/a-53135352?utm_source=akna&utm_medium=email&utm_campaign=20042020-Newsletter-ClimaInfo. Accessed June 2020.

Rockefeller Foundation. (2013). *City Resilience Index*. https://www.arup.com/perspectives/publications/research/section/city-resilience-index. Accessed May 2020.

Rolnik, R., Marino, A., Klintowitz, D., Brito, G., & Mendonça, P. (2020). *Não se enfrenta a pandemia com leituras simplificadas do território* [The pandemic cannot be tackled with simplified readings of the territory]. UOL. https://raquelrolnik.blogosfera.uol.com.br/2020/06/04/nao-se-enfrenta-a-pandemia-com-leituras-simplificadas-do-territorio/. Accessed July 2020.

Sachs, J., Schmidt-Traub, G., Kroll, C., Lafortune, G., Fuller, G., & Woelm, F. (2020). *The sustainable development goals and COVID-19. Sustainable development report 2020*. Cambridge University Press.

Salehi, S., Reddy, S., & Gholamrezanezhad, A. (2020). Long-term pulmonary consequences of coronavirus disease 2019 (COVID-19). *Journal of Thoracic Imaging, 35*(4), W87–W89.

Silva, J., Silva, R., Freitas, F., & Waltenberg, F. (2020). *Políticas socioeconômicas de reação à crise da covid-19 no município de Maricá, Rio de Janeiro* [Socioeconomic policies in response to the covid-19 crisis in the municipality of Maricá, Rio de Janeiro]. Instituto de Pesquisa Econômica Avançada (IPEA). http://repositorio.ipea.gov.br/handle/11058/10198. Accessed Aug 2020.

Stern, J. (2020). *Estudo aponta relação entre bairros com mais casos de Covid-19 e o uso de transporte público* [A study shows a relationship between neighborhoods with more cases of Covid-19 and the use of public transport]. EcoDebate. https://www.ecodebate.com.br/2020/07/08/estudo-aponta-relacao-entre-bairros-com-mais-casos-de-covid-19-e-o-uso-de-transporte-publico/. Accessed Sept 2020.

Toledo, K. (2020). *Risco de morrer por COVID-19 em São Paulo é 50% maior em áreas de menor nível socioeconômico* [The risk of dying from COVID-19 in São Paulo is 50% higher in areas of lower socioeconomic status]. Agência FAPESP. https://agencia.fapesp.br/risco-de-morrer-por-covid-19-em-sao-paulo-e-50-maior-em-areas-de-menor-nivel-socioeconomico/33880/. Accessed Sept 2020.

UOL. (2020, May 21). *Covid-19 escancarou a desigualdade na cidade de São Paulo* [Covid-19 opened up inequality in the city of São Paulo] [Video]. https://www.youtube.com/watch?v=o549eHRh0p8. Accessed June 2020.

United Nations [UN]. (2015). *Transforming our world: The 2030 Agenda for sustainable development*. https://sustainabledevelopment.un.org/content/documents/21252030%20Agenda%20for%20Sustainable%20Development%20web.pdf. Accessed July 2020.

UN. (2019). *World urbanization prospects: The 2018 revision (ST/ESA/SER.A/420)*. United Nations.

UN. (2020). *Sustainable development goals report 2020*. https://www.un.org/development/desa/publications/publication/sustainable-development-goals-report-2020. Accessed Aug 2020.

United Nations Conference on Trade and Development [UNCTAD]. (2020a, July 9). *COVID-19 stalls progress on global goals*. https://unctad.org/news/covid-19-stalls-progress-global-goals. Accessed Aug 2020.

UNCTAD. (2020b). *UNCTAD takes the pulse of the SDGs*. https://sdgpulse.unctad.org/. Accessed Aug 2020.

United Nations Educational, Scientific and Cultural Organization [UNESCO] & ECLAC. (2020). *Education in the time of COVID-19*. https://repositorio.cepal.org/bitstream/handle/11362/45905/1/S2000509_en.pdf. Accessed Sept 2020.

World Economic Forum [WEF]. (2020, June 3). *Colombia's Medellin boosts its 'eco-city" aims during coronavirus recovery*. https://www.weforum.org/agenda/2020/06/colombias-medellin-eco-city-coronavirus-covid19-recovery. Accessed Aug 2020.

Zerega, G., Pires, B., Criales, J., & Montes, R. (2020, August 1). A geração que pagará a conta da crise na América Latina [The generation that will foot the bill for the crisis in Latin America]. *El País*. https://brasil.elpais.com/internacional/2020-08-01/a-geracao-que-pagara-as-contas-da-crise-na-america-latina.html?utm_source=Facebook&ssm=FB_BR_CM&fbclid=IwAR2RPp2dYi1X7vR59O_Uub4zfzyMkHsdiQb4MQGYiBvL2jSnsrj7jyFK_g4#Echobox=1596327728. Accessed Sept 2020.

Chapter 8
Re-signifying Domestic Space in Times of Confinement Based on Biophilic Design

Carlos Cobreros, Mariana Flores-García, Stefania Biondi, Mariana Maya, and Elsa N. Ontiveros-Ortíz

Introduction

In 2020, the novel coronavirus disease—officially named 'COVID-19' by the World Health Organization—reached the level of a pandemic. The pandemic called for a period of social isolation and social distancing during the global contingency. This was an opportunity to question the role of designers and to rethink new alternatives of habitability. Designers seemed to have been absent in the COVID-19 discourses so unable to propose strategies or actions during the first period of the contingency when the need for creative and relevant design in health sectors was evident (Allam & Jones, 2020). This chapter is intended to be a training guide for professionals of the twenty-first century. The interdisciplinary project reflects on experimentation for social innovation in order to explore the topic of domestic spaces in times of confinement as a way to re-imagine resilient cities.

The environment has a direct impact on human perception. Different authors note the relationship between health, well-being, adaptation, and interaction with the built environment, physical space, and the pathological consequences that space can have on a human being (Doménech Gómez, 2015; Granda-Cango, 2016; Lotito Catino, 2009; Moser, 2009). Between a human being and the environment, there will always be an interaction that provides circumstances that influence behavior (Mercado-Domenech et al., 2016). In the context of confinement during the COVID-19 pandemic, it is necessary to generate environments that promote the well-being of human beings.

C. Cobreros (✉) · M. Flores-García · S. Biondi · M. Maya
Tecnologico de Monterrey, Escuela de Arquitectura, Arte y Diseño, Querétaro, Mexico
e-mail: ccobreros@tec.mx

E. N. Ontiveros-Ortíz
Tecnologico de Monterrey, Escuela de Ciencias Sociales y Gobierno, Querétaro, Mexico

© The Author(s), under exclusive license to Springer Nature Switzerland AG 2021

M. A. Montoya et al. (eds.), *COVID-19 and Cities*, The Urban Book Series,
https://doi.org/10.1007/978-3-030-84134-8_8

For the experiment, biophilia will be an important variable for the context of confinement and the user experience. Biophilia refers to the existence of an innate biological connection between human beings and nature and is the natural and hereditary human inclination to natural processes and systems (Wilson-Edward, 1984), promoting the idea that people's physical well-being depends on contact with nature and its processes (Kellert Stephen et al., 2008). Therefore, Biophilic Design (BD) is promoted to improve built environments, focusing on the connection between human beings and nature itself (García Pérez, 2015; Jones, 2013; Magos-Ramírez et al., 2016), incorporating natural elements that benefit physical and emotional health (Krasny & Delia, 2015; Ling & Chiang, 2018; Mangonea et al., 2017; Yin et al., 2018) in indoor environments (Krasny & Delia, 2015) as well as in public and outdoor spaces (Johnson, 2014). BD can reduce stress, enhance creativity, and improve mental clarity if analogous natural associations or nature itself is incorporated within a space (Browning et al., 2014).

Our health seems to be directly related to our proximity to nature. Outdoor views, having access to exterior landscapes (Ebrahimpour, 2020; Johnson, 2014), allowing natural light in (Ortega-Andeane et al., 2019), nature patterns, biomimicry, space diversity, fractals, native elements, plants, plant patterns, simulation of natural features, or water (Ebrahimpour, 2020) all perform (Mangonea et al., 2017) to constitute restorative healthy environments (Ortega-Andeane et al., 2018) and restorative functions (Gilchrist et al., 2015; Ozgen, 2018). BD represents a response to our need for healthy spaces, especially in the context of confinement.

Contact and visualization of natural beauty in an open environment (OE) can develop pro-social behavior and bring benefits such as empathy, generosity, trust, and collaboration (Zhang et al., 2014). Relating to nature can improve our physical and mental health (Charles et al., 2008; Chawla, 2015; Clayton et al., 2016; Corraliza et al., 2006; Engemann et al., 2019; Howell et al., 2011; Preuß et al., 2019) and provide psychological benefits, especially in children and adolescents (White et al., 2019). These benefits are perceived also in urban environments with some limited 'doses' of nature (Cox et al., 2017; Shanahan et al., 2015; White et al., 2019). With the context of the lack of contact with nature in open public spaces during the confinement restrictions of a pandemic, the chapter analyzes the potential BD in indoor domestic spaces, considering that domestic houses are key elements in our cities through which the pandemic is experienced (Garber, 2020).

This chapter has the objective to compile, compare, and explain the processes and results around the characterization of the domestic space from the point of view of biophilia and the relationship with nature, putting people at the center during the time of confinement through the ethnographic methodology. This was achieved through examining the perception of users and their experiences related to their daily life activities as well as exploring the physical characteristics of the domestic spaces and the influence of natural elements in the city of Querétaro / Mexico.

Methodology

Experimental research was used in the qualitative ethnographic methodology. This type of methodology design provides depth and contextualization as well as bringing out specific details and unique experiences while actively entering social situations, and a constant reflection (Hernández-Sampieri et al., 2006). A micro-ethnography and auto-ethnography were carried out using ethnographic tools, such as interviews, social cartographies, cognitive-body mapping, and experience mapping, in order to get a closer relationship with the people and their situations (Wilson & Zamberlan, 2015). The close relationship allows for discovering the particular needs of the users (Maya et al., 2019) as they immerse in an individual reality (Emerson et al., 2011) in their daily activities (Majoor, 2018). In particular, the micro-ethnography focuses on particular aspects in a short period of time (Bryman, 2008) to locate the social problem. Additionally, it allows for a spatial dimension to be added in order to discover the particularities within a global pattern, as well as full immersion (Hammersley & Atkinson, 2007), visualizing an added value based on personal motivations (Wilson & Zamberlan, 2015). An auto-ethnography allows for the prospect of a qualitative research strategy (Atkinson, 1996; Coffey & Atkinson, 1996; Marshall & Rossman, 1995) suitable for confinement. In order to approach the context from the researchers-actors' subjective perspective (Espinosa, 2007), we took advantage of the affective and cognitive "experiences" of the people who developed knowledge based on reality through their direct participation (Scribano & De Sena, 2009). In an auto-ethnography, the researcher has the privilege and responsibility of being the subject and object, and s/he is an active participant capable of narrating the scene in which he or she works and has distinguished access to the field of observation, implying the connection between the personal and the social (Scribano & De Sena, 2009). The researcher relates his or her reflection to the unknown as an approach between the personal and the interpretations, solely based on self-observation (Montero-Sieburth, 2006) and self-evaluation, and focuses on relationships with the others as the processes that involve a personal experience (Scribano & De Sena, 2009).

New avenues of reflection open up from the digital media used to obtain qualitative data in order to establish relationships between the researcher and the researched (Estalella & Ardèvol, 2007). Communication plays a key role that demands a series of theoretical and methodological adaptations (Arriazu-Muñoz, 2007). A virtual ethnography was associated with a cultural background reflection of the Internet in a dialogue of experiences and social interactions, posing a challenge that opened new fields within qualitative methodologies (Domínguez Figaredo, 2007). It proposes the translation of the virtual space of interaction that used to be exclusive to the present (Callén et al., 2007). The aforementioned requires the resizing of concepts in the adaptation of its basic principles, mediated by digital technologies, in order to be able to study social relations in this context (Villegas & Andrés, 2008). The specific ethnographic tools used (interview and self-interview, spatial and open social cartographies, and cognitive and experience maps) allowed analyzing the researcher's own experience and their relationship with the immediate domestic context.

Interview and Self-Interview

The interview and self-interview give way to an open, flexible, and intimate conversation to get and exchange information between the interviewer and the interviewee from a semi-structured format, following an open guide (Hernández-Sampieri et al., 2006) that yields quantitative and qualitative evaluation. There is also a 'free first' approach to the problem which deepens with the usage of other auto-ethnographic tools. For the preparation and application of the interview, a documentary analysis was initiated for the construction of a conceptual framework. 128 interviews and self-interviews were obtained. The survey consisted of quantitative comparable questions and qualitative questions, from which it was possible to draw specific conclusions about the analyzed domestic problem. There was a set of general questions to characterize the interviewed or self-interviewed person and their domestic context, another set to identify their experience during confinement, and, finally, a series of specific questions related to their experiences of living during confinement regarding biophilic elements such as access to nature (Table 8.1).

The instrument designed to identify the aspects of BD that represented the opportunity for users to have new experiences during confinement consisted of a structured interview based on 42 questions. The survey integrated open, categorical, and 5-point Likert scale responses; nine are directly associated with aspects of BD and biophilic elements.

The qualitative data analysis was developed with the MAXQDA2020 software, applied to the answers of the 16 open questions, and considered as an analysis criterion for the association of concepts and experiences during the confinement. The quantitative analysis was developed with the SPSS software from 26 categorical questions, through a correlational descriptive analysis where 26 variables were identified.

Social Cartographies

Social cartographies, derived from participatory and collaborative methodologies, were used to characterize socio-environmental conflicts that strengthened the link between humans and the physical environment (Vélez-Torres et al., 2012). It is a

Table 8.1 Variables included in the survey

Variables included in the survey	
Socio-demographic profile	Age, gender, occupation
Context	Urban environment, typology, size, house occupants
Biophilic elements	Natural light, natural ventilation, natural views, indoor plants, outdoor plants, terraces, or private patios
Temporality	Time spent at home (weekly stay, weekend stay)
Personal perception	Pleasure of being at home, initial feeling, current feeling, future feeling

dialogic technique using shared narratives (Iconoclasistas, 2011), that identifies and analyzes social relations from the temporal and the collective in a specific physical and social space, representing its borders as a material or symbolic division (Vélez-Torres et al., 2012).

In the face of the COVID-19 pandemic, the importance of mapping a spatiotemporal analysis was necessary to integrate the spatial and temporal dimensions (Franch-Pardo et al., 2020), as well as the interaction between biophysical and human factors (Turner, 2002 CR). Social cartographies allow the identification of spaces as social priorities and are sensitive to the context (Samuelsson et al., 2020), with the possibility of measuring, representing, and analyzing spatial information from the perception of the inhabitants (Barrera- Lobatón, 2009).

For this research, architectural representations of domestic spaces were carried out, as well as urban contextualization at the scale of the neighborhood, as a base for social cartographies built by the inhabitants themselves in order to understand the problem of inhabiting a domestic space in the confinement of COVID-19.

Cognitive—Body Mapping

Cognitive maps are a way of telling stories where events are organized through visual, textual, auditory, or other means (Hohenthal et al., 2017; McLees, 2013). This is a powerful way of communicating spatial information (Caquard, 2011). The narrative is fundamental for knowledge about a way of finding the relationships between place and time (Ingold, 2011). Narrated events, expressions, and interpretations of maps (Caquard & Cartwright, 2014) are a critical reflection (Cameron, 2012; Molden, 2020). Dissemination of findings, data visualization, communication of information, and the exchange of stories (Antoniou et al., 2018; Berendsen et al., 2018; Egiebor & Foster, 2018) are moments in the construction of collective knowledge through cognitive mapping.

The elaboration of body mapping, body cartographies, or "body-territory-space" maps, derived from a feminist and gender perspective background, is based on the idea that when there is conflict in the lived-in territories or spaces, we feel the pain that materializes directly in the body. Understanding bodies is the first frontier between the self and the other(s), as everything we do is spatially located and embodied in different hierarchical ledgers (Cruz et al., 2017).

Experience Mapping

Finally, the creation of experience maps is an effective method to understand and improve the user experience. This technique facilitates collaboration between stakeholders and designers, giving way to co-creation processes (Samson et al., 2017). In the present project, experience maps were used as a research technique that incorporated multiple methods and data sources in order to build visual narratives of individual and collective experiences, aiming for collection, analysis, and representation of spatial information, as well as visual and textual information (Drysdale et al., 2020).

The tools described above were applied within 2 months, with two working groups of student-researchers, and with a total number of 17 people. The group was made up of undergraduate students (industrial design and architecture undergraduates at Tec de Monterrey) and graduate students of architecture at the Autonomous University of Querétaro. The group was composed of ten women (five undergraduates and five graduates) and six men (all of them graduates). Most of them belonged to a medium-high socioeconomic group and they lived in medium-to-large-sized houses which allowed for open spaces, such as patios or terraces. Five of the women and two of the men lived by themselves, and the rest shared the inhabited space with their family, therefore having different relational dynamics within the group.

Results

This section presents the results of the mixed methods of the interviews and self-interviews, as well as the examples and graphic results of the ethnographic tools presented above. Only the most significant are shown, as well as a synthesis of the results and conclusions, regarding the conclusions obtained from this part of the research.

Interview and Self-Interview: Qualitative and Quantitative Data Analysis

The level of response associated with the typology of housing was concentrated on terraced houses with a terrace, patio, or private garden at 54.7% (Fig. 8.1).

Eight main variables associated with the BD were identified where, from the results of the survey, a weighting was made between the total responses and the correlation of the variables identified, with the perception of well-being, structuring the results on an evaluation scale from 1 to 10 to identify the importance of each variable and its impact during the period of confinement.

In relation to the qualitative analysis, the people surveyed mentioned experiences during confinement associated with new activities and their domestic environment. The responses were categorized regarding their association with the BD variables and well-being, either by the possibility that they were part of their environment, the possibility of making adjustments, or the desire to integrate new elements into their home to improve their level of well-being (Fig. 8.2).

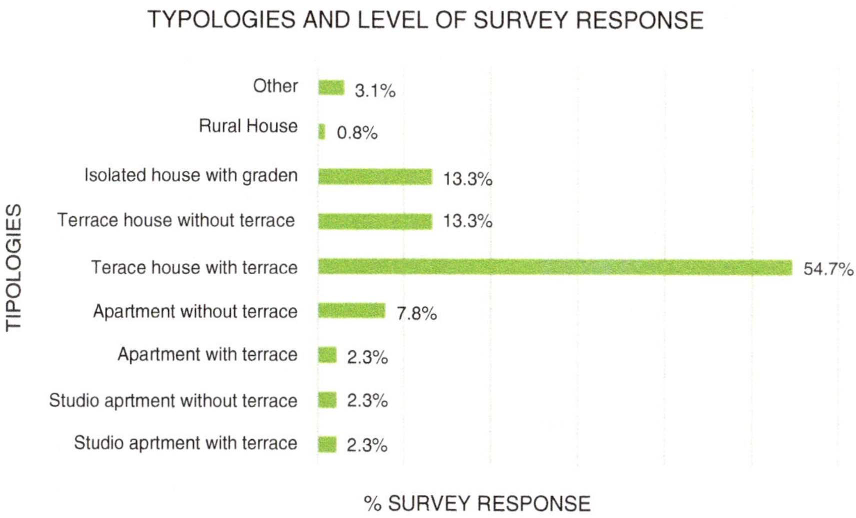

Fig. 8.1 Typologies and level of survey response

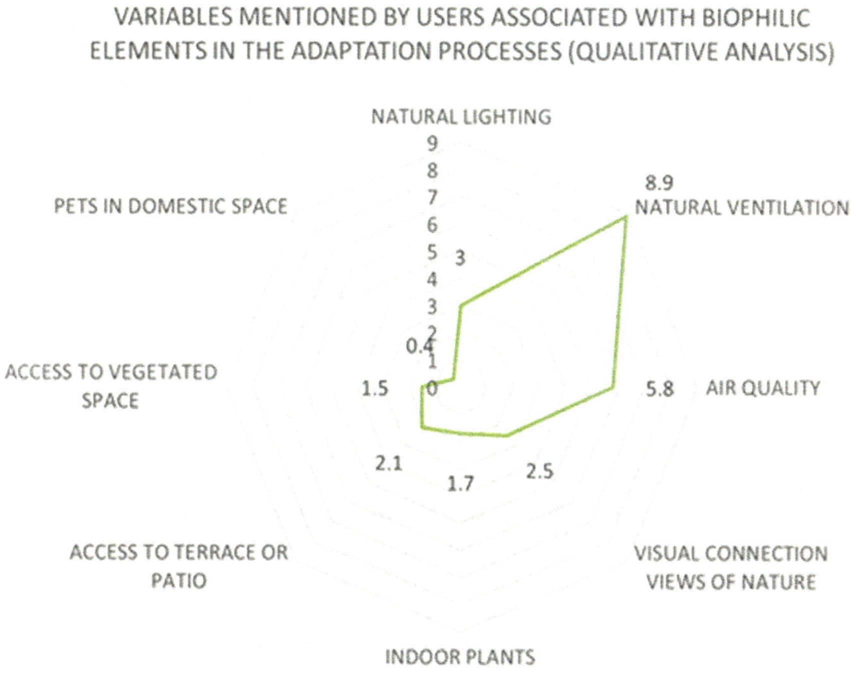

Fig. 8.2 Variables mentioned by users associated with biophilic elements in the adaptation processes (qualitative analysis)

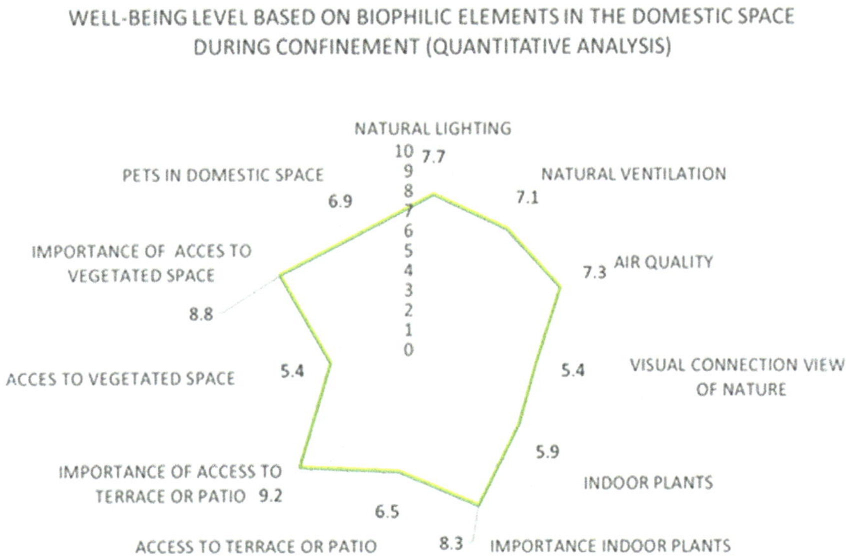

Fig. 8.3 Well-being level based on biophilic elements in the domestic space during confinement (quantitative analysis)

As a result, on a scale of 1–10, where 10 represents all aspects related to the habitability of the dwellings, aspects related to natural ventilation were mentioned 8.9 times, emphasizing the possibility of having large windows with fresh air circulation, or having very small windows that limited the comfort conditions inside the house. This aligned with the first aspect of air quality, mentioned 5.8 times on a scale of 1–10. It's important to mention that 54.7% of all respondents lived in houses with a terrace, and sometimes, the only possibility of interaction is on a terrace or patio, with or without vegetation. The third variable is natural lighting. The recurrent aspects are associated with problems derived from new uses or limitations in the adaptation of existing spaces, looking for alternatives that improve the living conditions in the face of new needs.

In the quantitative analysis, on an evaluation scale of 1–10, with respect to the level of well-being from the perception of the users, it appears to be a priority to have spaces with natural light (7.7), followed by good air quality (7.3) and natural ventilation (7.1), which coincides with the results of the qualitative analysis. It is relevant that the importance of having access to a private patio or terrace (9.2), or having plants inside (8.3), especially if there is no possibility of having a garden or terrace as part of the house, as well as how important it is to have access to a vegetated space, is mentioned 8.8 times (Fig. 8.3). The importance of having a terrace or vegetated space is mentioned the most, mainly by those who do not have that possibility.

Social Cartographies

Architectural plans were developed to identify open/exterior domestic spaces and their characteristic elements (vegetation, animals, natural light, natural ventilation, views of natural exteriors in the interior space, and its relationship with the direct exterior space). These were based on the social cartographies, personal, graphic, and photographic representations, exposing the emotional visuals as the experience of the domestic space and its transformations during confinement. Figure 8.4 shows an example of an architectural representation based on the social cartography of domestic spaces from one of the case studies.

Figure 8.5 shows an example of a social cartography showing the different intensity uses and routes between the different family members. The lines represent the flow of each member according to different colors.

In Fig. 8.6, you can see another example of social cartographies where new spatial relationships by home areas are under confinement. It can be seen how exterior spaces become fundamental in this period.

The first finding of social cartographies, repeated in some cases, is that the size of the house becomes somewhat relevant, and these small spaces can provoke depressive feelings and anxiety. These sensations are increased when there is no adequate ventilation and when there is a lack of an outdoor view.

Another finding is that during confinement, there was a tendency to use more spaces more often; the kitchen and the living room were commonly visited places within a house, for example. However, everyone also used their room or study room much more than before confinement. The aforementioned is represented in Fig. 8.7. We can read from different social cartographies that confinement has given way to the dynamic use of spaces and the disruption of roles and traditional relationships between the space and the person who inhabits it. During confinement, in these case studies, undesigned spaces were revisited as spaces that have to be rethought and re-designed to develop more activities within the same areas.

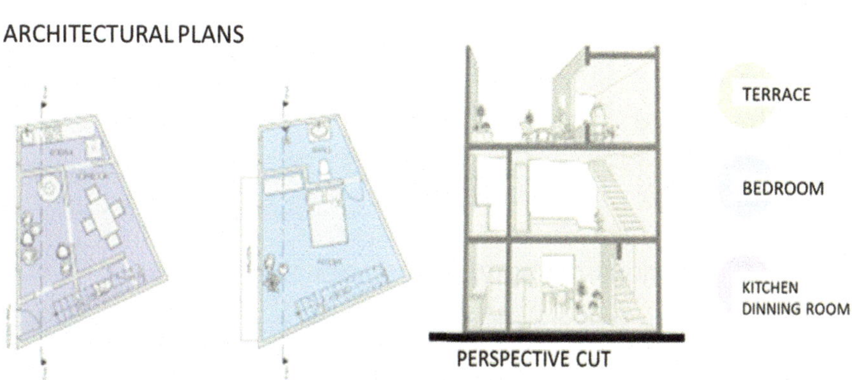

Fig. 8.4 Architectural representation: plans and perspective of a case study

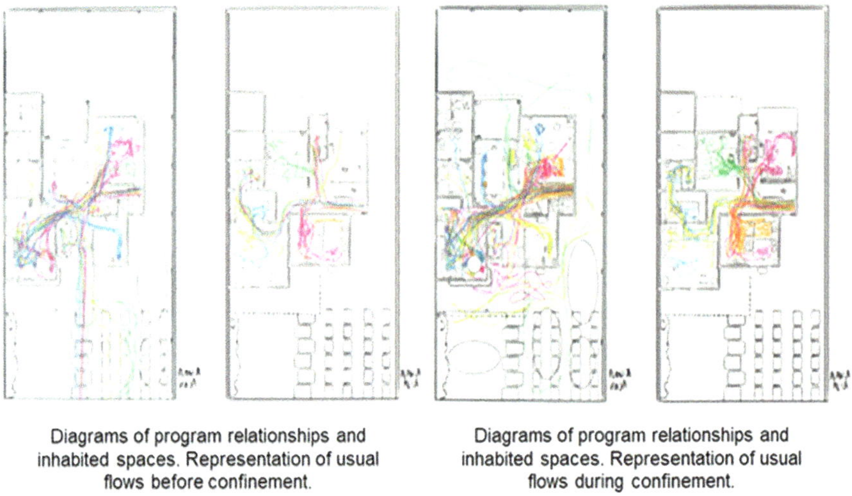

Fig. 8.5 Diagrams of program relationships and inhabited spaces. Representation of usual flows before and during confinement

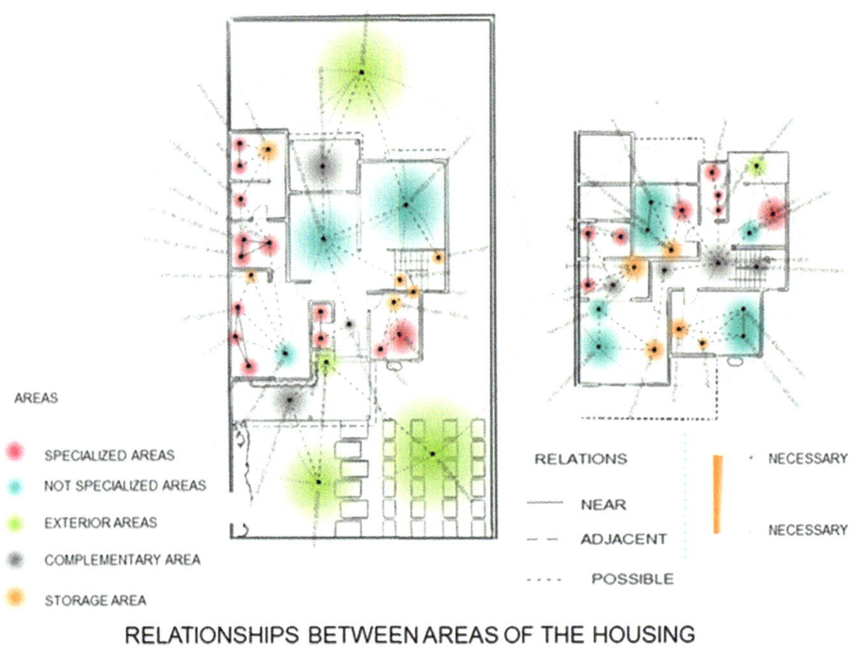

Fig. 8.6 Social cartographies: diagrams of new spatial relationships by areas of the home during confinement

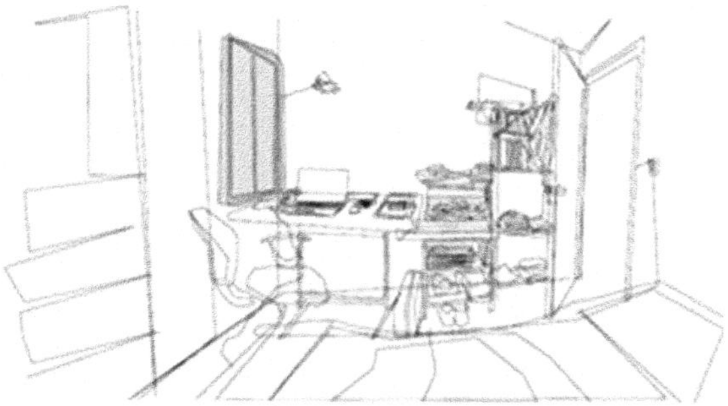

Fig. 8.7 Social cartographies: representations of relationships and uses of spaces by users

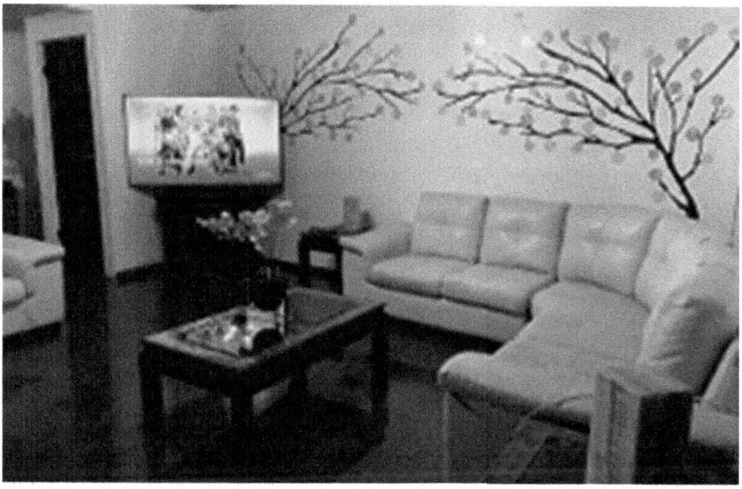

Fig. 8.8 Photographic documentation of the search for plant decoration in interior spaces

From the research project samples, issues such as acoustics, furniture, or light quality were highly requested. Furthermore, it was noted that the work–leisure balance was broken by spending too much time in the same spaces. The problem becomes more acute if the living spaces are small and uncomfortable. In the same way, cleanliness and hygiene became very relevant. The theme of the colors on the walls of the rooms was reviewed, as it became relevant in order to generate pleasant environments. Even new decorations with motifs inspired by nature were used in some case studies (Figs. 8.8 and 8.9).

Something that was recurrent in the cartographies and the photographic records used in them was the importance of outer spaces and vegetated spaces.

Gardens and terraces became a merging and coexisting place. People used the areas to develop activities such as exercising and playing. The spaces became a family gathering place. The use of roofs and terraces was intensified, as observed in different cartographies.

The lack of access to outdoor or green vegetated spaces is something that was assumed as something negative by different actors, as we can see in some

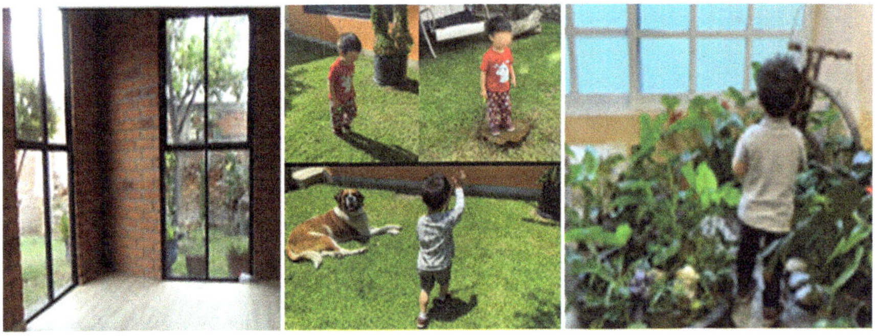

Fig. 8.9 Relation to interior and exterior spaces as vegetation became important in confinement, especially for children

cartographies. Views, natural light, and adequate lighting became important during the time of confinement for the researchers and other co-habitants. Gardening, whether indoors or outdoors, had become common and that was felt like something that improved emotional well-being. There were other cases where we saw houses filled with plants. The care for plants was a pattern that actively emerged in confinement.

Greater interaction with pets was detected, as caring for them was an activity that promoted family cohesion.

Cognitive Mapping–Body Mapping

There was a diversity in emotion detected by cognitive-body mapping, from positive to mixed and negative feelings, related to the spatial characteristics. More interpersonal relationships emerged during confinement, influenced according to who the spaces were shared with and with what intensity, more than due to the direct space. Issues around privacy arose (Fig. 8.10).

Emotions of liberation, tranquility, and peace were expressed in relation to open spaces, outdoor activities, rooftops, and terraces in general. There was again a clear relationship between positive emotions and the possibility of living in outdoor spaces, the open air, and being in contact with naturalized spaces, plants, natural light, animal sounds, and in a natural atmosphere.

Experience Mapping

The experience maps helped to understand how life had changed on a day-to-day basis in confinement, detecting positive or negative experiences happening within a day (Figs. 8.11 and 8.12). There were a variety of results; a common result was

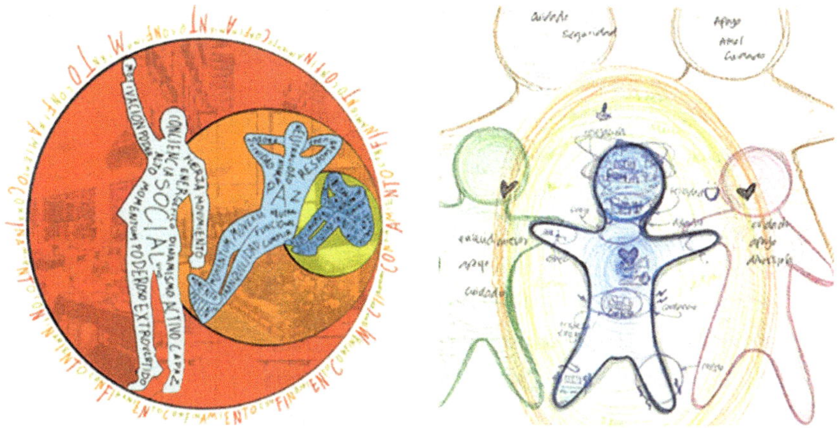

Fig. 8.10 Examples of cognitive-body mapping

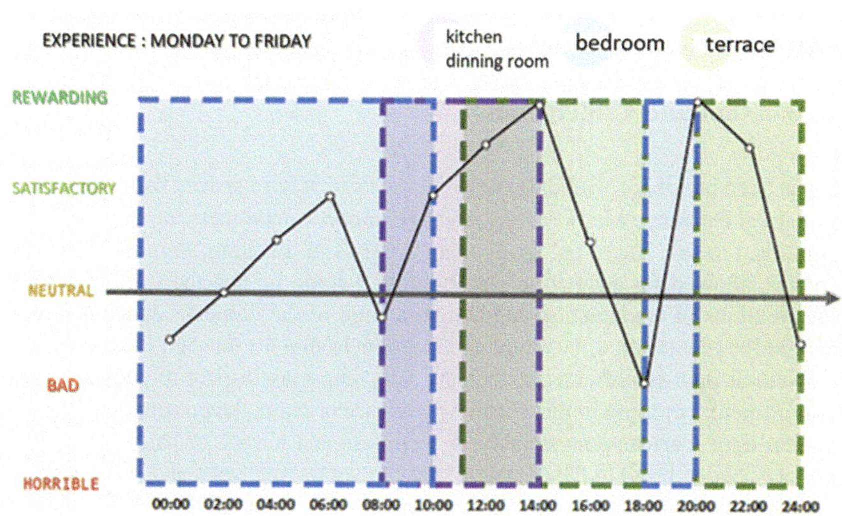

Fig. 8.11 Example of experience map

positive experiences in vegetated outdoor spaces, or simply outdoors, and those moments in which you have access to natural light and direct sunlight. With experience maps, the overlap of activities in the same spaces is highly marked, particularly regarding how this could reflect on a negative experience. It was seen that if you shared the same space to sleep, eat, and work, your intimacy was violated and mixed, or related to work stress, for example.

The experience maps, in some cases, showed how certain daily household activities became more burdensome than normal in confinement, with a possible gender issue behind it that should be analyzed in greater depth.

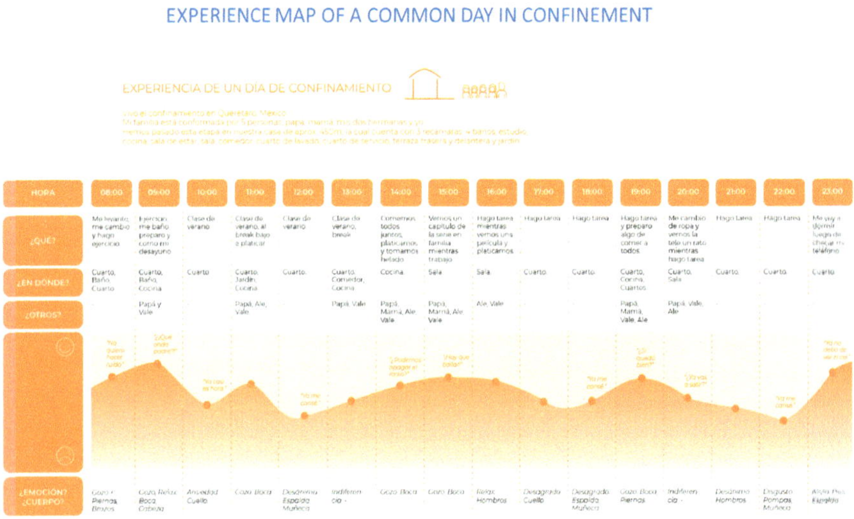

Fig. 8.12 Example of experience map

Discussion and Conclusions

It has been possible to validate the preferences to stay in spaces with the presence of natural elements. Many felt the negative impact of confinement on physical and emotional health. The typological characteristics of dwelling, in most of the cases studies, allowed for adaptation possibilities. It could be that the starting point for interventions of readaptation and resignification of the domestic space is directed toward the promotion of healthier and safer environments through BD.

Natural light is presented as being a very important aspect to consider during confinement. For those homes that have a terrace or patio, the possibilities of having natural light increase considerably. A well-designed terrace or patio is something that we have to bring to the domestic space as something basic and necessary.

Ventilation was always a prominent aspect of comfort and health. The confinement has revealed the importance of clean, hygienic, and well-ventilated spaces, mainly in those areas where we spend the longest time or where we develop our daily activities. In the case of the presence of spaces such as terraces or patios, it is easier to induce cross-ventilation. It is necessary to rethink important aspects in the conceptualization of housing in this way, as well as prioritize actions to be carried out in houses already built. Regarding pollution, it has been an aspect frequently mentioned, and vegetated areas or spaces have the possibility of filtering the air of pollutants that can affect the lung health of the population. In risky conditions, this aspect requires prioritizing.

Indoor plants represent a simple and inexpensive strategy to modify bad perceptions in closed environments. Plants can be highly valued when there is no access to urban green areas or when there is no possibility to have a terrace or patio space within the home itself. They also represent easily accessible resources, flexibility in their integration, and a very wide diversity in colors, textures, sizes, or smells, as well as offering the possibility of improving the domestic experience at any time.

The importance of having a private space, such as a terrace, patio, or balcony, represented possibilities for better health conditions. In addition, if it was vegetated, the experience was considerably more positive and healthier. The views and pleasant natural environments within the house through microenvironments promoted various dynamics of habitability that reduced tensions. It was identified in the survey results that those people who did not have access to natural elements were considering integrating them soon.

The ethnographic approach to the study of domestic space during a pandemic was ideal because of the isolation circumstances. The micro-ethnography, auto-ethnography, and virtual ethnography enriched the process as an innovation tool within the context. Some tools of these sub-disciplines, such as the self-interview and the various forms of cognitive and emotional mapping, had made it possible to obtain the necessary data for ethnographic analysis even in conditions lacking physical approximation. They have also been valuable instruments of self-reflection that, applied to the researcher's own spatial experiences, have allowed both the generation of a greater self-awareness of the body–space relationships and the development of a more acute and empathetic sensitivity toward the experiences of others. The evaluations, based on the mapping and the experience of the students, coincide with concepts identified in the results of the survey, particularly that the respondents were knowledgeable of Architecture and Design, potentiating the sensitivity and attention span of professionals in construction regarding regenerative strategies based on BD for well-being.

This study is an approach to resilience practices that, based on confinement, provides an opportunity to influence design and architecture as adaptive mechanisms toward healthier and more sustainable urban conditions. The authors hope to contribute to the understanding of urban resilience at a housing scale. The experience of habitability is seen as a minimal expression in a process of adaptation. The revaluation of natural environment aspects at the housing and neighborhood scale provide contact with nature and maintain the promotion of social development and landscape resilience to face climate change situations, natural disasters, and uncertain scenarios, as well as economic failures, including, in its conceptual evolution, more human and welfare aspects (Beatley & Newman, 2013).

Currently, there is little understanding of the minimum required level of nature, or access to it, that is required to have adequate health and well-being, so the study builds an approximation to identify those aspects that demand a greater presence in the domestic environment. In this case, the term "urgent biophilia" is present in the face of processes of revaluation of living spaces (Instituto Humboldt and PNUD, 2018). The search for urban resilience has been considered of vital importance in the survival of city structures, both in the short and long term, as they help vulnerable regions to resist impacts on various spatial scales, such as housing and neighborhood (Allam et al., 2020).

We can conclude that including greener elements and allowing contact with natural environments in the surroundings of domestic space undoubtedly reduces the stress on the emotional, mental, and physical aspects of the inhabitant while improving health. It is key to resignify the domestic environment, as the interaction with the outside was considered highly valued. Architectural aspects and spaces related to balconies, gardens, terraces, and patios, as well as spaces with ventilation, natural light, and pleasant views, represent great possibilities to generate healthier environments. The study represents an approach to understanding the interaction and influential processes of biophilic spaces based on the perception and experience of the user, and even on the researcher.

Hopefully, other studies can be carried out in the future, with the possibility to work with more information to evaluate the different aspects of biophilic design and how it can affect the user in their experience with domestic space. The findings are many and empirical, so we encourage others to venture into ethnographic methods within their own research. However, from the results obtained from this ethnographic approach to the problem, it can be considered that biophilic designers can contribute to the resignification of domestic spaces, making the experience of living a healthier and more rewarding experience, even during times of confinement.

Acknowledgments The work, as well as the graphics and images on which this research is fundamentally based, comes from the Master's Degree Architecture students at the Autonomous University of Querétaro: Edgar Barranco, Oscar Soto, Valentyn Kotsarenko, Mónica Rodriguez, Farit Acosta, Jorge Flores, Jonatan Shomar, Andrea Arenas, and Ricardo Zaraguas. Also from students from the School of Architecture, Art and Design at Tecnológico de Monterrey: Ximena Sánchez, Jessica Llamas, Jessica Coronas, Danya Escamilla, Daniela Suarez, and Elizabeth Medellín. We are grateful for the support of the directors and coordinators from both the Master's Degree in Architecture at the Autonomous University of Querétaro and the School of Architecture, Art and Design at the Tecnológico de Monterrey, for their support in carrying out the courses and research stays in which the present work is framed.

References

Allam, Z., & Jones, D. (2020). Pandemic stricken cities on lockdown. Where are our planning and design professionals [now, then and into the future]. *Land Use Policy, 97*. https://doi.org/10.1016/j.landusepol.2020.104805

Allam, Z., Jones, D., & Thondoo, M. (2020). *Cities and climate change: Climate policy, economic resilience and urban sustainability*. Palgrave Macmillan.

Antoniou, V., Ragia, L., Nomikou, P., Bardouli, P., Lampridou, D., Ioannou, T., Kalisperakis, I., & Stentoumis, C. (2018). Creating a story map using geographic information systems to explore geomorphology and history of Methana peninsula. *ISPRS International Journal of Geo-Information, 7*(12), 484. [Cross Reference].

Arriazu-Muñoz, R. (2007). On new means or new forms of investigation. A methodological proposal for online social investigation through a virtual forum. *Forum: Qualitative Sozialforschung/ Forum: Qualitative Social Research, 8*(3). https://doi.org/10.17169/fqs-8.3.275

Barrera- Lobatón, S. (2009). Reflexiones sobre Sistemas de Información Geográfica Participativos (sigp) y cartografía social [reflections about the participative geographic information systems

(PGIS) and social cartography]. *Cuadernos de Geografía: Revista Colombiana de Geografía, 18*, 9–23. https://www.redalyc.org/articulo.oa?id=2818/281822001002. Accessed 29 Aug 2020

Beatley, T., & Newman, P. (2013). Biophilic cities are sustainable, resilient cities. *Sustainability, 5*(8), 3328–3345. https://doi.org/10.3390/su5083328

Berendsen, M. E., Hamerlinck, J. D., & Webster, G. R. (2018). Digital story mapping to advance educational atlas design and enable student engagement. *ISPRS International Journal of Geo-Information, 7*(3), 125. [Cross Reference].

Browning, W., Ryan, C., & Clancy, J. (2014). *14 Patterns of Biophilic Design. Improving health & Well-being in the built environment.* Terrapin Bright Green LLC. https://www.hcm2.com/wp-content/uploads/Browning-2014-Patterns-of-Biophilic-Design-Terrapin.pdf. Accessed Aug 2020.

Bryman, A. (2008). *Social research methods* (3rd ed.). Oxford University Press.

Callén, B., Balasch, M., Guarderas, P., Gutierrez, P., León, A., Montenegro, M., Montenegro, K., & Pujol, J. (2007). Riereta.net: Epistemic and political notes from a techno-activist ethnography. *Forum Qualitative Sozialforschung/Forum: Qualitative Social Research, 8*(3). https://doi.org/10.17169/fqs-8.3.276

Cameron, E. (2012). New geographies of story and storytelling. *Progress in Human Geography, 36*(5), 573–592. [Cross Reference].

Caquard, S. (2011). Cartography I: Mapping narrative cartography. *Progress in Human Geography, 37*(1), 135–144. [Cross Reference].

Caquard, S., & Cartwright, W. (2014). Narrative cartography: From mapping stories to the narrative of maps and mapping. *The Cartographic Journal, 51*(2), 101–116. [Cross Reference].

Charles, C., Louv, R., Bodner, L., & Guns, B. (2008). *Children and nature. A report on the movement to reconnect children to the natural world.* Children and Nature Network.

Chawla, L. (2015). Benefits of nature contact for children. *Journal of Planning Literature, 30*(4), 433–452. https://doi.org/10.1177/0885412215595441

Clayton, S., Colleony, A., Conversy, P., Maclouf, E., Martin, L., Torres, A.-C., & Prevot, A.-C. (2016). Transformation of experience: Toward a new relationship with nature. *Conservation Letters, 10*(5), 645–651. https://doi.org/10.1111/conl.12337

Coffey, A., & Atkinson, P. (1996). *Making sense of qualitative data: Complementary research strategies.* Sage. [Cross Reference].

Corraliza, J. A., Berenguer, J., & Martín, R. (2006). *Medio ambiente, bienestar humano y responsabilidad ecológica [Environment, human Well-being, and ecological responsability].* Editorial Resma.

Cox, D. T. C., Hudson, H. L., Shanahan, D. F., Fuller, R. A., & Gaston, K. J. (2017). The rarity of direct experiences of nature in an urban population. *Landscape and Urban Planning, 160*, 79–84. https://doi.org/10.1016/j.landurbplan.2016.12.006

Cruz, D. T., Vázquez, E., Ruales, G., Bayón, M., & García-Torres, M. (2017). *Mapeando el cuerpo-territorio. Guía metodológica para mujeres que defienden sus territorios [Mapping the body-territory. Methodological guide for women who defend their territories].* Ed. Clacso. ISBN-978-9942-30-334-9.

Doménech Gómez, N. (2015). *Aplicación de técnicas cualitativas y cuantitativas Para recoger la respuesta del usuario frente a un espacio arquitectónico [application of qualitative and quantitative techniques to gather the user respoonse regarding an architectonic space].* Universidad Politécnica de Valencia. Escuela Técnica Superior de Gestión en la Edificación - Escuela Técnica Superior de Gestión en Edificación. https://riunet.upv.es/handle/10251/49871

Domínguez Figaredo, D. (2007). Sobre la Intención de la Etnografía virtual. *Revista Electrónica Teoría de la Educación. Educación y Cultura en la Sociedad de la Información, 8*(1), 42–63. [Cross Reference].

Drysdale, K., Newman, C. E., Persson, A., & Gray, R. M. (2020). Mapping experiences of Serodiscordance: Using visual methodologies to construct relationality in families living with or affected by stigmatized infectious disease. *Qualitative Health Research, 30*(5), 793–808. https://doi.org/10.1177/1049732319890304. [Cross Reference].

Ebrahimpour, M. (2020). Proposing a framework of biophilic design principles in hot and arid climate of Iran by using grounded theory. *Civil and Environmental Engineering, 16*(1), 71–78. https://doi.org/10.2478/cee-2020-0008
Egiebor, E. E., & Foster, E. J. (2018). Students' perceptions of their engagement using GIS-story maps. *Journal of Geography, 118*(2), 51–65. [Cross Reference].
Emerson, R. M., Fretz, R. I., & Shaw, L. L. (2011). *Writing ethnographic fieldnotes* (2nd ed.). University of Chicago Press.
Engemann, K., Pedersen, C. B., Arge, L., Tsirogiannis, C., Mortensen, P. B., & Svenning, J.-C. (2019). Residential green space in childhood is associated with lower risk of psychiatric disorders from adolescence into adulthood. *Proceedings of the National Academy of Sciences of the United States of America, 116*(11), 5188–5193. https://doi.org/10.1073/pnas.1807504116
Estalella, A., & Ardèvol, E. (2007). Field ethics: Towards situated ethics for ethnographic research on the internet. *Forum Qualitative Sozialforschung / Forum: Qualitative Social Research, 8*(3). https://doi.org/10.17169/fqs-8.3.277
Franch-Pardo, I., Napoletano, V., Rosete-Verges, F., & Billa, L. (2020). Spatial analysis and GIS in the study of COVID-19. A review. *Science of the Total Environment, 739*. https://doi.org/10.1016/j.scitotenv.2020.140033
Garber, M. (2020). Homes actually need to be practical now: One of the ironies of social distancing is that it can put privacy in short supply. *The Atlantic*. https://www.theatlantic.com/culture/archive/2020/03/finding-privacy-during-pandemic/608944/. Accessed 11 April 2020.
García Pérez, L. (2015). Intención creativa del diseño, hacia una arquitectura emocional. *Revista Legado de Arquitectura y Diseño, 17*, 9–20.
Granda-Cango, K. G. (2016). *El condicionamiento operante como estrategia dentro del proceso de enseñanza en la actualidad educativa ecuatoriana*. Universidad Técnica de Machala.
Gilchrist, K., Brown, C., & Montarzino, A. (2015). Workplace settings and wellbeing: Greenspace use and views contribute to employee wellbeing at peri-urban business sites. *Landscape and Urban Planning journal, 138*, 32–40.
Hammersley, M., & Atkinson, P. (2007). *Ethnography: Principles in practice*. Taylor & Francis Ltd..
Hernández-Sampieri, R., Fernández-Collado, C., & Baptista-Lucio, P. (2006). Recolección y análisis de los datos cualitativos. In *Metodología de la investigación* (pp. 581–683). McGraw-Hill Interamericana.
Hohenthal, J., Minoia, P., & Pellikka, P. (2017). Mapping meaning: Critical cartographies for participatory water management in Taita Hills, Kenya. *The Professional Geographer, 69*, 383–395. [Cross Reference].
Howell, A. J., Dopko, R. L., Passmore, H. A., & Buro, K. (2011). Nature connectedness: Associations with Well-being and mindfulness. *Personality and Individual Differences, 51*(2), 166–171.
Ingold, T. (2011). *Being alive: Essays on movement, knowledge and description*. Routledge. [Cross Reference].
Iconoclasistas. (2011). *Reflexiones cartográficas II*. http://iconoclasistas.com.ar/2011/05/19/reflexiones-cartograficas-ii/ [Cross Reference]. Accessed April 2020.
Instituto Humboldt, & PNUD. (2018). Transiciones socioecológicas hacia la sostenibilidad. Gestión de la biodiversidad en los procesos de cambio de uso de la tierra del territorio colombiano. In G. I. Andrade, M. E. Chaves, G. Corzo, & C. Tapia (Eds.), *Transiciones socioecológicas hacia la sostenibilidad. Gestión de la biodiversidad en los procesos de cambio en el territorio continental colombiano. Primera aproximación*. Instituto de Investigación de Recursos Biológicos Alexander von Humboldt.
Johnson, N. (2014). Why biophilic architecture works: Five reasons and case studies. *Architecture and Design*. https://www.architectureanddesign.com.au/features/features-articles/why-biophilic-architecture-works-five-reasons. Accessed April 2020.
Jones, D. R. (2013). 'The Biophilic university': A de-familiarizing organizational metaphor for ecological sustainability? *Journal of Cleaner Production, 48*, 148–165.
Kellert S. R., Heerwagen J. H. & Mador M. I. (2008) *Biophilic design.: The theory, science, and practice of bringing buildings to life*. Hoboken, New Jersey. ISBN 978-0-470-16334-4.

Krasny, M. E., & Delia, J. (2015). Natural area stewardship as part of campus sustainability. *Journal of Cleaner Production, 106*, 87–96.

Ling, T. Y., & Chiang, Y. C. (2018). Well-being, health and urban coherence-advancing vertical greening approach toward resilience: A design practice consideration. *Journal of Cleaner Production, 182*, 187–197.

Lotito Catino, F. (2009). Arquitectura psicología espacio e individuo. *Revista AUS, 6*. http://www.redalyc.org/articulo.oa?id=281723479003

Magos-Ramírez, S., Serrano-Arellano, J., Dávila-Núñez, M., & Trejo Torres, Z. (2016). Estudios de psicología ambiental en hospital general de Huichapan: elementos sensoriales y bioclimáticos. *Revista de Investigación y Desarrollo, 2*(6), 52–56. https://www.ecorfan.org/spain/research-journals/Investigacion_y_Desarrollo/vol2num6/Revista_de_Investigación_y_Desarrollo_V2_N6_5.pdf

Mangonea, G., Capaldi, C. A., van Allen, Z. M., & Luscuerea, P. G. (2017). Bringing nature to work: Preferences and perceptions of constructed indoor and natural outdoor workspaces. *Urban Forestry & Urban Greening, 23*, 1–12. https://www.sciencedirect.com/science/article/pii/S1618866715301230

Marshall, C., & Rossman, G. (1995). *Designing qualitative research*. Sage. [Cross Reference].

Majoor, S. (2018). Coping with ambiguity: An urban megaproject ethnography. *Progress in Planning, 120*, 1–28.

Maya, M., Cobreros, C., Ontiveros, E., & Biondi, S. (2019). Community Collaboration for Product Design (Co-Co Design): An Academic Alternative for Social Innovation. *Proceedings of the International conference on engineering and product design education 12–13 September 2019, University of Strathclyde, Glasgowm United Kingdom*. https://doi.org/10.35199/epde2019.20

McLees, L. (2013). A postcolonial approach to urban studies: Interviews, mental maps, and photo voices on the urban farms of Dar Es Salaam, Tanzania. *The Professional Geographer, 65*, 283–295. [Cross Reference].

Mercado-Domenech, S., Urbina-Soria, J., & Ortega-Andeane, P. (2016). *Relaciones hombre-entorno: la incursión de la psicología en las ciencias ambientales y del diseño*. UNAM.

Molden, O. C. (2020). Short take: Story-mapping experiences. *Field Methods, 32*(2), 131–139. https://doi.org/10.1177/1525822X19877381

Montero-Sieburth, M. (2006). La auto-etnografía como una estrategia para la transformación de la homogeneidad a favor de la diversidad individual en la escuela. *UNED*. http://www.uned.es/congreso-inter-educacion-intercultural/Grupo_discusion_1/74.pdf [Cross Reference]. Accessed April 2020.

Moser, G. (2009). *Psicología ambiental, Aspectos de las relaciones individuo-medioambiente*. Eco Ediciones.

Ortega-Andeane, P., Estrada, C., Toledano, F., & Campos, J. (2018). Calidad ambiental, carga y estrés en cuidadores primarios informales de un hospital pediátrico. In P. Ortega & C. Estrada (Eds.), *Ambientes hospitalarios y estrés* (pp. 65–96). UNAM.

Ortega-Andeane, P., Galindo-Vázquez, O. R., & Meneses-García, A. (2019). Factores ambientales y estrés en salas de espera: comparación en cuidadores primarios informales de pacientes con Cáncer. *Revista Latinoamericana de Medicina Conductual, 9*(1).

Ozgen, E. (2018). An evaluation on the change of healing perception at healthcare facilities the royal children's hospital. *International Journal of Emerging Trends in Health Sciences, 2*(1), 7–13. https://doi.org/10.18844/ijeths.v2i1.3423

Preuß, M., Nieuwenhuijsen, M., Marquez, S., Cirach, M., Dadvand, P., Triguero-Mas, M., & Zijlema, W. (2019). Low childhood nature exposure is associated with worse mental health in adulthood. *International Journal of Environmental Research and Public Health, 16*(10), 1809. https://doi.org/10.3390/ijerph16101809

Samuelsson, K., Barthel, S., Colding, J., Vetenskapsakademien, K., & Giusti, M. (2020). Urban nature as a source of resilience during social distancing amidst the coronavirus pandemic. OSF Preprints. https://doi.org/10.31219/osf.io/3wx5a. [Cross Reference].

Samson, S., Granath, K., & Alger, A. (2017). Journey mapping the user experience. *College & Research Libraries, 78*(4), 459. https://doi.org/10.5860/crl.78.4.459

Scribano, A., & De Sena, A. (2009). Construcción de Conocimiento en Latinoamérica: Algunas reflexiones desde la auto-etnografía como estrategia de investigación. *Cinta Moebio, 34*, 1–15.

Shanahan, D. F., Fuller, R. A., Bush, R., Lin, B. B., & Gaston, K. J. (2015). The health benefits of urban nature: How much do we need? *Bioscience, 65*(5), 476–485. https://doi.org/10.1093/biosci/biv032

Turner, B. L. (2002). Contested identities: Human-environment geography and disciplinary implications in a restructuring academy. *Annals of the Association of American Geographers, 92*(1), 52–74. [Cross Reference].

Vélez-Torres, I., Rátiva-Gaona, S., & Varela-Corredor, D. (2012). Cartografía social como metodología participativa y colaborativa de investigación en el territorio afrodescendiente de la cuenca alta del río Cauca. *Cuadernos de Geografía, Revista Colombiana de Gegrafía, 21*(2), 59–73. ISSN 0121-215X.

Villegas, M., & Andrés, M. (2008). De la Etnografía antropológica a la Etnografía virtual. Estudio de las relaciones sociales mediadas por Internet. *Fermentum. Revista Venezolana de Sociología y Antropología, 18*(53), 532–549. ISSN: 0798-3069. https://www.redalyc.org/articulo.oa?id=705/70517572006

White, M. P., Alcock, I., Grellier, J., Wheeler, B. W., Hartig, T., Warber, S. L., & Fleming, L. E. (2019). Spending at least 120 minutes a week in nature is associated with good health and wellbeing. *Scientific Reports, 9*(1), 7730. https://doi.org/10.1038/s41598-019-44097-3

Wilson-Edward, O. (1984). *Biophilia*. Harvard University Press.

Wilson, S., & Zamberlan, L. (2015). Design for an unknow future: Amplified roles for collaboration, new design knowledge and creativity. *Design Issues, 31*(2), 3–15.

Yin, J., Zhu, S., MacNaughton, P., Allen, J. G., & Spengler, J. D. (2018). Physiological and cognitive performance of exposure to biophilic indoor environment. *Building and Environment, 132*, 255–262.

Zhang, J. W., Piff, P. K., Iyer, R., Koleva, S., & Keltner, D. (2014). An occasion for unselfing: Beautiful nature leads to prosociality. *Journal of Environmental Psychology, 37*, 61–72. https://doi.org/10.1016/j.jenvp.2013.11.008

Chapter 9
Feeding, Solidarity, and Care: The Grassroots Experiences of Latin American Soup Kitchens in a Global Pandemic

Salvador Leetoy and Tommaso Gravante

Introduction

Latin American countries are struggling to contain the COVID-19 pandemic while facing serious challenges to their national economies. The deterioration of public services has pushed people into poverty, especially the vulnerable, due to extreme inequality. Our discussion is mainly focused on the resurgence of soup kitchens in the region (in Spanish, ollas comunitarias or ollas populares). These community kitchens are organized by volunteers, sharing what they have to try to cope with unemployment and the absence of public policies and aimed at ameliorating the harsh economic conditions produced by the pandemic. Usually, they receive the help and support of activists, philanthropic organizations, NGOs, and sometimes trade unions and local government institutions. However, here, we pay special attention to grassroots and activist self-organized groups to provide free or very low-cost meals to low-income and homeless individuals who are hard hit by the shutting down of economic activities to slow the virus spread.

In the 1980s and 1990s, soup kitchens proliferated all over large cities in South America, such as Lima, Montevideo, Buenos Aires, and Santiago. These *ollas comunitarias* were a response to the difficult economic circumstances of poor urban individuals, especially those living in periphery neighborhoods devastated by the financial crisis produced by neoliberal policies, the privatization of public services, cuts to social expenditure by the government, and the general disdain toward anything related to the construction of a welfare state (Roberts & Portes, 2006; Hicks

S. Leetoy (✉)
Escuela de Humanidades y Educación, Tecnológico de Monterrey, Guadalajara, México
e-mail: sleetoy@tec.mx

T. Gravante
Centro de Investigaciones Interdisciplinarias en Ciencias y Humanidades, Universidad Nacional Autónoma de México, Ciudad de México, México

© The Author(s), under exclusive license to Springer Nature Switzerland AG 2021

M. A. Montoya et al. (eds.), *COVID-19 and Cities*, The Urban Book Series,
https://doi.org/10.1007/978-3-030-84134-8_9

& Wodon, 2001). In light of the current COVID-19 pandemic, the inadequate and unaffordable access to health care and weak public services have aggravated the living conditions of the poor, daily waged, and informal workers in the area (OXFAM, 2020).

Accordingly, contrary to prevailing individualistic and utilitarian dynamics, we state that the pandemic has made evident the urgent necessity to restore the city's collectivistic social imagination as a locus for solidarity, social interactivity, and empathy. The design of contemporary cities has been based on an instrumental reason permeating the architecture of urban spaces. It flows in forms of exclusion based on discriminatory practices, such as ghettoization and gentrification; socio-economic privilege notoriously appears on the maps of the city, connecting areas and not individuals (Harvey, 2012; Lefebvre, 1996). Billboards, highways, urban landscapes, and public and private transit policies and strategies define how people commute and the city communicates, but not necessarily how they interact with one another. On the contrary, they are alienated and disconnected from public discussions related to their well-being and common social situation (Martín Barbero, 2001). Thus, soup kitchens are considered exemplary sites of connecting subaltern individuals, a reminder of the importance of restoring networks of care when societies are in turmoil. These forms of communitarian practices emphasize and make visible people's needs, as well as the imperative responsibility to act in consequence. After all, if nothing else, the presence of soup kitchens serves to uncover the cracks of the façade of modern, urban individualism, one based on the absence of public discourse and engagement. As stated by Richard Sennet (1994):

> Navigating the geography of modern society requires very little physical effort, hence engagement… as roads become straightened and regularized, the voyager needs account less and less for the people and the buildings on the street in order to move, making minute motions in an ever less complex environment (p. 18).

Therefore, we establish that the COVID-19 pandemic is a harsh reminder that we need to take seriously the route of ethics of care for promoting community resilience and the transformation of the city as a collaborative space. First, we posit a critical discussion of collective action and participatory publics to review the notions of care, otherness, and emotions. We consider these three concepts quintessential to challenging dominant instrumentality in Latin American politics, one that regards care as solely pertaining to the private realm, apart from in public life discussion. Taking the feminist maxim of "the private is public," we consider it crucial to rethink the concept of citizenship and social justice in the light of extreme conditions, such as the current pandemic. In the second part, we focus on issues of solidarity and empathy. Based on the review of grassroots soup kitchen initiatives in Latin America, we discuss social capital creation through civic participation.

The old and long tradition of soup kitchens in the region has had a resurgence because of the pandemic, turning their actions into potential citizen labs where people are not just fed but interact, collaborate, and help one another. We conclude that citizenship and ethics of care must not be separated concepts but an integral part of one another. Feeding the other by intervening in the city, is not merely an act of solidarity against market-driven policies, it may also be a strategy for agency formation through the consideration of care as a key element of civics, one embedded in notions of kindness, reciprocity, and compassion.

The analysis is based on a digital ethnography of more than 50 grassroots experiences that have emerged throughout the pandemic in Latin America between March and August 2020. We integrate the terms of our elaboration from digitally mediated field notes, derived from online participant observation in blogs and social media sites of soup kitchen collectives, as well as online and offline contributions from activists.[1]

Better Never Means Better for Everyone: Neoliberalism, Poverty, and COVID-19

In one of the most shocking passages of Margaret Atwood's "Handmaid's Tales" (1985), the protagonist of the novel, a woman called June, starts a conversation with the commander to whom she is serving as a "handmaid." In Atwood's narrative, a handmaid is a fertile woman who is submitted to state-engineered rape to give birth to children for Gilead's regime. This theocratic government is in command of what was once the United States. June, renamed as Offred after her commander (i.e., Of-Fred or belonging to Fred), is asked for her opinion on Gilead's regime and how things have worked out. In this strange moment of leniency between the despotic master and the subordinate handmaid, a bewildered June answers that she is not entitled to have an opinion on those subject matters.

Nonetheless, the answer seems obvious. Gilead has only produced benefits for a few, and despair and oppression for most, all in the name of progress and under the pretext of saving society from a sharp fertility decline. She does not dare to say it out loud, even though her disheartened countenance makes it evident. "You can't make an omelette without breaking eggs," the commander says, "we thought we could do better." "Better?" June responds softly. "How can he think this is better?" she thought to herself. "Better never means better for everyone," the commander answers, seeming to guess June's thought, "it always means worse, for some," concludes his statement (Atwood, 2017, Ch. 32).

"The Handmaid's Tale" is a dystopian text based on speculative fiction, meaning that it theorizes about possible futures, warning about how societies can set themselves, or interpretations of events that have actual precedents. In this case, it depicts a negative scenario warning about the dangers of authoritarian and egotistical practices. Novels, poems, stories, all cultural narratives, suffer from what is called "Cassandra's Curse," the Greek priestess to whom Apollo granted the gift of prophecy on condition that no one would believe her (Manguel, 2007, p. 20). Stories like

[1] We have interviewed 16 activists from the CDMX Ayuda Mutua project: https://cdmxayudamutua.org

Atwood's novel present gloomy predictions of a future picture of present conditions. However, societies are sometimes reluctant to believe in the risks of events that are considered just part of the path of progress and development. In this case, "better never means better for everyone" fits precisely within the logic of neoliberalism: a narrative engendered under the tenets of the Washington Consensus, which is founded on an economic and social model based on privatization, liberalization, and the prioritization of market relations over the welfare of the general public (de Sousa Santos, 2006). However, crisis and social unrest expose discourses behind the contradictions of power relations like neoliberalism, permeating all aspects of everyday life. Individualism over collectivism, privatization against public goods, utilitarianism over cooperativism, all these prerogatives are propelling the structural functioning of globalization suited to the indicators and requirements of dominant institutions such as the International Monetary Fund, the World Bank, and the political interests of the so-called developed countries (Chomsky, 1998; Harvey, 2005).

The COVID-19 pandemic that is afflicting the world is not only a public health problem. The different responses by states to the hundreds of thousands of infected people, the increasing death toll, and the confinement of entire populations worldwide demonstrate and exponentially magnify the neoliberal model's consequences that have guided public policy over the last 4 decades. Like all domination systems, neoliberalism is not only an economic doctrine, and it expands its domination to other spheres of social life, provoking diversification and a multiplicity of antagonisms derived from these domination logics (Laclau & Mouffe, 1985, p. 161). It is characterized by its adherence to social Darwinism principles, not on those of sympathy and co-responsibility. It is a model in which the natural order of things is based on the teleological conception of progress, one centered on the idea of mastering nature and the domination of Man over all living things. Of course, we intentionally use the concept of "Man": neoliberalism follows a patriarchal ideology that encourages the formation of hierarchies, extreme individualism, market authoritarianism, egoism, and narcissism, among other aspects. That is why ethics of care, a notion influenced by feminist approaches (Tronto, 1993), is at odds with neoliberal policies because the latter values domination and selfishness to climb the social ladder rather than altruistic or biospheric goals. Feminist theory, according to Iris Marion Young (1996), politicizes "the social by questioning a dichotomy of public and private and thereby proposing that family relations, sexuality, and the gendered relations of the street, school and workplace are properly political relations" (p. 487). Carol Pateman (1988) argues that caretaking must be at the center of all political discussions and a theme to be included in the Social Contract, not taken for granted, because someone else has to do it. Feeding the other and caring for the other is a political statement that brings everyday social interaction and culture into the formation of participative and responsible citizenship, one beyond the mere election of representatives and the law's observance.

In this landscape of authoritarianism, individualism, and despair, social movements continue to play a fundamental role in building social alternatives. As collective mobilization grows, the hope for change ensues for another world that is still possible and all the more needed (della Porta, 2020). Since the beginning of the pandemic, we have witnessed how social movements, at the national and transnational levels, have canceled and suspended their public actions. However, they have quickly adapted to the new social circumstances we live in, and they are adopting creative tactics for protests in the era of social distancing (Bringel & Pleyers, 2020; Faiola et al., 2020). Most of them have followed technopolitical advancements: the encompassing of connective and collective digital actions merging multiple identity vanguards; the innovation in the design of public policy arisen from collective intelligence and hacktivism; and collaborative productions for restoring the public space, among many other forms of digital and agency civics aimed at developing strategies for communicative action in the middle of the current pandemic (Chattopadhyay et al., 2020).

There are several examples of this adaptation: webinars, virtual strikes, conferences, teach-ins, assemblies, and other online initiatives and digital protests. From an emotional point of view, these activities allow participants to connect with other people worldwide and feel united and stronger, instead of isolated and powerless. Therefore, social justice movements have not just been particularly active during this pandemic period; they have developed original and innovative strategies to reclaim the public space virtually and by some selective physical means. These movements are mostly due to the systemic destruction of well-being policies aimed at the amelioration of human needs, such as health, feeding, housing, education, and leisure. As stated by Geoffrey Pleyers (2020, p. 2), "[a]round the world, activists focused their energy in implementing five roles: protests (that re-emerged in some countries despite sanitary risks); defending workers' rights; mutual aid and solidarity; monitoring policymakers and popular education."

Indeed, at the local level, many grassroots groups are organizing themselves to deal with the pandemic's social costs and cope with the needs that the most underprivileged communities are experiencing. We are not talking about associations of social workers, NGOs, or other groups using public and private funds to solve needs created by the neoliberal system itself. The grassroots activism we have in mind is born of autonomous, self-organized groups that carry out direct action at protest events and everyday practices.

Undoubtedly, sociological imagination is required to dig into the human potential to solve a crisis. This imagination enables the realization of alternative and critical reasoning to challenge domination and oppression. Charles Wright Mills (2000 [1959], p. 5) explains this concept as follows:

> The sociological imagination enables its possessor to understand the larger historical scene in terms of its meaning for the inner life and the external career of a variety of individuals. It enables him to take into account how individuals, in the welter of their daily experience, often become falsely conscious of their social positions. Within that welter, the framework of modern society is sought, and within that framework the psychologies of a variety of men and women are formulated. By such means the personal uneasiness of individuals is focused upon explicit troubles and the indifference of publics is transformed into involvement with public issues.

Accordingly, we consider that the resurgence of ollas comunitarias is in line with a sociological imagination acting as a catalyzer to civic involvement and participation in critical circumstances and survival emergencies. It follows a pragmatic strategy to help people feel supported and soothed in times of uncertainty and distress. Following a similar pragmatic perspective as Wright Mills, Richard Rorty (1989) proposes his notion of the liberal ironist, defined as those people who hope that suffering will be diminished, that humiliation of human beings by other human beings may cease. Rorty (1989, p. xvi) presents a route for both sociological imagination and agency, and splendidly states:

> In my utopia, human solidarity would be seen not as a fact to be recognized by clearing away "prejudice" or burrowing down to previously hidden depths but, rather, as a goal to be achieved. It is to be achieved not by inquiry but by imagination, the imaginative ability to see strange people as fellow sufferers. Solidarity is not discovered by reflection but created. It is created by increasing our sensitivity to the particular details of the pain and humiliation of other, unfamiliar, sorts of people. Such increased sensitivity makes it more difficult to marginalize people different from ourselves by thinking, "They do not feel it as we would," or "There must always be suffering, so why not let them suffer?"

Latin American countries have failed to assist the most vulnerable families. Among the problems that plague Latin America are the precariousness of large sectors of its population, mostly informally employed, the collapse of the social services due to decades of government oblivion, and the weak leadership of politicians who downsized the severity of the pandemic to protect their political interests (Enriquez et al., 2020). For this reason, citizens have had to seize the initiative to act by themselves. Accordingly, in the following section, we review caring collective actions via the organization of *ollas comunes*, which are created to palliate the suffering caused by this global health emergency.

Urban Grassroots Activism During the Pandemic

Since the first half of March 2020, the health crisis has become a deep social crisis too. We have observed in several cities the emergence of many different grassroots groups whose primary goal is to deal with the needs of the most underprivileged urban communities. In the United States, more than 300 local groups and mutual support networks had been set up by April 2020. In Spain, even during the highest peak of the pandemic in March, around 188 groups had already been formed in 57 towns and cities. In the United Kingdom, about 4000 groups across the country were supporting people through different social initiatives. In Chile, Argentina, Uruguay, Peru, and Colombia, hundreds of soup kitchens were set up by groups of volunteers to feed the local population. As mentioned above, ollas populares are spaces organized by neighbors and activists where food is collected and cooked for those most in need. In Mexico, Guatemala, Ecuador, Peru, and Brazil, among other countries, tens of mutual aid groups involved in different social activities had already been formed.

There is nothing like a homogenous experience of soup kitchen establishments in Latin America. Although it varies among countries, they follow a common cause on the continent, marked by severe inequality and weak public services caused by decades of neoliberal policies. These, at times, spontaneous and diverse surges of solidarity are part of social practices challenging the states' incapacity to respond quickly to a humanitarian crisis due to the market-driven design of public policies, in addition to the high levels of corruption at all levels of government institutions. Moreover, these spaces do not only provide hunger relief. Some of them have been able to organize different collaborations with social service workers, medical personnel, artists, and local public officials to offer psychological support, help to female victims of domestic violence and sex workers, art workshops, and more.

Accordingly, these experiences are exemplary practices of community resilience. In this case, it integrates the participation and collaboration of diverse publics and subaltern subjects to deal with risks compromising their well-being. Resilience is also a matter of creativity and co-creation of alternatives for survival in times of crisis, prompting forms of civic agency to actively connect networks of publics focused on mitigating calamities aggravated by prior systemic conditions.

These interventions in the public space represent a challenge to egotistic and one-dimensional policies governing the city's communication. They are focused instead on practices that encourage social capital creation; those forms of social solidarity, reciprocity, and interplaying of citizens interested in democratizing the public space (Putnam, 2000, Ch. 1). Moreover, social capital provides resources to soothe distress in disaster situations (Aldrich & Meyer, 2015) and stimulates adaptative capacities to mitigate suffering through collaboration and association (Berkes & Ross, 2013). In the same vein, Victoria Held (2006, p. 10) attests, "the central focus of the ethics of care is on the compelling moral salience of attending to and meeting the needs of the particular others for whom we take responsibility." The pandemic has made evident that the exacerbated individualism proper to exclusion practices neglects the urban poor of better conditions for dealing with this health and economic crisis. In Latin America, the vulnerability of those communities is particularly severe. For example, according to the Oxford Poverty and Human Development Initiative, three indicators capture the risk of COVID-19 infection: lack of access to safe drinking water, use of noxious fuels inside homes, and malnutrition (UNDP, 2020). This initiative reports that one-quarter of the region, about 142 million people, are at risk of contracting COVID-19.

The practices proposed by these grassroots experiences are mainly characterized by direct action in their everyday life. In this case, the immediate action aims at producing improvements to human conditions within a specific oppressed community (illegal migrants, nomads, prisoners, groups in extreme poverty, ethnic groups, etc.). Another prominent characteristic of these mutual support groups is that they do not see themselves as, nor do they have ties to, NGOs, volunteer associations, charities, or other bodies funded by public or private funds. As highlighted by one of the mutual support networks in England: "We are not an organization or charity, and local groups are not officially affiliated with us. We are not affiliated with any political or religious groups, though we are united by a belief that social exclusion increases individual and community vulnerability."[2] Thus, the soup kitchen experiences provide a grassroots scenario for *extitutional* creativity based on community resilience: a series of practical actions derived from solidary networked efforts developed by citizen collaborations transcending institutional prerogatives and directives.

A qualitative mapping carried out in these months in different cities around the world[3] allowed us to establish the various activities that define this grassroots activism in the COVID-19 era. In some cases, this information showed that groups and networks focus on just one of these activities, while others present more than one:

1. Collection and distribution of food and essential supplies.
2. Support for health matters, such as free appointments or collection and free distribution of medicines.
3. Support on civil rights, labor, or abuse matters, such as dealing with domestic violence, violation of labor rights, legal aid for illegal migrant communities, or prison communities.
4. Support for highly vulnerable people or those with illnesses who cannot risk going out, including shopping, walking pets, paying for services, and sometimes keeping them company and providing emotional support.

Regardless of the activities, these experiences show that one of the main objectives has been to show that another world is possible, outside the logic of the neoliberal model, i.e., a (potential) world characterized by mutual aid, solidarity, respect, fraternity, and anti-authoritarianism. Unlike simple actions that impact just near or proximate individuals or relatives (for example, shopping for a neighbor who cannot go out, sharing information on social networks, etc.), this form of activism has disruptive potential. It reveals the failure of a system founded on individualism and competition, generating a response based on compassion and solidarity. This process is fundamental to create mobilization. It makes it possible to transform fear, anger, and pain into collaboration; its discontent motivates the creation of collective actions, encouraging the identification of those to make accountable for the past and present dismantling of welfare institutions.

The pandemic has worsened inequality in the current food system, promoted by an economic model based on social injustice and exploitation. For some countries, such as Latin America, the halt of productive activity, the lack of public health and social measures, as well as poverty and structural inequality, have meant the loss of jobs (formal and informal) for millions of people, and access to food for themselves and their families has been put at stake. The Latin American "dormitory suburbs," in addition to being areas of social inequality, have been turned into real deserts of despair and misery; urban places where thousands of people find access to a healthy daily diet difficult. For this reason, the groups and networks which are collecting

[2] https://covidmutualaid.org/faq/

[3] We have mainly observed cities in the US, Italy, Spain, UK, Mexico, Argentina, Chile, Brazil, Guatemala, Colombia, and Peru.

and freely distributing food and essential supplies have become among the primary experiences of collective action present in the Latin American countries. As an activist of the project *CDMX, Ayuda Mutua* said: "Everyone deserves to feed their families and stay safe. We will get through this together" has been the *leitmotif* of dozens of these experiences of coping with these social interventions in the public space.

These *ollas comunitarias* (also called fondas comunitarias, ollas populares, comedores populares, depending on the country) have taken on a broader social significance. They can be transformed into citizen labs due to the diversity of publics they attend and the different subaltern groups participating. Thanks to the presence of new social actors, such as collectives of the recent wave of Latin American feminism and climate activism, anti-speciesist groups, urban gardens, LGTBQ collectives, libertarian groups, among others, these soup kitchens have been redesigned to actively strengthen the social fabric and the creation of social capital in the community. It creates a new understanding of the city as a locus of diversity and empathy.

For example, in Argentina, the *La Toma* group cooks without animal products; that is, they promote a diet without animal suffering, trying to expand the circle of compassion to non-human living beings. In Chile, the soup kitchen in Mostazal known as the Olla en Resistencia, and the one in Los Angeles, the Olla común, are organized around a feminist frame, proposing workshops and talks against female violence. In Uruguay, these expediencies connect peasant cooperative networks to claim the people's right to food sovereignty, as in the case of the *Mercado Popular de Subsistencia* (MPS), a network of 50 self-managed territorial groups coordinated to purchase outside of supermarkets. To sum up, these experiences are characterized by a response to the crisis based on compassion and solidarity which counters a hegemonic pandemic response based on individualism and cynicism.

Besides mitigating social problems generated by the crisis at a local level, soup kitchens collectively work on a series of emotions, such as powerlessness, despair, shame, or sadness, and encourage the emergence of other collective *resistance* emotions (Whittier, 2001). Those are necessary to emphasize the social injustice experienced by COVID-19 and eventually reconstitute their degraded urban social fabric.

Based on the mottos of *Collective care is our best weapon against COVID-19* and *Solidarity not charity*, these soup kitchen experiences are challenging the dominant social and cultural model, proposing, through their practices, a resilient process that involves values and emotions. In solidarity, support from grassroots groups can break through this feeling of guilt and stigma thanks to a collaborative framing process that manages trauma due to resistance emotions. In the case of soup kitchens organized throughout the pandemic, the trauma emotions include, for example, the pain of losing a loved one, fear and distress about getting ill or infecting others, the shame of not having the economic resources to feed themselves, the humiliation of not being able to provide financial security to their loved ones, and the sadness and resignation of living in poverty.

As a result, to manage these emotions, these grassroots experiences promote collaborative strategies, such as sharing emotions like pain, fear, sadness, etc., without feeling weak and defeated; framing these emotions as consequences of a crisis for which some dominant groups are politically responsible and are losing guilt about feeling these emotions and the implications of this situation in their lives. The management of these emotions provides space to build a political discourse around trauma (Champagne, 1996). In other words, sharing and accepting trauma emotions enable the exposing of personal experience as a collective injustice in the entire social arena (Gamson, 1992). It allows one to overcome guilt and stigma and provides an opportunity to look for those socially responsible for the consequences experienced, for example, government authorities and corporations.

Another collective process that is taking place in Latin American soup kitchens involves resistance emotions (Whittier, 2001). These are hope, moral anger, indignation, pride, and reciprocal emotions such as love and respect, which help people cope with trauma and produce emotional energy (Collins, 2001, 2012; Jasper, 2011, 2018). This category of emotions permits people affected by the pandemic to recover from grief and overcome powerlessness and the sentiment of helplessness and vulnerability emerging through traumatic situations. One consequence of this emotional work is that people who received help are empowered and participate in their self-recuperation projects. It is sometimes evident in the experiences presented here, that some of those who benefited from the soup kitchens helped organize them afterward. Moreover, evoking resistance emotions enables people to overcome powerlessness and creates an injustice frame around their social vulnerability (Poma & Gravante, 2019). By generating feelings of empowerment (Drury & Reicher, 2009), resistance emotions go beyond the event itself, producing an impact on people's lives in the present, and probably in the future, by getting involved in new projects (Drury & Reicher, 2009, p.714).

Emotions are a fundamental characteristic observed in soup kitchens. It is a feature embraced in the ethics of care. As mentioned above, even anger and anxiety are components of moral indignation that trigger social justice and equality claims. It also values individuals' interdependence, avoiding isolation and exclusion, contrary to the city's market-oriented architecture. In a nutshell, being helped and being worthy of compassion is not an anti-value but a common human condition. Joan Tronto (2015, p. 8) states that "a functioning democracy is full of people who are attentive, responsible, competent and responsive." "Caring about" makes us attentive, says the author, because as soon as we witness others' unmet needs, we pay attention to the sort of problems causing that problem. "Caring for" makes us responsible, because we encourage ourselves and others to perform in case of any given required action. "Caregiving" makes us competent because we gain knowledge and experience in serving others. Finally, "care-receiving" makes us responsive, because we ask for responses to know the given care's quality and identify new needs (Tronto, 2015, pp. 4–7). Care, then, should be an essential component of citizenship, one formed on meeting needs and the co-responsibility of actively participating in helping those in distress. It recognizes our finitude and the inauthentic existence based on selfishness and narcissism. It emphasizes the importance of active collaboration to fashion a more democratic space for all citizens to enjoy. Of course, it is always a work in progress, but it needs to be done to make the city a more just place for all. The soup kitchen initiatives are a good reminder of this.

To conclude, in this time of the pandemic, soup kitchens lead to debating not only the causes of this food crisis or the discussing of other social problems, such as the climate crisis, racism, or female violence, they also offer grassroots responses based on altruistic emotions and values. Thanks to this prefigurative approach, they are building resilient social alternatives that could face economic and social crises in the future.

Conclusions: The Political Prefiguration of Alternative Futures for Our Cities

As we wrote earlier, the presence of emotions linked to social stigma is connected to a demand for specific values concerning others, such as collectivism over individualism, commons against privatization, and cooperativism over utilitarianism. It also involves experimentation in innovative practices and discourses for community resilience experiences, such as in the case of soup kitchens as described here. One of the significant impacts of this type of grassroots activism is the opening of a debate on current forms of food production, distribution, access, and consumption.

At the same time, they are practicing a possible diet without animal suffering. They organize workshops on feminism and the different sexualities, the environment and the climate crisis, self-management practice, and the possibility of a solidarity economy. These experiences have surpassed their "kitchen" boundaries, because they are connected to other neighborhood projects, such as community bakeries, urban gardens, peasant cooperatives, and artistic projects. In this way, they create mutual solidarity networks to strengthen the social fabric of these disadvantaged urban community spaces. These networks are transformed into a political expression of their everyday lives, shaping a resilient political identity. A collective identity, on one hand, serves to strengthen the circle of "we" (the poor, the marginalized, the sick, the supported, etc.), and on the other hand, serves to build the circle of "they" (the powerful, the elite, the individualists, etc.).

We can see that these experiences of grassroots activism seek coherence between means and ends, practices and values; that is, the soup kitchens emerging throughout this global pandemic are prefigurative experiences. The activists connect social change to their everyday lives to develop new social relationships and experiences in their local dimension. The feminist slogan, "the personal is political" has been reinterpreted as "the everyday life is political." The commitment for those who promote these experiences is the coherence between their direct action and their values, such as respect for nature, solidarity, trust, and mutual aid. A commitment therefore has a prefigurative character in values and beliefs. These social experiences do their best to choose the strategies and practices that fit the type of society that they claim and propose for themselves and others (Gravante, 2019; Maeckelbergh, 2009; Yates, 2014). The means–ends relationship is not only structured on the commitment assumed by everyone, but the prefigurative orientation is also developed around values, beliefs, and moral emotions, and very significantly, on ethics of care.

The prefigurative character of the soup kitchens in Latin America during this pandemic is building a new form of political action that is not only capable of creating new alternative food geographies; it can also promote alternative futures for our cities and open a range of possibilities and desires in opposition to the current neoliberal system. This prefiguration is a particular way of bridging, on the one hand, the temporal distinction between the immediacy of the here and now, and an alternative future society, practice, or organization, on the other hand. The tendencies and performances of these experiences consist of attempting to confront and transform the status quo. In other words, Latin American soup kitchens are not a proposed alternative to social struggle, but rather "'future ends" of this struggle.

The politicization process of everyday life allows the protagonists to redefine how they see the world. In this process, the activists are searching for alternative practices that are coherent with their goals and resilience to crisis. This prefigurative characterization includes the possibility of imagining the construction of alternatives linked to activities of everyday life, such as care.

In Latin America, the urban grassroots activism of soup kitchens is not only facing the problem of daily sustenance, but also breaking the borders that confined the concept and practice of care, one generally conceived as an individualistic practice (especially if we talk about urban contexts), and a patriarchal one, because it is considered a woman's task. The experiences lived in these aid networks, the collectivization of resistance emotions, and the prefigurative practices characterized by values such as solidarity, friendship, love, and respect make caring a fundamental democratic concept. People who participate in these experiences feel that the only way to protect themselves is to protect their community and their social and natural environment. The dual expression of rationality and emotion, the feeling-thinking process (Jasper, 2018), breaks down gender, age, and social status roles, and the differences between human and non-human living beings. It is all-inclusive collective care, where the ethical premises and respect for nature and people (the circle of us) play a prominent role.

We are still only at the beginning of a much broader and more painful crisis than we see now, and we do not know all of the consequences yet. We can already feel the impact of individualistic practices because of the human catastrophe the pandemic is causing. We consider that our hope is again sustained in life's everyday struggles, in the politicization of identities that act through grassroots activism, mobilizing thousands of people worldwide to open up positions for propelling and promoting civic agency and restoring the public space.

There will likely be no return to normality for people who participate in these soup kitchens. The crisis will leave profound social wounds and fractures, but we also know that normality has brought us to where we are now. Moreover, we do not yet know if these experiences will strengthen this feeling of collective care and weaken the neoliberal system's cultural component. However, we think that everything that is being done will be needed to build other conceptions of living in the city, demonstrating that there is no possible civilization without care and that establishing a moral economy is a global priority.

References

Aldrich, D. P., & Meyer, M. A. (2015). Social capital and community resilience. *American Behavioral Scientist, 59*(2), 254–269. https://doi.org/10.1177/0002764214550299

Atwood, M. (2017). *The Handmaid's Tales*. Vintage. [Kindle Edition].

Berkes, F., & Ross, R. (2013). Community resilience: Toward an integrated approach. *Society & Natural Resources, 26*(1), 5–20. https://doi.org/10.1080/08941920.2012.736605

Bringel, B., & Pleyers, G. (Eds.). (2020). *Alerta global. Políticas, movimientos sociales y futuros en disputa en tiempos de pandemia [Global Alert: Policies, Social Movements, and Futures in Dispute during Pandemic Times]*. CLACSO.

Champagne, R. (1996). *The politics of survivorship*. New York University Press.

Chattopadhyay, S., Wood, L., & Cox, L. (Eds.). (2020). Special issue: Organizing amidst Covid-19. *Interface: A Journal For and About Social Movements, 12*(1), 1–400.

Chomsky, N. (1998). *Profit over people: Neoliberalism and global order*. Seven Stories Press.

Collins, R. (2001). Social movements and the focus of emotional attention. In J. Goodwin, J. M. James, & F. Polletta (Eds.), *Passionate politics: Emotions and social movements* (pp. 27–44). University of Chicago Press.

Collins, R. (2012). C-escalation and D-escalation: A theory of the time-dynamics of conflict. *American Sociological Review, 77*(1), 1–20.

Drury, J., & Reicher, S. D. (2009). Collective psychological empowerment as a model of social change: Researching crowds and power. *Journal of Social Issues, 65*(4), 707–726. https://doi.org/10.1111/j.1540-4560.2009.01622.x

Enriquez, D., Rojas, S., & Centeno, M. (2020, September 1). Latin America's COVID-19 nightmare lessons from the World's hardest-hit region. *Foreign Affairs*. https://www.foreignaffairs.com/articles/americas/2020-09-01/latin-americas-covid-19-nightmare. Accessed Nov 2020.

Faiola, A., Wessel, L., & Mahtani, S. (2020, April 20). World health crisis forces activists to innovate. *The Guardian*, A 26. Accessed Sep 2020.

Gamson, W. (1992). *Talking politics*. Cambridge University Press.

Gravante, T. (2019). Prácticas emergentes de activismo alimentario en la Ciudad de México [Emerging Practices of Alimentary Activism in Mexico City]. *Iberoforum, Revista de Ciencias Sociales de la Universidad Iberoamericana, 14*(28), 105–125.

Harvey, D. (2005). *A brief history of neoliberalism*. Oxford University Press.

Harvey, D. (2012). *Rebel cities: From the right to the city to the urban revolution*. Verso.

Held, V. (2006). *The ethics of care: Personal, political, and global*. Oxford University Press.

Hicks, N., & Wodon, Q. (2001). Social protection for the poor in Latin America. *CEPAL Review, 73*, 93–113.

Jasper, J. M. (2011). Emotions and social movements: Twenty years of theory and research. *Annual Review of Sociology, 37*, 285–303. https://doi.org/10.1146/annurev-soc-081309-150015

Jasper, J. M. (2018). *The emotions of protest*. University of Chicago Press.

Laclau, E., & Mouffe, C. (1985). *Hegemony & socialist strategy*. Verso.

Lefebvre, H. (1996). *Writings on cities*. Wiley-Blackwell.

Maeckelbergh, M. (2009). *The will of the many: How the alterglobalisation movement is changing the face of democracy*. Pluto Press.

Manguel, A. (2007). *The city of words*. Anansi.

Martín Barbero, J. (2001). *Al sur de la modernidad. Comunicación, globalización y multiculturalidad* [South to Modernity. Communication, Globalization, and Multiculturalism]. IILI-Serie Nuevo Siglo.

OXFAM. (2020). *How the coronavirus pandemic exploits the worst aspects of extreme inequality*. https://www.oxfam.org/en/how-coronavirus-pandemic-exploits-worst-aspects-extreme-inequality

Pateman, C. (1988). *The sexual contract*. Stanford University Press.

Pleyers, G. (2020). The pandemic is a battlefield. Social movements in the COVID-19 lockdown. *Journal of Civil Society*. https://doi.org/10.1080/17448689.2020.1794398

Poma, A., & Gravante, T. (2019). 'Nunca seremos las mismas de antes'. Emociones y empoderamiento colectivo en los movimientos sociales: el Colectivo Mujer Nueva (Oaxaca, México) ['We'll never be the same as before'. Feelings and collective empowerment in social movements: The new woman collective (Oaxaca, Mexico)]. *Desafíos, 31*(2), 231–265. https://doi.org/10.12804/revistas.urosario.edu.co/desafios/a.7308

della Porta, D. (2020). Movimientos sociales en tiempos de COVID-19: Otro mundo es necesario [Social movements in COVID-19 times: Another world is necessary]. In B. Bringel & G. Pleyers (Eds.), *Alerta global. Políticas, movimientos sociales y futuros en disputa en tiempos de pandemia* (pp. 175–180). CLACSO.

Putnam, R. (2000). *Bowling alone. The collapse and revival of American community*. Simon & Schuster [Kindle Edition].

Roberts, B., & Portes, A. (2006). Coping with the free market city. Collective action in six Latin American cities at the end of the twentieth century. *Latin American Research Review, 41*(2), 57–83.

Rorty, R. (1989). *Contingency, irony, and solidarity*. Cambridge University Press.

Sennet, R. (1994). *Flesh and stone. The body and the city in Western civilization*. W. W. Norton & Company.

de Sousa Santos, B. (2006). Globalizations. *Theory, Culture & Society, 23*(2–3), 393–399. https://doi.org/10.1177/026327640602300268

Tronto, J. (1993). *Moral Boundaries*. Routledge.

Tronto, J. (2015). *Who Cares. How to Reshape a Democratic Politics*. Cornell University Press.

UNDP. (2020, July 14). In Latin America, COVID-19 infections surge as virtually every country faces recession. *United Nations Development Programme*. https://www.undp.org/content/undp/en/home/news-centre/news/2020/LAC_COVID19_infections_surge_as_countries_face_recession.html. Accessed Aug 2020.

Whittier, N. (2001). Emotional strategies: The collective reconstruction and display of oppositional emotions in the movement against child sexual abuse. In J. Goodwin, J. M. James, & F. Polletta (Eds.), *Passionate politics: Emotions and social movements* (pp. 233–250). University of Chicago Press.

Wright Mills, C. (2000 [1959]). *The sociological imagination*. Oxford University Press.

Yates, L. (2014). Rethinking prefiguration: Alternatives, micropolitics and goals in social movements. *Social Movement Studies, 14*(1), 1–21. https://doi.org/10.1080/14742837.2013.870883

Young, I. M. (1996). Political theory. An overview. In R. Goodwin & H. D. Klingerman (Eds.), *A new handbook of political science* (pp. 479–502). Oxford University Press.

Chapter 10
The Impact of COVID-19 on Informal Settlements in Buenos Aires, Argentina

Ana Laura Azparren Almeira

Introduction

The COVID-19 pandemic has revealed the vast and longstanding territorial inequalities that persist in Latin American cities. Although it has been said that the virus does not discriminate between social classes, its spread from March to October 2020 has had a differential impact on the working-class neighborhoods and the informal urban settlements of the region's largest cities.[1]

According to UN-Habitat data (2015), one in four urban dwellers in Latin America resides in an informal settlement. These neighborhoods are characterized by poor access to basic services (running water, electricity, and sanitation), poor housing conditions, and high levels of overcrowding in households.

In this chapter, we aim to analyze the characteristics of the impact of COVID-19 on the informal settlements of the City of Buenos Aires, as well as the public policies implemented in these neighborhoods and the work developed by territorial organizations to reduce the social, health, and economic consequences of the pandemic.

As we will analyze in this chapter, the work carried out by these territorial organizations has been fundamental for the sustainability of life in these neighborhoods

[1]Although these characterizations have not gotten the same meaning, here we are looking to emphasize the transformation of many working-class neighborhoods since the 1970s in Latin America, which took place at the same time as some urban spaces were occupied by rural migrants. This conversion of traditional working-class neighborhoods and these internal migrations concurred in what is often called "informal settlements." In Latin America, there are several native names for these urban settlements: "cantegriles" in Uruguay, "favelas" in Brazil, "callampas" in Chile, "pueblos jóvenes" in Peru, "invasiones" in Ecuador and Colombia, and "villas" in Argentina.

A. L. Azparren Almeira (✉)
Facultad de Ciencias Sociales, Universidad de Buenos Aires, Buenos Aires, Argentina

© The Author(s), under exclusive license to Springer Nature Switzerland AG 2021

M. A. Montoya et al. (eds.), *COVID-19 and Cities*, The Urban Book Series,
https://doi.org/10.1007/978-3-030-84134-8_10

during the pandemic, so it can be defined as a form of resilience in the terms in which it has been defined in the introduction of this book, that is, as "a dynamic process of 'bouncing forward' which provides for the adaptation and constant reinvention needed to innovate and to do new things" (Shaw, 2012, p. 309).

At the methodological level, we recovered a qualitative strategy based on semistructured interviews with key informants from the eight informal settlements with the largest number of inhabitants in the City of Buenos Aires.[2] These are Villa 21-24 (Barracas), Padre Carlos Mugica (previously called Villa 31, Retiro), Padre Rodolfo Ricciardelli (previously called Villa 1-11-14, Bajo Flores), Villa 20 (Lugano), Villa 15 (Ciudad Oculta), Villa 3 (Villa Fátima), Playón de Chacarita, and Rodrigo Bueno[3] (see Tables 10.1 and 10.2). In addition, we have analyzed several official documents and journalistic notes on the subject.[4]

Table 10.1 Data from the villages analyzed

Neighborhood	Commune	Number of inhabitants[a]	Positive cases of COVID-19 on March 31, 2021[b]
21-24	4	31.018	5.626
Padre Mugica (31)	1	27.013	2.427
Padre Ricciardelli (1-11-14)	7	26.295	6.542
20	8	22.563	3.110
15 (Ciudad Oculta)	8	16.937	3.404
Villa Fatima	8	9.914	1.476
Playón de Chacarita	15	2324	410
Rodrigo Bueno	1	1960	257

[a]These data correspond to the last National Population, Household and Housing Census available, conducted by the National Institute of Statistics and Censuses in 2010
[b]Source: Website GCBA

[2] Interviews have been done over the phone because of the decree on Compulsory Preventive Social Isolation ("Aislamiento Social Preventivo y Obligatorio" or ASPO in Spanish) that has ruled the public space in Argentina since March 20th, 2020. We chose a delegate from each of the eight larger informal settlements, where the only condition was that they were actively participating in their local COVID-19 crisis committee. We interviewed three men and five women. Their names have been modified to preserve their identity.

[3] Informal settlements from Buenos Aires were identified with a number during the last military dictatorship in Argentina (1976–1983) under the ambition of their eradication. The City of Buenos Aires laws 6.129 in 2018 and 6.219 in 2019 changed their usual name "Villa 31" and "Villa 1-11-14" to "Padre Carlos Mugica" and "Padre Rodolfo Ricciardelli" after the priests who were members of the "Equipo de Sacerdotes para la Pastoral de las villas de emergencia".

[4] At the end of this chapter, a small chart has been attached which summarizes the total number of inhabitants and the total cases of COVID-19 in each informal settlement. The information provided has been updated up until March 31, 2021.

Table 10.2 Interviews conducted

Pseudonym	Neighborhood	Interview date
Agustin	Villa Fátima	August 10th, 2020
Yamila	Villa 15	August 11th, 2020
Mauro	Villa 20	August 12th, 2020
Adriana	Villa 21-24	August 13th, 2020
Ernesto	Padre Mugica	August 14th, 2020
Fabiana	Padre Ricciardelli	August 15th, 2020
Patricia	Playón de Chacarita	October 13th, 2020
Romina	Rodrigo Bueno	October 14th, 2020

The Impact of COVID-19 on the Informal Settlements in the City of Buenos Aires

Informal urban settlements can be defined as neighborhoods whose housing groups form an irregular urban grid (not a square-shaped one) that have deficiencies in formal access to basic services and have an irregular situation in relation to land tenure (Cravino, 2009). Lack of regular income, lack of formal documentation required to access a rental, and the absence of public policies on these issues hinder some inhabitants of the largest cities in having access to housing on the formal market. As Arqueros et al. (2011) state, informal settlements can be defined as a popular mode of access to urban land in capitalist cities; a mode which is determined by a *logic of necessity*.[5] Therefore, informal settlements constitute a strategy of lower-income households to address their housing needs (Carmona Barrenechea & Messina, 2015).

Currently, in the City of Buenos Aires, there are 15 *villas*, 24 settlements, and 2 transient housing units, where approximately 300,000 people reside. This number equals almost 10% of the total population of the city (Asociación Civil por la Igualdad y la Justicia [ACIJ], 2016). As Eduardo Lépore (2012)[6] affirms, informal settlements present more precarious housing, education, labor, and health conditions than other neighborhoods in Buenos Aires. Half of the people live in overcrowded conditions (in contrast to the 8% who live in overcrowded conditions in the city as a whole) and 60% live in inadequate housing. In relation to the highest educational level achieved, the author affirms that 78% of the adult residents of these neighborhoods have not completed their compulsory education, which contrasts

[5] Pedro Pírez (1995) defines three different ways in which the capitalist city is constructed: the state or public logic, the private logic or guided by economic benefit, and the logic of necessity.

[6] This paper collects information from the National Population, Household and Housing Census carried out by INDEC in 2010 (Censo Nacional de Población, Hogares y Viviendas, in Spanish), and from the 2009 Annual Household Survey of the City of Buenos Aires (Encuesta Anual de Hogares, in Spanish). The next Census and Survey are expected to be taking place in 2021, so demographic information provided in 2009 and 2010, and used by Lépore, is the most appropriate to illuminate territorial inequalities in the city of Buenos Aires today.

with 36.6% of the overall population of the city. Unemployment and underemployment are also higher than average in these neighborhoods than those in the rest of the city, and most of the residents who are employed (two out of three) have been incorporated into the informal economy. In addition, 90% of the working men and women who live in informal settlements have an income below the minimum wage. With regard to health coverage, while only 18% of the population in the city depends exclusively on the public system, in these neighborhoods this percentage rises to up to 80%.[7] Lépore (2012, p. 107) states after the evaluation of this demographic data: "multidimensional poverty in informal settlements is 12 times greater than in the rest of the city."[8]

Informal settlements can also be defined as segregated territories. The concept of residential segregation is the degree of spatial proximity in households that belong to the same social group, whether in ethnic, age, religious, and/or socioeconomic terms (Sabatini et al., 2001). Leading Argentinian experts, Mercedes Di Virgilio and Mariano Perelman (2014), have demonstrated that urban segregation in Latin American cities occurs mainly because of socioeconomic reasons, with the subsequent concentration of lower-income populations in certain neighborhoods and their segregation from those in which the most favored sectors converge. Social inequalities thus acquire a territorial dimension, which in turn reinforces and deepens these inequalities. As Patricia Ramírez and Alicia Ziccardi (2008, p. 23) state, the territory constitutes:

> (...) a source of exclusion and inequality, and not just a spatial expression of the processes of accumulation of economic, social, cultural and environmental disadvantages that characterize the different social groups that inhabit the city.

Since the beginning of the COVID-19 pandemic and the implementation of the measures of Compulsory Preventive Social Isolation (ASPO) decreed by the national government on March 20th 2020 (Executive Decree 297/20), these territorial inequalities affected the impact of the virus in the towns of the City of Buenos Aires in a differential way, which was reflected in the high rates of contagion presented by these neighborhoods compared to the rest of the city during the first months of the pandemic.[9]

These differences can be explained through the structural dimensions of the settlements. In the first place, people living in informal urban settlements in the city

---

[7] With reference to the Argentinian health system, it must be said that it is composed of three subsectors: a public (universal access) health system, compulsory social security provided by registered employers and unions, and private or prepaid health insurance or coverage.

[8] As can be seen in the Bibliographic References, this quote is originally in Spanish. Unless specifically stated, all quotes originally in Spanish have been translated.

[9] In the first months of the pandemic, the informal urban settlements of the City of Buenos Aires presented the highest number of positive cases and deaths compared to the rest of the neighborhoods. This gap has narrowed over time as the virus spread. For example, while on June 26th 2020 36% of the total positive cases corresponded to people living in the settlements studied here, on March 31st 2021 that percentage decreased to 7%. Similarly, while on June 26th 2020 18% of deaths due to COVID-19 corresponded to these settlements, by March 31st 2021 the percentage had decreased to 4%.

found it very difficult to accomplish the requirements of the ASPO, linked to precarious living conditions, high levels of household overcrowding, the decrease in or complete halt of their economic activities, and limited or no Internet access. As one of the interviewees points out:

> It's hard to keep up with the isolation in the neighborhood. It's a lot of people living in a very small house; no internet, no TV, no job. We've been here a long time and people need to go outside. (Agustín, Villa Fátima, August 10th, 2020)

Secondly, the lack of regular access to water in some of these neighborhoods, which was denounced by referents and social and religious organizations, made it almost impossible to respect the necessary hygiene measures and, therefore, increased the possibility of contagion. The lack of water was mostly evident in Padre Carlos Mugica, Padre Ricciardelli, Playón de Chacarita, and Villa 21-24, some of the most emblematic and overpopulated neighborhoods, and continues to be a persistent problem in the city's informal settlements. In the words of a delegate from the Padre Carlos Mugica:

> We are living in a pandemic without water. When the first infections of COVID-19 began, the neighborhood had no water and that is the responsibility of the City Government. In many blocks there is no water. (...) We have been complaining about the lack of water for over a year. The summer ended, there was dengue fever, the pandemic arrived, and we were still without water. An extreme [contagion] peak and extreme social pressure had to take place for them (the city authorities) to intervene in a problem as structural as water. And it has not been fixed yet. Families are still without water. The pandemic isn't over yet. (Ernesto, Padre Carlos Carlos Mugica, August 14th, 2020)[10]

Besides the problems of overcrowding, precarious housing, and lack of access to basic services, neighbors also suffer discrimination in many key public services, such as ambulances, as they do not enter these settlements. On May 30th, 2020, a 54-year-old woman from the Villa 21-24, Ramona Collante, died after waiting for more than 2 h for the ambulance to arrive:

> Our first death from COVID was Ramona. It took the ambulance two hours to get here. That's what we've been asking for many years. (...) When something happens in the neighborhood, it is necessary that thirty people call at the same time, because if not, the ambulance does not arrive. (Adriana, Villa 21-24, August 13th, 2020).

Additionally, the economic crisis had a particular impact on the informal settlements of the City of Buenos Aires, as many people lost their jobs, mainly in the informal economy. As one of the interviewees mentions:

> Most of the people here work in informal jobs, they live from hand to mouth. Many make a living as informal traders, others are bricklayers or street sellers. Many women work as housemaids and are paid by the hour. They pay you when you go to work and if you can't

[10] Dengue is a viral infection transmitted through the bite of infected female mosquitoes of the genus Aedes. It often occurs in tropical and subtropical climates, especially in urban areas. Symptoms are high fever (around 40 °C) and some of the following: very intense headache, pain behind the eyeballs, muscle and joint pain, nausea, vomiting, and enlargement of lymph nodes (World Health Organization website).

> make it, they don't pay you at all. Due to the pandemic, people in the neighborhood were unable to work and had no income. (Patricia, Playón de Chacarita, October 13th, 2020)

In addition to the economic difficulties of the pandemic, those who live in the settlements of the city suffer discrimination and stigmatization because of the place where they live:

> The truth is people are out of work. Most of them here in the neighborhood work as housemaids, masons, and in clothing houses. Most lost their jobs because of the pandemic. There's a lot of discrimination, too. I know cases of women working as housemaids whose employers discriminated against them because they lived in the neighborhood. They told them, 'don't come back anymore, you can infect my family.' (Yamila, Villa 15, August 11th, 2020)

As a result of the loss of employment, many families were forced to resort to community kitchens in the neighborhoods, which saw a substantial increase in their demand. In this way, and as we will analyze in the last section of this chapter, it was the community organizations that had to respond to this problem, opening new community kitchens in the neighborhoods to be able to provide food assistance to their neighbors.

An inequality issue that has gained a new magnitude in this context is the lack of access to Internet service in these neighborhoods. Since public schools began demanding students participate in online classes or access their educational activities via the Internet, the lack of service, or its high cost in those neighborhoods where it is available, has caused many neighborhood children to lose the possibility to continue studying online:

> The right to education was totally violated here in the neighborhood. The vast majority could not connect; it is difficult, it is expensive. And the pedagogical continuity was lost, which will have consequences in years to come. It´s going to have consequences for all kids because of how virtuality changes things. But those who were 'left to their own devices' ('les soltaron la mano,' lit. 'let go of the hand') will take a long time to recover. (Agustin, Villa Fátima, August 10th, 2020)

Besides its impact on school-age children and those pursuing a formal education, limited connectivity has had other consequences for the populations of these neighborhoods. Under the ASPO, Internet connectivity became a fundamental need to access the various social programs implemented by the national government, whose procedures must be executed online in all cases. This has resulted in many people being excluded from the economic aid provided by the government, such as the Emergency Family Income (IFE),[11] which has in turn resulted in an increase in the exclusion of the population living in informal settlements.

Finally, one of the consequences of the economic crisis has been the increase in evictions and in the number of people on the street in these neighborhoods. Although the national government presented a decree that prevents evictions (Executive Decree 320/20), the informality of the real estate market in these settlements makes

[11] Ingreso Familiar de Emergencia, in Spanish.

it impossible to ensure its enforcement, so many people have seen their right to housing violated. As one of the interviewees mentions:

> Legality hasn't taken place in the neighborhood for a long time, and even less in that sense. Even if you tell the landowner of a room that he will not be able to evict his tenant because there is an executive decree, he will get away with it anyway. There is no decree preventing any eviction. They take people out of their homes all the time. (Fabiana, Padre Ricciardelli, August 15th, 2020)

In this way, the pandemic has highlighted the enormous social and territorial inequalities that exist in the City of Buenos Aires, where those who live in these informal settlements face discrimination and stigmatization on a daily basis. To add insult to injury, they lack essential public services, such as water or electricity; they face difficulties in accessing Internet providers; and they are always one step away from being thrown out of their homes due to the informality of the housing market. Although these various problems have been denounced by residents and social organizations in these neighborhoods, they remain a major challenge to the implementation of efficient public policies in the context of the pandemic.

Territorial Inequalities as a Challenge for Public Policies

When the World Health Organization (WHO) declared the coronavirus a pandemic on March 11th, 2020, Argentina recorded 21 positive cases of COVID-19 and only one death due to the virus. A little more than a month later, on April 20th, 2020, the neighborhood Padre Carlos Mugica registered its first positive case of COVID-19 and by May 20th there were already approximately 1000 people infected and four dead, including two neighborhood delegates.[12] Thus, the neighborhood of Padre Mugica had a very high rate of contagion in the first months of the pandemic, which was reflected in the estimation that more than half of its residents were infected with coronavirus (*Diario Clarín*, August 24th, 2020).

Accordingly, on May 5th, 2020, the national government, in coordination with the Buenos Aires City Government,[13] inaugurated in this neighborhood the first Strategic Test Device for Coronavirus in the Terrain of Argentina (DETeCTAr),[14] with the aim of carrying out an active search for people with febrile symptoms to achieve the early detection of positive cases of COVID-19. However, this first device presented

[12] The cases were Ramona Medina, delegate from the organization La Poderosa, and Víctor "El Oso" Giracoy, delegate from the community kitchen "Estrella de Belén". Ramona had repeatedly denounced in the media the lack of running water in the neighborhood. See: https://www.pagina12.com.ar/266446-murio-ramona-vocera-de-la-poderosa-y-vecina-de-la-villa-31

[13] It is important to clarify that there are two different political parties governing both districts. While "Frente de Todxs" is in charge of the national government, the City of Buenos Aires is governed by a center-right party called "Propuesta Republicana" (PRO).

[14] Dispositivo Estratégico de Testeo para Coronavirus en Terreno de Argentina, in Spanish.

a lot of problems since people had to wait in the same place for many hours for their test results, which increased the chances of contagion:

> There were many very serious failures. At first there were all the families that had symptoms in the same place as the families that had no symptoms but were isolated because they were close contacts. When they were going to take the test, they mixed them all in the same place. (Ernesto, Padre Mugica neighborhood, August 14th, 2020)

Because of the difficulties in being able to carry out the isolation in their homes, the city government ordered people who were positive with COVID-19 to be transferred to hotels for 10 days to comply with the isolation. However, as one of the interviewees points out, the transfer was carried out in school buses, where people who were COVID-19 positive were mixed with those who only had to wait in hotels for the results of their test:

> People were transferred to hotels on school buses. If a person was going to take the test, the same DETeCTAr already put it together with people who had symptoms, so it exposed them to the contagion. Then it got better because the crisis committee called many times. (Fabiana, Padre Rodolfo Ricciardelli, August 15th, 2020)

Based on the claims of the neighbors, the DETeCTAr program improved its operation and new devices were opened in other neighborhoods which began to present a lot of contagions. In this way, DETeCTAr operations were inaugurated in the neighborhoods of Padre Ricciardelli, Playón de Chacarita, Rodrigo Bueno, and in the villas 21-24, 15, 20, and in the neighborhood Ramón Carrillo, near Villa Fátima. As of August 2020, the City of Buenos Aires has 24 DETeCTAr operation centers, eight of which are located in informal settlements.

Another policy implemented by the national government to deal with the pandemic in the informal settlements is "The Neighborhood Takes Care of the Neighborhood Program,"[15] an operation developed by the Ministry of Social Development in conjunction with popular organizations, through which the community promoters travel to the neighborhoods and distribute elements of personal hygiene and perform disinfection activities in the common spaces. However, according to the interviewees, this program was implemented in only a few settlements in the city.

Finally, to address the economic consequences of the pandemic, the national government implemented two main programs: Emergency Family Income (IFE) and Emergency Assistance to Work and Production Program (ATP).[16] The IFE is aimed at workers from private households, social and lower-income categories, unemployed people, and unregistered workers, and consists of an income of 10,000 Argentinian pesos (approximately 100 dollars) granted to date on three occasions. The ATP program is aimed at women or men working in the formal economy, whether they work in the private sector or as single-tax workers in the lowest-income categories. In the first case, the state pays the worker part of his/her salary, and in the second, it grants bank loans at a zero rate.

[15] "El barrio cuida al barrio," in Spanish.

[16] "Programa de Asistencia de Emergencia al Trabajo y la Producción," in Spanish.

In the case of people living in settlements, and as we analyzed from Lépore's study (2012), two-thirds of those who are employed work in the informal sector, so the vast majority should have applied for the IFE. However, due to a lack of access to the Internet and computers (since registration was done online), many people found great obstacles to access this emergency income.

On the other hand, the Government of the City of Buenos Aires (GCBA) provided food assistance to the most affected families. However, as the people interviewed pointed out, this food aid was not sufficient for the great need that existed in the neighborhoods:

> The assistance that the GCBA gave to the families was not enough. They gave a bag every 15 days and they only gave it to adults over 65. In that period of the pandemic, at the beginning, when everyone had to stay at home, everyone needed food as they couldn't work at all. (Patricia, Playón de Chacarita, October 13th, 2020)

Furthermore, the pandemic revealed the noncompliance of the city government with the urbanization laws, which have been in force for more than two decades.[17] In addition to the deficient urbanization of these neighborhoods, the lack of hospitals in their neighborhoods, a historical demand from the residents which has never been properly addressed, made matters worse in the context of the pandemic.

> The fact that we do not have a hospital, with the situation in Commune 8, which are the neighborhoods where there are the most cases of COVID-19, is very serious. Especially because we have been demanding one for many years. (Mauro, Villa 20, August 12th, 2020)

Due to the lack of policies by the Buenos Aires City Government, community-based organizations decided to take over some of the key tasks to manage the crisis. Since then, they have played a central role in dealing with the social, health, and economic consequences of the pandemic. In the following section, we analyze the work carried out by these organizations, within the framework of the crisis committees.

The Importance of Community Care Work in Informal Settlements

When the first positive cases of COVID-19 began to be registered in the informal settlements, the organizations and neighbors organized themselves into crisis committees with the aim of articulating the different tasks of assistance and of making

[17] In 1998, the Legislature of the City of Buenos Aires passed Law 148. This law provides priority attention to the social and housing problems in the city's informal settlements. Subsequently, specific urbanization laws were enacted for each settlement: Law 403 in 2000 for the Padre Ricciardelli neighborhood, Law 1770 in 2005 for Villa 20, Law 3343 in 2009 for the Padre Carlos Mugica neighborhood, Law 5799 in 2017 for Playón de Chacarita, and Law 5798 in 2017 for Rodrigo Bueno, among others. At present, the Government of the City of Buenos Aires is executing some urbanization projects in the Padre Carlos Mugica, Padre Ricciardelli, Playón de Chacarita and Rodrigo Bueno neighborhoods, but they have not been completed yet.

their claims visible in the public agenda. In some neighborhoods, such as Villa Fátima or Villa 20, these crisis committees were based on previous organizing experiences, such as the *Mesas por la Urbanización*:[18]

> In 2016, when the urbanization process of the neighborhood began, we created the 'Mesa Técnica por la Urbanización,' where we discussed different topics related to the neighborhood: health, education, public services, etc. So, when the pandemic started, we were already organized. (Mauro, Villa 20, August 12th, 2020)

In other neighborhoods, such as Villa 21-24, the crisis committee was formed a few months before the coronavirus pandemic to respond to another very serious health problem in this informal settlement: dengue.

> The crisis committee started before COVID-19. We were a group of health promoters and self-hosted neighbors who were fighting dengue. In less than four months we had more than thirty neighbors with dengue fever. We had to mourn four deaths. We were already very organized. So, in March, when COVID-19 appeared, we started working on it and social organizations joined in, such as the Catholic Church, civil associations, schools, and health centers. (Adriana, Villa 21-24, August 13th, 2020)

Finally, in other cases, such as the Padre Mugica, Padre Ricciardelli, Playón de Chacarita, or Ciudad Oculta neighborhoods, the crisis committees were formed specifically to deal with the consequences of the coronavirus pandemic:

> When the pandemic began, we formed a group in the neighborhood that we called 'comunidad organizada.'[19] We are approximately 11 organizations that come together, working in facing the consequences of the pandemic. We are between 2 and 5 referents per block and we are in charge of distributing the food and assisting the neighbors. (Yamila, Villa 15, August 11th, 2020)

In each of the neighborhoods, the crisis committees acquire different names, are made up of different organizations and institutions (community kitchens, social organizations, territorial delegates, health promoters, schools, public organisms, etc.), and are organized in various ways (WhatsApp groups or face-to-face meetings). However, they all perform five main tasks: (1) the development of community kitchens to provide food to the families of the neighborhood; (2) the delivery of food bags provided by the city government to the most affected families of the economic crisis and to persons that belong to risk groups;[20] (3) the accompaniment and support of "close contacts"[21] of COVID-19 confirmed cases that must observe isolation in their homes;

[18] These groups meet in open spaces where neighbors are allowed to discuss and make decisions about the urbanization of their settlement.

[19] "Organized community" in English.

[20] People over 60 years old, pregnant women, and people with previous chronic diseases belong to this risk group according to the Ministry of Health of the Nation.

[21] A "close contact" is "any person who, without adequate personal protection measures, has been less than two meters away from a confirmed case for 15 min or more during the 48 hours prior to the start of the symptoms of that confirmed case". It is also a "close contact" if you share a room, bathroom or kitchen with a positive case of COVID-19. As close contacts have a high risk of having acquired the disease, they must complete 14 days of preventive isolation, even if they do not have symptoms (Ministry of Health of the Nation website. Date of consultation: August 25th, 2020).

(4) the prevention of coronavirus and the spread of information; and (5) the development of activities to raise awareness of the different problems in the neighborhood (lack of water, Internet access, DETeCTAr operations, etc.).

Food assistance and support provided by the organizations to the most affected families, such as close contacts of confirmed cases and the elderly in the neighborhood, are essential tasks that are not recognized in that way by the city government. As one of the interviewees specified:

> The city government comes, literally throws the food bags in a store, and tells us to 'take care.' Here in Villa Fátima we have 106 older adults to carry the bags to, and they are big, heavy sacks. They don´t provide us with vans or personnel. We have to transport them in wheelbarrows. You don't get gloves. When they arrive, we usually stay from 13hrs to 22hrs and sometimes we do not complete the distribution, so we have to continue the next day. (...) I mean, we are working for the city government for free. We believe that the work of our fellow workers ('compañerxs' in Spanish) should be recognized because it is a job they are doing. (Agustin, Villa Fátima, August 10th, 2020)

As the interviewees put forward, the tasks performed by these crisis committees can be defined as "community care work." *Care* is defined as the set of activities, paid or unpaid, that are necessary for the daily survival and well-being of people (Zibecchi, 2013). The tasks of care include different dimensions: the direct care of other people, the provision of the preconditions for that care to be carried out (cleaning, cooking), and the management of the care (coordination of schedules, transfers, etc.) (Rodríguez Enríquez, 2015). In this way, the crisis committees in the neighborhoods develop these different tasks, they take care of the elderly and close contacts, carry out the cleaning and cooking tasks, and manage the care, as well as coordinating the delivery of the food bags to the neighborhood families.

On the other hand, they are defined as *community* care work teams since they are developed by *territorial organizations*. The organization of care activities is performed in a way that can be represented as a diamond (Razavi, 2007) as it is built by the interaction of four main actors: families, market, state, and community organizations. In the informal settlements, the pandemic has revealed the importance of community organizations for ensuring the sustainability of life. Because of insufficient state action and the lack of economic income in the market, the community organizations are those that carry out the tasks necessary for the continuation of life. However, as Norma Sanchís (2020) points out, the care work done by community organizations is the least studied and recognized dimension in the provision of care in this pandemic.

In this way, the people who participate in the crisis committees and perform the main part of the assistance tasks in the neighborhoods, not only go unpaid for the work they do, but they are also the most exposed to the virus. In fact, a large number of delegates from the community care teams have been infected with coronavirus, which meant that the community kitchens in which they worked had to close for a while. As a neighborhood spokesperson points out:

> Many members of the crisis committee became infected, the people who work in the community kitchens, the people we were accompanying from the organizations, we all became infected. (Ernesto, Padre Carlos Mugica, August 14th, 2020)

The pandemic has shown that community care work developed by organizations is essential for health care and, therefore, for the sustainability of life in informal settlements. Food preparation and distribution, care for vulnerable people (older adults, close contacts), cleaning of common spaces, etc., all of these tasks have been carried out historically by community organizations, but they have gained greater visibility in the context of the current COVID-19 pandemic. As Fabiola Carcar (2020) suggests, although the pandemic is an extraordinary situation, the care work provided by the inhabitants of the informal settlements is not unprecedented. Another community spokesperson expressed her views on the matter as follows:

> I don't know what would have happened without the work of social organizations in our neighborhood. (…) We, the neighbors, were already used to community work. That commitment that we have with our community, walking from one block to another, certainly has had an extra value. That is what the city government rarely recognizes. Their silliness does not allow them to take notice of the fact that, through social organizations, they are being covered. Many functions that the state should perform and guarantee are being covered by these organizations and by neighbors' community work. It is unfair that they do not recognize our work. Without social organizations, our life here would have been very different. (Romina, Rodrigo Bueno, October 14th, 2020)

The community organizations, articulated in a "crisis committee," have been a central actor in dealing with the consequences of the pandemic in the informal settlements of the City of Buenos Aires. The tasks they have performed have not been properly recognized as work by the city authorities; therefore, they do not receive any kind of economic compensation, nor have they been provided with the adequate conditions to carry them out (health coverage, hygiene and biosecurity elements, appropriate training, etc.). Nonetheless, the social and community networks developed by these organizations in informal settlements and neighborhoods have allowed their residents to substantially reduce the sanitary and economic effects of the current COVID-19 crisis.

Conclusions

The social and territorial inequalities that characterize the great urban centers of our region have always been noticeable, but they have become dramatically evident since the emergence of the coronavirus pandemic. The large number of people living in informal settlements in Latin America (more than 100 million according to UN-Habitat data), without access to basic services, who live in precarious conditions and in households with high rates of overcrowding, has shown itself to be a problem requiring an urgent response.

In the case of the City of Buenos Aires, the informal settlements have constituted the urban environment where the virus presented the highest rates of COVID-19 during the first months of the pandemic. Accordingly, the national government has implemented various measures to cope with this problem, like the DETeCTAr program. This has made it possible to detect positive cases more quickly and to isolate people in other areas (e.g., hotels) in order to prevent the spread of the virus and the increase in infections and fatal cases.

As we analyzed in this chapter, the DETeCTAr program has presented, in some cases, important difficulties in its implementation, which have been corrected by the demands of the crisis committees of each neighborhood. In addition, the assistance provided by community-based organizations has been essential, as they have been responsible for bringing the necessary food to the homes of people self-isolating, so that they could observe the isolation rules.

While these care efforts have increased under the pandemic, many of them (such as food assistance through community kitchens, daily accompaniment of people in situations of social vulnerability, etc.) have historically been carried out by these organizations, and they are the ones that allow, in many cases, the sustainability of life in these neighborhoods. As a result, the pandemic has made visible the fact that, in the face of state inaction, market discrimination, and the many other difficulties which resident families face on a daily basis, community organizations can become a central actor in the provision of care in these informal settlements. They have continued to provide support and assistance to their communities, contributing with their efforts and risking contagion and disease, despite not receiving adequate symbolic or economic recognition for their work.

With this chapter, we hope to have contributed to highlighting the importance of community care work performed by community organizations in the informal settlements of the City of Buenos Aires, so that they can be properly recognized and remunerated in the near future. May this recognition be a first necessary step in the development of more equal cities and societies in our region and in the world at large.

Acknowledgments I would like to thank Ignacio Villagrán, Santiago Cunial, and Tomás Ferreyra for reading this chapter and making comments on it, and to all the people interviewed, for their time and for sharing their experiences with me.

References

Administración Nacional de la Seguridad Social. (n.d.). *Emergency family admission*. https://www.anses.gob.ar/ingreso-familiar-de-emergencia. Accessed July 2020.

Arqueros, S., Calderón, C., Jauri, N., Ramos, J., Vitale, P., & Yacovino, M. P. (2011). Apuntes sobre la cuestión villera en la Ciudad de Buenos Aires [Notes about the Village Situation in the City of Buenos Aires]. *Herramienta, 48*, 169–181.

Asociación Civil por la Igualdad y la Justicia. (2016). Urbanización de villas y asentamientos en Buenos Aires [Urbanization of villages and settlements in Buenos Aires]. *Colección Es Nuestra la Ciudad N° 3.*

Boletín Oficial. (2005, September 22). *Ley 1770 2005* [Law 1770 2005]. https://boletinoficial.buenosaires.gob.ar/normativaba/norma/76906. Accessed July 2020.

Boletín Oficial. (2009, December 3). *Ley 3343, Buenos Aires, Argentina (Urbanización de villas 31 y 31 bis)* [Law 3343, Buenos Aires, Argentina (urbanization of villages 31 and 31 bis)]. http://www2.cedom.gob.ar/es/legislacion/normas/leyes/ley3343.html. Accessed July 2020.

Boletín Oficial. (2017a, March 23). *Ley 5798, Buenos Aires, Argentina (Urbanización barrio Rodrigo Bueno)* [Law 5798, Buenos Aires, Argentina (urbanization neighborhood Rodrigo Bueno]. http://www2.cedom.gob.ar/es/legislacion/normas/leyes/ley5798.html. Accessed July 2020.

Boletín Oficial. (2017b, March 23). *Ley 5799, Buenos Aires, Argentina (Reurbanización e Integración socio-urbana del barrio denominado "Playón Chacarita")* [Law 5799, Buenos Aires, Argentina (reurbanization and socio-urban integration of the neighborhood called "Playón Chacarita"]. http://www2.cedom.gob.ar/es/legislacion/normas/leyes/ley5799.html. Accessed July 2020.

Boletín Oficial. (2020a, March 20). *Decreto 297, Buenos Aires, Argentina (Aislamiento social, preventivo y obligatorio)* [Decree 297, Buenos Aires, Argentina (social distancing, preventfull and mandatory)]. https://www.boletinoficial.gob.ar/detalleAviso/primera/227042/20200320. Accessed June 2020.

Boletín Oficial. (2020b, March 29). *Decreto 320, Buenos Aires, Argentina (Suspensión de desalojos)* [Decree 320 Buenos Aires, Argentina (eviction suspension)]. https://www.boletinoficial.gob.ar/detalleAviso/primera/227042/20200320. Accessed June 2020.

Carcar, F. (2020). El trabajo de cuidados en los barrios populares [The work of caring for others in popular neighborhoods]. *Flacso.* https://www.flacso.org.ar/noticias/el-trabajo-de-cuidados-en-los-barrios-populares/. Accessed Nov 2020.

Carmona Barrenechea, V., & Messina, G. (2015). La problemática habitacional de la Ciudad de Buenos Aires desde la perspectiva de la provisión de bienestar [The habitational problem in the city of Buenos Aires from a well-being provision perspective]. In L. Pautassi & G. Gamallo (Eds.), *El bienestar en brechas. Un análisis de las políticas sociales en la Argentina de la post-convertibilidad* (pp. 201–236). Editorial Biblos.

Consejo de Derechos Humanos de la Defensoría del Pueblo de CABA [CDH]. (1999, January 29). *Ley M – N° 148: de atención prioritaria a la problemática social y habitacional en las villas y núcleos habitacionales transitorios* [Law M – N° 148: About the priority attention to the social and habitational problematic in villages and transitory habitational nucleuses]. https://cdh.defensoria.org.ar/wp-content/uploads/sites/3/2018/01/Ley-Ciudad-148-2.pdf. Accessed July 2020.

CDH. (2000, July 14). *Ley 403: Plan integral de urbanización Villa 1-11-14* [Law 403: integral plan of urbanization 1-11-14]. https://cdh.defensoria.org.ar/normativa/ley-403-plan-integral-de-urbanizacion/. Accessed July 2020.

Clarín. (2020, August 24). *Coronavirus en la Ciudad: afirman que en la villa 31 se contagiaron la mitad de los vecinos* [Coronavirus in the city: They affirm that in the village 31 half the neighbors got sick]. https://www.clarin.com/ciudades/coronavirus-ciudad-afirman-villa-31-contagio-mitad-vecinos_0_6QBjtr8JN.html. Accessed Sept 2020.

Cravino, M. C. (2009). *Vivir en la villa: relatos, trayectorias y estrategias habitacionales* [Living in the village: Stories, trajectories, and habitational strategies]. Universidad Nacional de General Sarmiento.

Di Virgilio, M. M., & Perelman, M. (2014). Ciudades latinoamericanas. La producción social de las desigualdades urbanas [Latin American cities. The social production of urban inequalities]. In M. M. Di Virgilio & M. Perelman (Eds.), *Ciudades latinoamericanas. Desigualdad, segregación y tolerancia* (pp. 9–26). CLACSO.

Government of the City of Buenos Aires. (n.d.). *Actualización de los casos de coronavirus en la Ciudad de Buenos Aires* [Update of the coronavirus cases in the city of Buenos Aires]: https://www.buenosaires.gob.ar/coronavirus/noticias/actualizacion-delos-casos-de-coronavirus-en-la-ciudad-buenos-aires. Accessed July 2020.

Instituto Nacional de Estadísticas y Censos. (2010). *Censo Nacional de Población, Hogares y Viviendas* [Nacional census of population, homes, and households]. https://www.indec.gob.ar/indec/web/Nivel4-Tema-2-41-135. Accessed June 2020.

Lépore, E. (Coord.). (2012). *Capacidades de desarrollo y sociedad civil en las villas de la ciudad* [Development and civil society capacities in the villages of the city]. EDUCA-Editorial de la Universidad Católica Argentina.

Ministry of Health. (n.d.). *Definition of close contact*. https://www.argentina.gob.ar/coronavirus/glosario/contacto-strait. Accessed July 2020.

Nueva Ciudad. (2020. June 2). *Otra vez Ramona: la ambulancia tardó dos horas y falleció por Covid-19 en la villa 21–24* [Ramona once again: The ambulance took two hours and she passed away due to Covid-19 in the village 21–24]. https://www.nueva-ciudad.com.ar/notas/202006/43824-otra-vez-ramona-la-ambulancia-tardo-dos-horas-y-fallecio-por-covid-19-en-la-villa-21-24.html. Accessed July 2020.

Página 12. (2020, May 17). *Murió Ramona, vocera de La Poderosa y vecina de la villa 31*. https://www.pagina12.com.ar/266446-murio-ramona-vocera-de-la-poderosa-y-vecina-de-la-villa-31. Accessed June 2020.

Pírez, P. (1995). Actores sociales y gestión de la ciudad. *CIUDADES, 28*, 8–14.

Ramírez, P., & Ziccardi, A. (2008). Pobreza urbana, desigualdad y exclusión social en la ciudad del siglo XXI. Una introducción [Urban poverty, inequality, and social exclusion in the city of the XXI century. An introduction]. In R. Cordera, P. Ramírez Kuri, & A. Ziccardi (Coord.), *Pobreza, desigualdad y exclusión social en la ciudad del siglo XXI* (pp. 23–50). Siglo XXI Editores.

Razavi, S. (2007). *The political and social economy of care in the development context. Conceptual issues, research questions and policy options*. Gender and Development Programme Paper Num. 1. https://repositorio.unal.edu.co/bitstream/handle/unal/47163/The%20Political%20and%20Social%20Economy.pdf?sequence=1&isAllowed=y. Accessed Aug 2020.

Rodríguez Enríquez, C. (2015). Economía feminista y economía del cuidado. Aportes conceptuales para el estudio de la desigualdad [Feminist economy and care economy. Conceptual contributions to study inequality]. *Revista Nueva Sociedad, 256*, issn: 0251-3552.

Sabatini, F., Cáceres, G., & Cerda, J. (2001). Segregación residencial en las principales ciudades chilenas: Tendencias de las tres últimas décadas y posibles cursos de acción [Residential segregation in the main Chilean cities: Tendencies in the past three decades and possible courses of action]. *Eure (Santiago), 27*(82), 21–42.

Sanchís, N. (2020). Ampliando la concepción de cuidado: ¿privilegio de pocxs o bien común? [Widening the care conception: priviledge of a few or common good?]. In N. Sanchís (Ed.), *El cuidado comunitario en tiempos de pandemia… y más allá* (pp. 9–21). Asociación Lola Mora. Red de Género y Comercio.

Shaw, K. (2012). "Reframing" resilience: Challenges for planning theory and practice. *Planning Theory & Practice, 13*(2), 308–333.

Conferencia de las Nacionales Unidas sobre la Vivienda y el Desarrollo Urbano Sostenible (2015). Hábitat III. Documento temático sobre asentamientos informales. https://uploads.habitat3.org/hb3/Issue-Paper-22_ASENTAMIENTOS-INFORMALES-SP.pdf

World Health Organization. (n.d.). *Dengue*. www.who.int/topics/dengue/en/s. Accessed July 2020.

Zibecchi, C. (2013). Organizaciones comunitarias y cuidadoras; reconfiguración de responsabilidades en torno al cuidado infantil [Communitary organizations and care takers; reconfiguration of responsabilities around child care]. In L. Pautassi & C. Zibecchi (Coord.), *Las Fronteras del Cuidado. Agenda, derechos e infraestructura* (pp. 317–352). Equipo Latinoamericano de Justicia y Género (ELA) y Biblos.

Chapter 11
Feeding Cities During COVID-19 Lockdowns: Responses from China and Latin America

Sofía Boza

Introduction

The COVID-19 pandemic has affected both the demand and supply of food markets. Food transmission channels include the end user's purchasing power, which has in many cases diminished due to unemployment. Measures taken to stop the spread of COVID-19 have impacted the availability of productive factors and disrupted food transport and distribution (Schmidhuber et al., 2020). Stay-at-home orders intensify those effects as most daily activities stop. Some of the drastic changes in the operation of food markets, such as the increase in online shopping and delivery services, are expected to remain even after the COVID-19 pandemic is controlled (Hobbs, 2020).

Due to their high population density, cities concentrate food demand. They depend, however, on food that is mostly grown and processed outside of their borders. Consequently, maintaining distribution channels to and within a city is essential for ensuring the well-being of its inhabitants. It is therefore necessary to implement strategies to help city dwellers access sufficient and nutritious food. These responses are originating not only from the public sector, but also from the private sector and civil society, increasing food system resilience against this pandemic and other current crises, like climate change, obesity, and malnutrition, which altogether are referred to as a "global syndemic" (Kanter & Boza, 2020; Swinburn et al., 2019). Building resilience will strengthen food systems against the global syndemic, which is already visible in the global south (Martorell et al., 2020).

In many cases, the actions that were implemented were insufficient in scope and were short-term, and food access in the most vulnerable populations has been truly

S. Boza (✉)
Faculty of Agricultural Sciences and Institute of International Studies, University of Chile, Santiago, Chile
e-mail: sofiaboza@u.uchile.cl

© The Author(s), under exclusive license to Springer Nature Switzerland AG 2021

M. A. Montoya et al. (eds.), *COVID-19 and Cities*, The Urban Book Series,
https://doi.org/10.1007/978-3-030-84134-8_11

threatened. Social distancing measures and the related economic recession are driving up food insecurity dramatically worldwide (Laborde et al., 2020). Food and Agriculture Organization [FAO] and Economic Commission for Latin America and the Caribbean [ECLAC] (2020) recently estimated that in Latin America, poverty and hunger could reach levels not seen in 20 years, turning the COVID-19 health crisis into a serious food crisis.

The objective of this chapter is to review the actions taken in mega cities in China and Latin America to guarantee food distribution and access during the mandatory and voluntary COVID-19 lockdown orders. In addition to describing the responses, we want to reflect on whether resilience was built into the system. That is, which of the responses to the lockdown orders, if any, might be translated into long-term innovations or improvements, as opposed to limited or short-term fixes. The most populated city in China, Shanghai, and two capital cities from different Latin American subregions, Mexico City, Mexico, and Santiago, Chile, are considered as case studies. Information was obtained from secondary sources, mainly reports, articles, and news media published between December 2019 and August 2020. The focus of our analysis will be on identifying and studying the strategies used to maintain food access and distribution during the shutdowns. The entities implementing these strategies are divided into three groups: the private sector, such as food distribution and sales companies; the public sector, especially local and regional governments; and formal and informal not-for-profit organizations.

Responses to Food Supply and Distribution During COVID-19 Lockdowns

The Case of Shanghai

Shanghai is the most populated city in China and the third most populated worldwide with more than 24 million inhabitants. Along with Tianjin, Chongqing, and Beijing, Shanghai is one of China's four municipalities, i.e., cities considered equivalent to provinces and under the direct administration of the central government. Shanghai is located on the banks of the Yangtze River, which increases the fertility of its land. Shanghai's peri-urban areas have a large amount of small-scale farming, which produces vegetables (especially leafy greens), cereals, poultry, pigs, and aquaculture. Urban sprawl results in a steady loss of this agricultural land. In response, there has been a growth in urban agriculture in Shanghai, using innovative methods such as hydroponics, indoor horticulture, and vertical farming to grow more food in less space (Hosseinifarhangi et al., 2019). Today in Shanghai, agriculture is fully accepted as an adequate use of urban space, especially environmentally conscious operations such as organic farms (Ding et al., 2018).

Shanghai represents the largest food market in mainland China and is therefore an important distribution hub, especially for the Eastern Region and the Yangtze

River Delta (Ng et al., 2016). Shanghai also has the most advanced retail system in China; however, traditional wet markets (of which there are nearly 1,000 in Shanghai) are still preferred for shopping for fresh foods (Maruyama et al., 2016). The fragmentation in production and in the wholesale system limits the supermarkets' ability to compete with wet markets, which offer a greater variety of products, fresher food, and lower prices than supermarkets (Cavish, 2020; Zhang & Pan, 2013). In contrast, with processed foods, supermarkets and hypermarkets have rapidly increased their market share. As Shanghai has the largest foreign population in China, there is an abundance of Western supermarkets, such as Carrefour, Tesco, Walmart, and Marks & Spencer. Local supermarkets and grocery stores of various sizes are also prevalent. With economic growth, the food consumption habits of Shanghai inhabitants are dramatically changing. There has been a notorious increase in eating out and, therefore, an expansion of the restaurant industry, including fast-food outlets from international franchises like McDonald's and Subway, and street food options. Students and workers in Shanghai often eat at company and school cafeterias (Zang et al., 2018). In Shanghai, there is a school lunch program which started in 1993 that feeds lunch to more than 95% of students (Huang et al., 2017).

On January 20th, 2020, the first case of COVID-19 was identified in Shanghai. The Municipal Government announced restricted entry to the city to reduce incoming cases. At the beginning of February, Shanghai launched a "closed management" strategy for residential communities. This meant entrance and exit restrictions, registration and temperature checks, and notification to the authorities of any abnormality. In coordination with police stations and community health centers, door-to-door interviews were conducted with residents to control the proliferation of COVID-19 within communities (Everington, 2020). In March, the restrictions were notably relaxed, even allowing the reopening of leisure establishments and tourist attractions, but some of these steps were quickly reversed when cases increased (Anstey, 2020). In the spring, Shanghai regained a certain normality in its activities, and students returned to classes at the end of April. The measures were refocused on travel restrictions and prevention. As of mid-August, Shanghai had 741 confirmed COVID-19 cases (mostly imported) and 7 deaths.

Retail markets in Shanghai were limited in their operations during the stay-at-home orders. Wet markets, meanwhile, were at the center of the controversy because the Huanan Market at Wuhan is assumed to be the most likely source of the COVID-19 outbreak. Sixty US senators and representatives even signed a letter calling for China to shut down wet markets (White, 2020). This shows a misunderstanding as not all wet markets sell wild animals. In fact, they are more like what is known as "farmers markets" in the United States (Cavish, 2020). The wet markets in Shanghai continued working during the lockdowns but avoided crowding. The Shanghai Municipal Government imposed regulations requiring disinfection stations and strict hygiene standards, as well as guidance to help all merchants follow the law properly (Yu, 2020).

Most supermarkets in Shanghai stayed open as well; however, customers were reluctant to shop in-person for fear of infection. Online grocery shopping, which was already a fast-growing market, increased during the lockdown. Major Chinese online retailers, such as JD.com and Alibaba, dramatically increased sales of groceries, but also of fresh foods like vegetables and meat, requiring employees to use protective equipment such as masks and goggles (The Economic Times, 2020). By the end of February, 100% of the supermarkets and 95% of the shopping malls in Shanghai had resumed activities (Xinhua, 2020).

Many Shanghai restaurants were closed at the beginning of the COVID-19 spread to avoid risk to the staff and because a very low number of customers were willing to eat out (Davis, 2020). Some restaurants, especially fast-food chains, offered delivery. Housing complexes restricted access to grocery and restaurant delivery men, asking them to leave orders in a specific area at the entrance. Delivery men carried ID cards showing that they and the people who packaged the food had no fever, and contactless pickup points were common at fast-food outlets (Russ & Yu, 2020). At the end of February, the Shanghai government allowed restaurants to open for dine-in services if they met certain criteria for preventing the spread of COVID-19 (ASEANPLUS NEWS, 2020). Surveys of 160 Shanghai restaurants and bar operators in April 2020, however, showed that more than half had a revenue of 40% or less than in April 2019, and less than 5% said they were back to normal. In addition to delivery, restaurants increased in-store promotions, reduced operation hours and menu options, reduced worker's salaries, and delayed payments to suppliers (Gouk, 2020).

Along with regulating sanitary conditions in wet markets and stores, local authorities were worried about price gauging. Shanghai's Market Supervision Administration recorded prices daily and fined supermarkets that increased them too much. For instance, Carrefour was fined two million Yuan (289,284 USD, August 27, 2020) for quintupling the price of cabbage (Wall Street Journal, 2020). More recently, the Shanghai government adopted a national strategy, supported by the central government as well as private companies, to reduce food losses and waste. Restaurants are giving information to clients, reducing the number of dishes served per group, encouraging clients to take home the leftovers, and offering smaller servings of delivery and takeaways. Supermarkets like Alibaba's Freshippo grocery stores have reduced produce package size (Shanghai Municipal People's Government, 2020). President Xi Jinping raised the alarm about food security, maintaining that food waste cannot be allowed in China (Kuo, 2020). In the same spirit, the Shanghai Green Food Bank, the first of its kind in mainland China, offers free food donated by supermarkets and restaurants, those products which would otherwise have been thrown away. After COVID-19 lockdowns, the Green Food Bank intensified its operations to alleviate food insecurity, also because supermarkets, and especially restaurants, had more food stored and thus donations increased (Qian, 2020).

The Case of Mexico City

The Mexico City Metropolitan Area (MCMA) is composed of Mexico City, which is divided into 16 municipalities, and 41 adjacent municipalities from the states of Mexico and Hidalgo. Mexico City is the second most populated capital in Latin

America with 8.98 million inhabitants, and the MCMA is one of the largest metropolitan areas in the world with more than 21.5 million inhabitants (18% of the national population). Mexico City is responsible for 15% of the gross domestic product (GDP) of Mexico. Its main sector is services, which makes up 63% of employment. As expected, agriculture has a very marginal presence in the GDP and employment within the MCMA; however, the food industry is the main manufacturing sector in Mexico City (Secretaría de Desarrollo Económico [SEDECO], 2020). Eighty percent of the food consumed in Mexico City is imported from other states or from abroad (FAO, 2014).

Given its large population and economy, the MCMA is the most important market for food demand and supply in Mexico. The Mexico City Wholesale Market (*Central de Abastos de Ciudad de México*), the largest of its kind worldwide, serves 500,000 visitors daily, distributing 35% of the national fruit and vegetable production. The most important retail food markets in the MCMA are the open-air, public markets called *tianguis*, municipal markets, small grocery stores, and, increasingly, supermarkets. A significant part of the population of Mexico City shops at the 1,700+ public markets (300 municipal markets and 1400 *tianguis*). They are open on certain days of the week on a public site designated by the municipal authorities, which requires the payment of a fee by each street vendor. They are popular for fresh produce purchases, especially in middle- and low-income areas of Mexico City (Ayala & Castillo, 2014). Municipal markets and *tianguis* in Mexico City are comprised of 72,000 tenants, and they employ 250,000 people (Reveles, 2020). According to the Mexican economic census, in Mexico City there are more than 220,000 small grocery stores (known as *tiendas de abarrotes*), which employ 900,000 people. They mainly sell packaged goods in small shopfronts with little storage capacity. Supermarkets have markedly increased their store count and share of retail food sales in major Mexican cities. Walmart is the dominant supermarket chain in central Mexico. It has sought high coverage in Mexico City, but has adapted and differentiated its stores depending on the socio-economic level of different areas (Casado-Izquierdo, 2018). The 58,000 restaurants in Mexico City are a huge business sector, catering to national consumption and tourism. The street and informal sale of food is also deeply rooted in the culture of Mexico City, representing an economic activity that generates income for the most vulnerable families, especially in times of economic difficulty and increased unemployment. The Mexico City government operates a network of more than 300 meal centers (*comedores comunitarios*) that offer a complete meal for only 10 Mexican pesos (0.45 USD, August 27, 2020). The federal government has other food programs for students (e.g., school breakfasts) and low-income citizens.

At the end of February 2020, Mexico City confirmed its first case of COVID-19. That March, preventive measures were implemented, including school closures, stay-at-home restrictions, and a campaign to promote social distancing. With COVID-19 cases and deaths increasing, the federal government declared a state of emergency at the end of March and tightened restrictions. They started what they called a "National Healthy Distance Schedule" (*Jornada Nacional de Sana Distancia*), which amounted to a voluntary lockdown. Nonessential activities were asked to stop. The aforementioned *Jornada Nacional de Sana Distancia* was supposed to finish at the end of May but was continually postponed in Mexico City due to a lack of clear and stable improvement in COVID-19 control. In mid-June, the city began to resume normal activity, though several districts were still on "red alert," especially poorer areas with conditions less conducive to the prevention of infections. By mid-August, Mexico had the third highest death count in the world, with over 60,000 COVID-19 deaths. In Mexico City, the pandemic has been especially tough.

During the times of the stay-at-home measures, food production and distribution in the MCMA were deemed essential, and it was a challenge to continue operating while reducing the risk of transmission. The Mexico City Wholesale Market stayed open, but took preventative measures like frequent hand washing, cleaning of stalls and utensils, mandating masks, and avoiding crowds by serving only two customers at a time. Likewise, the market's administration established a web page through which sellers and buyers could arrange home deliveries. The Mexico City Secretary of Economic Development worked with the municipal markets and *tianguis* to offer home sales services from the beginning. Local authorities enforced compliance with prevention and hygiene standards for in-person sales (Reveles, 2020). With the spread of COVID-19 in Mexico City, however, some outbreaks were associated with municipal markets, which led to the total or partial closure of several of them. The local government also declared the Mexico City Wholesale Market and various municipal markets to be "high contagion zones" (Delgadillo, 2020).

Since the end of March 2020, supermarkets in Mexico City have taken different measures to reduce the risk of transmission in their stores, including limiting entry to one person per family, recommending the use of masks, sanitizing shopping carts, or enforcing social distancing for customers in the checkout lines. Many supermarkets put purchase limits on some products to avoid shortages (Corro et al., 2020). Despite the restrictions, supermarkets had an abnormal increase in sales in the first quarter of 2020. This was due in part to the strengthening of home delivery services through digital platforms (Delgadillo, 2020). Many Mexican consumers have started shopping for groceries online for the first time to stay at home and avoid crowds (Asociación Mexicana de Venta Online [AMVO], 2020). Small grocery stores in Mexico City also had an increase in sales at the beginning of the health emergency (Carbajal, 2020). As the number of infections grew, however, sales stagnated and even decreased for this sector, and operations became difficult. In response, a group of grocery stores launched an initiative called "My Safe Shop" (*Mi Tienda Segura*). They implemented a communication campaign, installed 50,000 acrylic protection partitions, and improved point-of-sale practices (Morales, 2020).

Restaurants were especially limited in their operations during the lockdowns. Some restaurants continued serving customers with takeaway and delivery services, either independently or through applications such as Rappi and Uber Eats, while many small restaurants and food stalls preferred to close. On the first of July 2020, restaurants in Mexico City could reopen at 40% capacity. Many restaurants that reopened took precautionary measures, such as extreme cleanliness, waiters wearing masks, gloves, and a protective visor, and empty tables between occupied tables, and, in some cases, physical menus were replaced with digital versions using QR codes. In the first weeks of operation, the average occupancy did not exceed 20%. It is estimated that a quarter of Mexico City restaurants will not make it through this pandemic and will go out of business (Lozano, 2020). For street food, sales were severely impacted during stay-at-home measures due to the large decrease in passers-by. After the restrictions were lifted, street food vendors had to facilitate social distancing, and sales were only allowed 2 days a week in the center of Mexico City. In response, the street vendors' associations committed to a protocol to be allowed to expand their operations. This protocol includes takeaway-only food sales, mandatory mask use for vendors and customers, distance between vendors, regular temperature checks, frequent cleaning and disinfection, and hand sanitizer available for vendors and customers (Navarrete, 2020).

One of the major concerns of both the federal government and Mexico City's government is the closure of small businesses and its economic effects on low- and middle-income families. It is estimated that 170,000 micro and small businesses in Mexico City will close because of the COVID-19 crisis, many of them related to food distribution such as grocery stores, leading to the loss of 1 million jobs, 40% of which are formal and 60% informal. To alleviate this situation, the Mexico City government offered loans with a 0% interest rate (Infobae, 2020). The Mexico City government also launched the app "ComeCDMX" to connect restaurants, cafes, and bars with customers to bolster food delivery.

During the lockdown, 80 public meal centers in Mexico City maintained their operations, each serving between 100 and 350 meals daily. This effort was complemented by others from the private sector and civil society. For instance, the World Central Kitchen, a community kitchen initiative from the chef José Andrés in New York, arrived in Mexico City in partnership with local foundations. Participating restaurants offered meals for only 50 Mexican pesos (2.26 USD, August 27, 2020), covering the costs with donations. Other civil society and private sector initiatives in Mexico City were mostly promoting local businesses and facilitating delivery or receiving donations to help families buy food.

Despite this effort, a report from the United Nations Children's Fund [UNICEF], the Pan American Health Organization [PAHO], and the FAO warns that there is a high probability that food insecurity in Mexico will increase dramatically, especially in the lower economic strata. They recommended a multifaceted response which includes, among other things, an emergency fund and the expansion of public food programs like the one for students (UNICEF et al., 2020).

The Case of Santiago, Chile

Santiago is the capital of Chile and its most populous city with seven million inhabitants. It is in the center of the Santiago Metropolitan Region (SMR). The SMR accounts for 40% of the Chilean population and generates 45% of the national GDP

(Biblioteca del Congreso Nacional de Chile [BCN], 2020). It is divided into 52 districts, 34 of which form the urban center known as *Gran Santiago*. Encircling them is a belt of 18 peri-urban districts with lower population density and prevalent agriculture. In fact, the SMR is the main vegetable-producing region in Chile, with a third of the vegetable acreage of the nation (Instituto Nacional de Estadísticas Chile [INE], 2018).

Santiago is central to the food demand in Chile and, therefore, for food supply and distribution. The largest wholesale market for fresh produce in Chile, Lo Valledor, is in Santiago, with an area of 300,000 square feet and 30,000 daily visitors. Santiago also has the biggest open-air, fresh market in Chile, La Vega Central, with 1,200 stalls. Another 455 outdoor markets are spread throughout Santiago and are considered cheaper than supermarkets for fresh products, especially fruits and vegetables (Carreño & Silva, 2019). However, more than 60% of the retail value for food sales in Chile is collected by supermarkets, which are concentrated in Santiago and regional capitals. Small grocery stores have an important presence as well, especially for the middle- and low-income areas. Fast-food restaurants have expanded rapidly in recent years in Chile, with two thirds of them located in Santiago. The expansion of delivery services has furthered this growth (Gajardo, 2019). Santiago distributes the most food to students through school lunch programs.

In Chile, the first case of COVID-19 was identified at the beginning of March 2020. Two weeks later, President Piñera declared a Constitutional State of Disaster Emergency for the whole country for 90 days. Soon after, Santiago began a curfew from 22:00 to 05:00. In May, the number of infections accelerated. The SMR was the region with the most cases and deaths in both absolute and relative terms (per 100,000 inhabitants). First, the health emergency was addressed in Santiago through weekly rotating district lockdowns. By mid-May, however, rapidly rising cases in the *Gran Santiago* districts caused a complete lockdown. At the end of July, as the number of COVID-19 cases and deaths decreased, the Chilean government launched the *Plan Paso a Paso* (Step-by-Step Plan) to ease and eventually lift the lockdowns. In the first phase of the plan, the inhabitants of six districts in Santiago (mainly upper-income areas) could move freely inside their own districts on weekdays. By the end of August, the lockdown was eased in 26 of the SMR districts.

COVID-19 has had a clear impact on Santiago's food distribution system. In the days before and at the beginning of the lockdowns, there were long lines of customers at supermarkets. Some stores had shortages. Supermarkets limited the number of customers in stores and the quantity of each product that they could buy. Supermarkets also limited their hours, closing three or four hours earlier than normal and reserving the first hours of the day for elderly customers. Some supermarkets took customers' temperatures prior to entry, provided them with water for hand washing, and required them to wear a mask. One of the most relevant changes in supermarket operations in Santiago due to COVID-19 was the increase in online shopping and delivery services. The main supermarket chains rapidly ramped up their capabilities for both in-person and delivery services. They formed important partnerships with applications such as Rappi, CornerShop, and Uber.

Some districts in Santiago decided to temporarily suspend the open-air markets due to the transmission risk associated with large crowds. In the cases of Lo Valledor and La Vega Central, during the complete lockdown, they only supplied wholesalers and retailers, as well as people who shop for multiple families. Access was limited and controlled by police officers and private guards. Mask use was mandatory. Markets in Santiago, especially in upper and upper middle-income areas, have incorporated delivery services both independently and through applications such as Uber Eats. In some cases, independent farmers or merchants advertised on social media and delivered their products to their customers. Small grocery stores are operating relatively normally. The most common changes have been limiting the number of customers in the store at the same time and making masks a requirement.

The sanitary measures taken in Santiago prohibited dine-in services, limiting restaurants to delivery and takeaway. The curfew cut into restaurants' operating hours significantly. All this has inevitably had a negative impact on profitability. At the beginning of July 2020, it was estimated that 70% of restaurants in Providencia, one of the most traditional and touristy areas of Santiago, were on the verge of bankruptcy or massive layoffs. Another development in food distribution in Santiago has been the disruption, in many cases out of necessity, of informal activities in preparation and distribution of food.

In addition to health regulations, the government has tried to increase food access. Unemployment in Santiago increased during lockdowns at rates not seen for more than 30 years. This translates into a sharp decrease in family income and, therefore, in the ability to purchase goods, including food. In mid-May 2020, the Chilean government launched the *Plan Alimentos para Chile* (Food for Chile Plan). The plan involved the delivery of 2.5 million food boxes, valued at 35,000 CLP each (44.52 USD, August 27, 2020), to lower-income families, 80% of them in the SMR. The boxes included nonperishable foods such as rice, pasta, legumes, powdered milk, canned mackerel and tuna, sauce, jam, instant mashed potatoes, flour, sugar, tea, and oil. In mid-July, a second phase of the plan began, with 1.5 million food boxes delivered in the SMR. The access to food and basic goods has also been supported by direct payments to low- and lower-middle income families. Meanwhile, the School Lunch Program redirected its resources to deliver food bags or boxes through schools to the students who would otherwise be eating at school.

Civil society has also played a very active role in facing difficulties with food access. Since the beginning of the lockdowns, dozens of so-called "*ollas comunes*" (community soup kitchen) have emerged in Santiago. These are self-managed initiatives in which the residents of an area pool resources and cook together for their neighbors. The *ollas comunes*, common under military rule in the 1980s, are concentrated in low-income areas. At the beginning of June in La Pintana, the poorest district in Santiago, there were 50 *ollas comunes* operating. There are also similar initiatives in which civil society and the private and public sectors collaborate. A paradigmatic example is *Comida para Todos* (Food for Everyone) in which restaurants prepare lunches with funds from private donations that are distributed through charities to low-income families in Santiago with the cooperation of local governments.

Concluding Remarks

In this final section, we will compare the three different approaches taken to maintain food supply and distribution during COVID-19 lockdowns in the three cases presented and reflect on whether they might contribute to building resilience. Our procedure will be based on what, in policy analysis, is known as an "output" approach, i.e., a comparison based on the content of the immediate decisions made to confront a situation (Schmitt, 2012). This is because the information available on actors' responses to COVID-19 is mainly the description of actions, and to a much lesser extent, their impacts or outcomes. We will divide the comparison by the three groups of actors present in the cases: the private sector, the public sector, and formal and informal not-for-profit organizations.

In the three cities analyzed, private actors in the food supply and distribution business tried to adapt to COVID-19-related sanitary restrictions. There were some common actions, such as the increase in sanitary and hygiene precautions (i.e., masks, frequent cleaning, and temperature checks). Crowds were also avoided by limiting the number of customers at the stores and markets. Online shopping and delivery services grew during the stay-at-home orders, a trend that might endure as many consumers have learned how to do it and supply capacities have increased. In Shanghai, the existing Chinese online retail giants JD.com and Alibaba increased their food sales operations. In Santiago and Mexico City, meanwhile, the supermarkets intensified their own online sales and delivery services, independently or in collaboration with applications like Rappi and Uber Eats. Supermarkets and retail companies seemed to have the capacity to adjust to the situation, maintaining or even increasing their food sales.

On the other hand, traditional markets have seen their operations reduced. In China, wet markets have been questioned due to their probable relationship with the origin of COVID-19, and in Santiago and Mexico City, some markets were closed during stay-at-home orders as they were identified with outbreaks. In Mexico City, the authorities supported vendors by facilitating home delivery. In Santiago, there were similar efforts made by online applications, especially through informal networks. Given that traditional markets are the most accessible source of fresh food for the population in the cities analyzed, limiting their operation may have negative effects on diet quality.

Restaurants were devastated by stay-at-home orders. In all three cities, they were limited to takeaway and delivery for at least some time. In Shanghai, delivery workers were held to stricter sanitary requirements than in Santiago and Mexico City, carrying identity cards and leaving deliveries at drop-off points to avoid any contact with the clients and their neighbors. Food delivery has narrow margins anyway, and many restaurants, especially independent restaurants, and informal street vendors, who also belong to low-income groups, are struggling to survive.

The public sector also had some common responses in all three cases, such as increasing the regulation of sanitation, hygiene, and social distancing, as well as increasing enforcement. A very relevant difference between Shanghai and the other cities is the major role played by decentralized structures like housing complexes in support of the authorities. This made detailed control of the situation and coordination of specific actions possible. In Mexico City, authorities focused on helping small businesses, often food suppliers, survive. The municipal government also maintained meal centers. In Santiago, food access was supported by distributing free boxes of food to low-income families and students. In Shanghai, no public policies aimed at increasing access to food for families in need during the lockdowns were identified by this research.

Nonprofit initiatives driven by civil society, in some cases in partnership with the public and private sectors, have also increased due to COVID-19, especially in Mexico City and Santiago. These include chefs serving meals for populations in low-income districts, donation campaigns, or, in the case of Santiago, the return of community potlucks. In Shanghai, a very interesting initiative is the Green Food Bank, which also uses food that otherwise would be discarded, in line with the Chinese government's fight against food waste. However, it seems that civil society actions in Shanghai during lockdowns were mostly related to the aforementioned cooperation by housing complexes with authorities. Initiatives like food banks are still not recognized by Chinese law.

The digitalization of the food system will continue long-term. Schroeder et al. (2021) state that COVID-19 has exposed serious inefficiencies in the food system, such as information asymmetries and high transaction costs, for which digital technologies are a promising solution. The authors say, however, that this rapid development of digital technologies has two sides. On the one hand, it can overcome market and policy failures, but, investment allowing, it can also accelerate food system transformation. It is therefore very relevant, especially in cities with a large, low-income population, to promote digital solutions that democratize access to healthy food instead of widening existing gaps. As these three cities show, for some food suppliers, digital technology incorporation is much more difficult than for others, which was evident in the differences between supermarkets and traditional open-air markets. However, open-air markets are the most common place where middle- and low-income citizens buy fresh and nutritious food. The government should facilitate digitalization of traditional markets and ensure the inclusion of low-income consumers.

Another pandemic response that might be maintained over time is the use of protective equipment like face masks, goggles, hand sanitizer, temperature checks, improved sanitization practices, and limited store capacity. As the World Health Organization has repeatedly stated, the COVID-19 vaccination roll out is a slow process, especially for developing countries, so other preventative measures must be maintained. While supermarkets again might be better able to implement these measures, open-air markets may have advantages for disease control since they are held outdoors.

Finally, another promising, resilience-building solution is the increase in civil society initiatives aimed at improving food access in low-income areas of these cities. As we have seen, these initiatives generate positive externalities like the diffusion of homemade and traditional recipes, reduced food waste, and in some cases, increased local employment. To continue, however, they require stable governmental support.

Maintaining food security in cities is a big challenge. In fact, it is a challenge that will continue beyond the stay-at-home orders, given rising unemployment and poverty. It is essential, therefore, for city governments to prioritize access to sufficient, nutritious, and culturally appropriate food. It is also vital to develop coordinated and synergic strategies between public, private, and civil society actors, as was seen in the actions taken to contribute to the food supply during COVID-19 lockdowns.

References

Anstey, T. (2020, March 31). U-turn in Shanghai as reopened attractions close again. *Leisure Opportunities*. https://www.leisureopportunities.co.uk/news/U-turn-in-Shanghai-as-reopened-attractions-close-again/345196. Accessed May 2020.

ASEANPLUS NEWS. (2020, February 29). *Shanghai commerce businesses resuming operation as epidemic eases*. https://www.thestar.com.my/news/regional/2020/02/29/shanghai-commerce-businesses-resuming-operation-as-epidemic-eases. Accessed May 2020.

Asociación Mexicana de Venta Online. (2020). *Reporte 3.0 Impacto COVID-19 en venta online México* [Report 3.0 COVID-19 impact on online sales in Mexico]. https://www.amvo.org.mx/wp-content/uploads/2020/07/AMVO_Estudio3.0_ImpactoCOVID19_VP%C3%BAblica.pdf. Accessed May 2020.

Ayala, S., & Castillo, V. (2014). La distribución de alimentos y bebidas en México: una perspectiva desde el comercio tradicional [Food and beverages distribution in Mexico: A perspective from traditional commerce]. *Revista Espacio Abierto, 23*(4), 661–681.

Biblioteca del Congreso Nacional de Chile. (2020). *Indicadores sociodemográficos y económicos Región Metropolitana* [Sociodemographic and economic indicators in the Metropolitan Region]. https://www.bcn.cl/siit/nuestropais/region13/indica.htm. Accessed May 2020.

Carbajal, B. (2020, April 21). Covid-19 dispara en marzo ventas en tienditas: ANAM. *La Jornada*. https://www.jornada.com.mx/ultimas/economia/2020/04/21/covid-19-dispara-en-marzo-ventas-en-tienditas-anam-1738.html. Accessed May 2020.

Carreño, P., & Silva, A. (2019). Fruit and vegetable expenditure disparities: evidence from Chile. *British Food Journal, 121*(6), 1203–1219.

Casado-Izquierdo, J. M. (2018). Supermercados en México: expansión y espacios de inserción [Supermarkets in Mexico: Expansion and spaces of reinsertion]. *Estudios Geográficos, 74*(284), 167–190. https://doi.org/10.3989/estgeogr.201807

Cavish, C. (2020, March 11). No, China's fresh food markets did not cause coronavirus. *Los Angeles Times*. https://www.latimes.com/food/story/2020-03-11/coronavirus-china-wet-markets. Accessed April 2020.

Corro, N., Campuzano, J., Meneses, N., Tula, M., Blancas, E., Velásquez, E., & Ojeda, R. (2020, April 22). Compras sin la familia y productos limitados: así es ir al 'súper' en días de covid-19 [Purchases without the family and limited stock: That's how going to the 'supermarket' is like in Covid-19 days]. *Milenio*. https://www.milenio.com/politica/comunidad/como-es-ir-al-supermercado-durante-coronavirus-en-cdmx-y-edomex. Accessed May 2020.

Davis, C. (2020, February 26). Shanghai restaurant owners and chefs share outlooks on the coronavirus. *TimeOut Shanghai*. http://www.timeoutshanghai.com/features/Restaurants-Restaurants/72336/Shanghai-restaurant-owners-and-chefs-share-outlooks-on-the-coronavirus.html. Accessed April 2020.

Delgadillo, V. (2020, May 27). La covid-19 golpea los mercados de abasto en Ciudad de México [Covid-19 strikes the wholesales markets in Mexico City]. *El País*. https://elpais.com/elpais/2020/05/19/seres_urbanos/1589871781_940994.html. Accessed June 2020.

Ding, D., Liu, P., & Ravenscroft, N. (2018). The new urban agricultural geography of Shanghai. *Geoforum, 90*, 74–83. https://doi.org/10.1016/j.geoforum.2018.02.010

Everington, K. (2020, February 10). Shanghai, Chongqing also locked down as Wuhan virus spreads. *Taiwan News*. https://www.taiwannews.com.tw/en/news/3874064. Accessed April 2020.

FAO & Economic Commission for Latin America and the Caribbean. (2020). *Cómo evitar que la crisis del COVID-19 se transforme en una crisis alimentaria: acciones urgentes contra el hambre en América Latina y el Caribe* [How to avoid that the COVID-19 crisis turns into a food crisis: Urgent actions against hunger in Latin America and the Caribbean]. https://www.cepal.org/es/publicaciones/45702-como-evitar-que-la-crisis-covid-19-se-transforme-crisis-alimentaria-acciones. Accessed July 2020.

Food and Agriculture Organization [FAO]. (2014). *Ciudades más verdes en América Latina y el Caribe* [Greener cities in Latin America and the Caribbean]. Author.

Gajardo, C. (2019). *Modelo de negocio para implementar una empresa de comida rápida en Talca* [Business model to implement a fast food company in Talca]. Bachelor thesis, Universidad Técnica Federico Santa María, Chile. https://repositorio.usm.cl/bitstream/handle/11673/46473/3560903501096UTFSM.pdf?sequence=1&isAllowed=y. Accessed April 2020.

Gouk, R. (2020, April 20). Impact of COVID-19 on restaurants in Shanghai (April 2020). *Shanghai Food & Drink News*. https://rachelgouk.com/impact-of-covid-19-on-restaurants-in-shanghai/. Accessed May 2020.

Hobbs, J. E. (2020). Food supply chains during the COVID-19 pandemic. *Canadian Journal of Agricultural Economics, 68*(2), 171–176. https://doi.org/10.1111/cjag.12237

Hosseinifarhangi, M., Turvani, M. E., Van der Valk, A., & Carsjens, G. J. (2019). Technology-driven transition in urban food production practices: A case study of Shanghai. *Sustainability, 11*(21). https://doi.org/10.3390/su11216070

Huang, Z., Gao, R., Bawuerjiang, N., Zhang, Y., Huang, X., & Cai, M. (2017). Food and nutrients intake in the school lunch program among school children in Shanghai, China. *Nutrients, 9*(6), 582. https://doi.org/10.3390/nu9060582

Infobae. (2020, August 28). *Coronavirus en la CDMX: 170,000 negocios no sobrevivirán, son el equivalente a 1 millón de empleos, aproximadamente* [Coronavirus in Mexico City: 170,000 businesses will not survive, they are the equivalent of 1 million jobs, approximately]. https://www.infobae.com/america/mexico/2020/08/09/coronavirus-en-la-cdmx-170000-negocios-no-sobreviviran-son-el-equivalente-a-1-millon-de-empleos-aproximadamente/. Accessed Sept 2020.

Instituto Nacional de Estadísticas Chile. (2018). *Encuesta de superficie hortícola* [Horticulture area survey]. https://www.ine.cl/estadisticas/economia/agricultura-agroindustria-y-pesca/hortalizas. Accessed May 2020.

Kanter, R., & Boza, S. (2020). Strengthening local food systems in times of concomitant global crises: Reflections from Chile. *American Journal of Public Health, 110*(7), 971–973. https://doi.org/10.2105/AJPH.2020.305711

Kuo, L. (2020, August 13). 'Operation empty plate': Xi Jinping makes food waste his next target. *The Guardian*. https://www.theguardian.com/world/2020/aug/13/operation-empty-plate-xi-jinping-makes-food-waste-his-next-target. Accessed Sept 2020.

Laborde, D., Martin, W. J., & Vos, R. (2020). Poverty and food insecurity could grow dramatically as COVID-19 spreads. In J. Swinnen & J. McDermott (Eds.), *COVID-19 and global food security* (pp. 16–20). International Food Policy Research Institute, IFPRI.

Lozano, L. F. (2020, July 12). Restaurantes tienen 'hambre' de comensales en la nueva normalidad. *Forbes México*. https://www.forbes.com.mx/negocios-restaurantes-hambre-comensales-cdmx/. Accessed Aug 2020.

Martorell, M., Ulloa, N., González, M. E., Martínez-Sanguinetti, M. A., & Celis-Morales, C. (2020). Obesidad, desnutrición y cambio climático: una sindemia que Chile deberá enfrentar [Obesity, malnutrition, and climate change: A syndemic that Chile will have to face]. *Revista Médica Chilena, 148*, 881–886. https://doi.org/10.4067/S0034-98872020000600882

Maruyama, M., Wu, L., & Huang, L. (2016). The modernization of fresh food retailing in China: The role of consumers. *Journal of Retailing and Consumer Services, 30*, 33–39. https://doi.org/10.1016/j.jretconser.2015.12.006
Morales, A. (2020, May 14). Negocios de abarrotes peligran por COVID-19; por ello lanzan Mi Tienda Segura [Grocery stores in danger due to COVID-19; therefore, my safe store gets launched]. *El Contribuyente*. https://www.elcontribuyente.mx/2020/05/negocios-de-abarrotes-peligran-por-covid-19-por-ello-lanzan-mi-tienda-segura/. Accessed June 2020.
Navarrete, S. (2020, July 22). Vendedores ambulantes de la CDMX proponen un protocolo ante el COVID-19 [Street vendors in Mexico City propose a protocol against COVID-19]. *Expansión Política*. https://politica.expansion.mx/cdmx/2020/07/22/vendedores-ambulantes-de-la-cdmx-proponen-un-protocolo-ante-el-covid-19. Accessed Aug 2020.
Ng, E., Ximing, S., Woodhead, A., & Nugent, T. (2016). *Why China? Shanghai and food consumption trends*. University of Southern Queensland & Queensland Government. https://eprints.usq.edu.au/33152/1/Why%20China_Shanghai%20and%20food%20consumption%20trends%20technical%20report%20.pdf. Accessed July 2020.
Qian, L. (2020, August 19). *Shanghai's food banks have twin benefits*. Shine. https://www.shine.cn/news/metro/2008194509/. Accessed Nov 2020.
Reveles, C. (2020, March 26). Mercados y tianguis de CDMX no cerrarán por COVID-19, tendrán servicio a domicilio [Open markets in Mexico City will not close due to COVID-19, they will have delivery service]. https://www.animalpolitico.com/2020/03/mercados-tianguis-covid-19-no-cierran/. Accessed April 2020.
Russ, S., & Yu, H. (2020, February 16). Fast-food companies in China step up 'contactless' pickup, delivery as coronavirus rages. *Reuters*. https://www.reuters.com/article/us-china-health-fast-food-focus/fast-food-companies-in-china-step-up-contactless-pickup-delivery-as-coronavirus-rages-idUSKBN20A0RS. Accessed April 2020.
Schmidhuber, J., Pound, J., & Qiao, B. (2020). *COVID-19: Channels of transmission to food and agriculture*. FAO.
Schmitt, S. (2012). Comparative approaches to the study of public policy-making. In E. Araral, S. Fritzen, M. Howlett, M. Ramesh, & X. Wu (Eds.), *Routledge handbook of public policy* (pp. 29–43). Routledge.
Schroeder, K., Lampietti, J., & Elabed, G. (2021). *What's cooking: Digital transformation of the agrifood system*. World Bank.
Secretaría de Desarrollo Económico de la Ciudad de México. (2020). *Reporte económico de la Ciudad de México. Primer trimestre 2020* [Economic report of Mexico City. First Quarter 2020]. https://www.sedeco.cdmx.gob.mx/storage/app/media/uploaded-files/reporte-economico-1t-2020.pdf. Accessed June 2020.
Shanghai Municipal People's Government. (2020, August 18). *All eyes on eateries as blitz against food waste begins*. http://www.shanghai.gov.cn/shanghai/n46669/n48081/n48088/u22ai129877.html. Accessed Nov 2020.
Swinburn, B., Kraak, V., Allender, S., Atkins, V., Baker, P., Bogard, J., Brinsden, H., Calvillo, A., De Schutter, O., Devarajan, R., Ezzati, M., Friel, S., Goenka, S., Hammond, R. A., Hastings, G., Hawkes, C., Herrero, M., Hovmand, P. S., Howden, M., … Wolfenden, L. (2019). The global syndemic of obesity, undernutrition, and climate change: The Lancet Commission report. *Lancet, 393*(10173), 791–846. https://doi.org/10.1016/S0140-6736(18)32822-8
The Economic Times. (2020, February 8). *China scrambles to keep cities in virus lockdown fed*. https://economictimes.indiatimes.com/news/international/world-news/china-scrambles-to-keep-cities-in-virus-lockdown-fed/articleshow/74022218.cms. Accessed April 2020.
United Nations Children's Fund, Pan American Health Organization, & FAO. (2020). *Prevención de mala nutrición en niñas y niños en México ante la pandemia de COVID-19* [Preventing malnutrition in girls and boys in Mexico during the COVID-19 pandemic]. https://www.unicef.org/mexico/sites/unicef.org.mexico/files/2020-07/FINAL%20Posicionamiento%20Conjunto%20Nutricio%CC%81n%20COVID19.pdf. Accessed Nov 2020.

Wall Street Journal. (2020, February 4). *Chinese supermarkets fined, warned against price gouging amid outbreak.* https://www.wsj.com/articles/chinese-supermarkets-fined-warned-against-price-gouging-amid-outbreak-11580818854. Accessed April 2020.

White, C. (2020, April 14). US politicians call for shutdown of wet markets in China. *Seafood Source*. https://www.seafoodsource.com/news/supply-trade/us-politicians-call-for-shutdown-of-wet-markets-in-china. Accessed June 2020.

Xinhua. (2020, August 28). *Shanghai sees acceleration in work resumption*. http://www.xinhuanet.com/english/2020-03/01/c_138833010_3.htm. Accessed Nov 2020.

Yu, F. (2020, April 14). Wet markets critical in providing market supply to Shanghai residents. *Global Times*. https://www.globaltimes.cn/content/1185527.shtml. Accessed June 2020.

Zang, J., Luo, B., Wang, Y., Zhu, Z., Wang, Z., He, X., Wang, W., Guo, Y., Chen, X., Wang, C., Guo, C., Zou, S., Jia, X., & Fan, W. (2018). Eating out-of-home in adult residents in Shanghai and the nutritional differences among dining places. *Nutrients, 10*(7), 951. https://doi.org/10.3390/nu10070951

Zhang, Q. F., & Pan, Z. (2013). The transformation of urban vegetable retail in China: Wet markets, supermarkets, and informal markets in Shanghai. *Journal of Contemporary Asia, 43*(3), 497–518.

Chapter 12
A Typological Analysis of Nursing Home Environments During the COVID-19 Pandemic: Risks and Potential

Lucía Martín López and Rodrigo Durán López

Introduction

The Problem

According to studies conducted in Spain on 235,000 people, the COVID-19 mortality rate is higher in those people aged 70 years or older. The mortality rate is 14.5% in people aged between 70 and 79 years old, 21.2% in people aged between 80 and 89, and 22.2% in people 90 years or older, compared to 0.3% in people aged between 30 and 39 years old. The vulnerable nature of this population, combined with the inherent risks of close-living conditions in long-term care settings, has made nursing homes in countries like Spain greatly affected by coronavirus, with high rates of infection and mortality. As of April 19, 2020, at least 10,719 people have died from COVID-19 or similar symptoms in nursing homes in Spain, which represents half of the official deaths in the entire country. Madrid, Catalonia and Castile, and Leon were the autonomous communities with the most incidences (García Rada, 2020).

As of 2019, there were 5417 registered nursing homes in Spain. Of these, 71% (3844) are private and shelter 271,696 residents (García Rada, 2020). In Madrid, one of the regions most greatly affected by the pandemic, there are 710 nursing homes with 42,500 residents, which is 5% of people aged 70 and older in Madrid (TeleMadrid, 2020). Between March 8 and April 14, 2020, about 5000 people in Madrid's nursing homes died from coronavirus, 781 were confirmed to have the

L. Martín López (✉)
Tecnologico de Monterrey, School of Architecture, Art and Design, Querétaro, Mexico
e-mail: luciamartinlopez@tec.mx

R. Durán López
Universidad Anáhuac México, Naucalpan, Mexico
e-mail: rodrigo.duranlo@anahuac.mx

© The Author(s), under exclusive license to Springer Nature Switzerland AG 2021

M. A. Montoya et al. (eds.), *COVID-19 and Cities*, The Urban Book Series,
https://doi.org/10.1007/978-3-030-84134-8_12

disease, and 4172 had symptoms related to COVID-19, compared to 900 dead from other causes in nursing homes in March 2019 (García Rada, 2020).

According to the government of Catalonia, the community with the most nursing homes in Spain, between March 15 and April 15, 2020, 1810 people infected with coronavirus died in nursing homes in this region; 3920 were treated in isolation, 1214 were admitted to hospital, and 5755 workers in these facilities were isolated with confirmed symptoms. Castilla La Mancha, Valencia, Aragon, Extremadura, Basque Country, and Andalusia confirmed 636 323, 364, 287, 269, and 300 deaths from COVID-19, respectively (García Rada, 2020).

Spain's mainstream media indicated that this mortality rate was caused by a lack of medicalization in these residences, inadequate management from the authorities that control the admission of patients into hospitals, and the lack of resources for the protection of nursing homes' personnel and residents (TeleMadrid, 2020).

The impact of COVID-19 on nursing home residents has been varied on an international level, with some countries not informing deaths or infection rates in these facilities, like Hong Kong, Jordan, and Malta, while two countries informed that over 80% of COVID-19 deaths were of nursing home residents. In a study conducted in 26 countries, researchers concluded that 47% of deaths caused by COVID-19 were of nursing home residents. The percentage of elderly people that died in nursing homes during the pandemic ranges between 0% and 6.1%, which is highly correlated with the total number of deaths caused by COVID-19 in the entire population (Comas-Herrera et al., 2020).

Nursing homes are part of a citizens' network that consolidates the city and has not been taken into consideration when designing it (Valdivia, 2017). During the COVID-19 pandemic, it has become evident that there is a deficit in this citizens' network within the city. Large cities don't favor elderly people's autonomy and don't permit them to engage with the diverse spheres of everyday life. Thus, it is necessary to look into these infrastructures and services and adapt them, not only to solve public health-specific emergencies like the coronavirus pandemic, but also to provide a better quality of life to the entire population, which would result in an increment of resilience capacity in communities and, therefore, the cities themselves.

State of the Art

The approach to the propagation phenomenon of COVID-19 in nursing homes, from a typological point of view, was addressed from four aspects, as seen in Table 12.1.

Regarding the texts on nursing homes and cohousing from a morphotypological and functional point of view, two works are considered of special interest. The first one, "Die 5. Generation: KDA-Quartiershäuser" (Michell-Auli & Sowinski, 2012), for its typological classification of residences and for the detailed explanation of how they work and are organized. The second one, "The Co-Housing Phenomenon" (Giorgi, 2020), in which shared space becomes a topic of particular interest, as it is

Table 12.1 Texts on nursing homes and cohousing from a morphotypological and functional point of view; studies on how COVID-19 spreads in nursing homes; studies on how COVID-19 spreads in general and a graphical analysis on coronavirus spatial spread

Bibliography	Nursing homes & cohousing	COVID-19 & nursing homes	COVID-19 spreads	COVID-19 spatial analysis	Region
CDC (2020h, How…)			•		Worldwide
Florida (2020)			•		Worldwide
CDC (2020a, Infection Control…)			•		Worldwide
Anderson et al. (2020)			•		Worldwide
Fraser et al. (2004)			•		Worldwide
Zhang et al. (2020)			•		Worldwide
Murphy (2020)			•		Worldwide
Mass (2020b, Designing Spaces…)			•		Worldwide
Salas and Zafra (2020)			•	•	Worldwide
Mass (2020d, Spatial…)			•	•	Worldwide
Mass (2020a, Carceral…)			•	•	Worldwide
Mass (2020c, Rules…)			•	•	Worldwide
Mass (2020, Redesigning…)			•	•	Worldwide
Mass (2020b, Designing Senior…)	•	•	•	•	Worldwide
Ministerio de Sanidad (2020)		•	•		Spain
CDC (2020f, Responding…)		•	•		USA
CDC (2020d, Nursing…)		•	•		USA
CDC (2020b, Infection Prevention…)		•	•		USA
Center for Clinical Standards and Quality (2020)		•	•		USA
Gardner et al. (2020)		•			Worldwide
Comas-Herrera et al. (2020)		•			Worldwide
García Rada (2020)		•			Spain
Carreño and Allen (2020)		•			Spain
Bachega (2020)		•			Spain
BBC Radio (2020)		•			Spain
Rodriguez Martinez (2020)		•			Spain

(continued)

Table 12.1 (continued)

Bibliography	Nursing homes & cohousing	COVID-19 & nursing homes	COVID-19 spreads	COVID-19 spatial analysis	Region
Marcos and Sosa Troya (2020)		•			Spain
McMichael et al. (2020)		•			USA
Kimball et al. (2020)		•			USA
Roxby et al. (2020)		•			USA
Yourish (2020)		•			USA
Aiello (2020)		•			Canada
Osman (2020)		•			Canada
Michell-Auli and Sowinski (2012)	•				Germany
Giorgi (2020)	•				Worldwide
Valdivia (2018)	•				Spain
Rodríguez (2015)	•				Spain
Magdziak (2019)	•				Worldwide
Ossokina et al. (2019)	•				Worldwide
Abramsson and Andersson (2016)	•				Worldwide
Costa-Font et al. (2009)	•				Spain
Steels (2015)	•				Worldwide
Luciano et al. (2020)	•				Worldwide
Malik and Mikołajczak (2019)	•				Worldwide
Rusinovic et al. (2019)	•				Netherlands
Oliveira et al. (2019)	•				Worldwide
Yang and Fu (2019)	•				Worldwide
Pettigrew et al. (2020)	•				Worldwide
Mosquera et al. (2020)	•				Spain
Serrano-Jiménez et al. (2020)	•				Spain
Lee et al. (2020)	•			•	Worldwide
Kim and Kim (2020)	•				Worldwide

Own creation, 2020
•Represents that one of the main topics of the text is the one indicated in the column

characterized, typified, and its functioning is explained. The space of coexistence is extremely important when analyzing the spread of any airborne disease. It is important to highlight that in any of the framed texts in this group, there is a mention of the spread of this type of disease in these infrastructures.

Regarding the studies on how COVID-19 spreads in nursing homes, we have two subtypes of bibliography: one that only informs about the number of cases and its location, such as García Rada (2020), Bachega (2020), Yourish (2020), Carreño and

Allen (2020), Marcos and Sosa Troya (2020), Osman (2020), or Aiello (2020) among others; and the other that talks about how the virus spreads inside a nursing home and how to avoid it according to management and good behavioral practices such as texts from the Ministry of Health in Spain (2020), the Centers for Disease Control and Prevention (CDC) (2020a), or the Center for Clinical Standards and Quality of the USA.

Concerning the studies on how COVID-19 spreads in general, the bibliography from the Centers for Disease Control and Prevention (CDC) is noteworthy as it provides specific data about spread forms of COVID-19 (CDC, 2020h, How…), and Infection Control Guidance is presented in a clear and easy-to-apply way (CDC, 2020a, Infection…).

Finally, as it pertains to the graphical analysis on coronavirus spatial spread, the work from the Mass Design Group (2020d) and Salas and Zafra (2020) was revised. Both use the layout and the axonometry as diagnostic and phenomenon explanation tools. It is worth noting that the work by the Mass Design Group refers to Senior Housing for this work as it approaches the same problem and the same user (Mass, 2020b). However, that study is a behavior manual for Senior Housing design and not a diagnostic tool for nursing homes, which is the proposal of this investigation.

Hypothesis

During this pandemic, it has been demonstrated that a strong Infection Prevention and Control Program, which tackles space management and how we relate to it, is vital to protect residents and health personnel (CDC, 2020e, Preparing…). Therefore, it is considered as a hypothesis for this investigation that spatial configuration and its social logic (Space Syntax) can directly influence the propagation probabilities of airborne diseases like COVID-19 in nursing homes.

Research Question and Objectives

As a result of the hypothesis and based on the attention centered on the person concept, the objective of this investigation is to identify the type of nursing home that can present a lower propagation of COVID-19 based on its spatial structure.

Methodology Statement

The analysis will be done under four parameters that directly affect the virus propagation: density, social distancing, sectorization/isolation, and ventilation. The study of these parameters is based on the use of a comparative graphic method, for which same-scale layouts are used for each type of residence. In these layouts, people concentrations per square meter are mapped, as well as distances, areas, and movements previously mentioned, so they can be measured and correlated with each other. In addition to these maps that allow an intuitive understanding of each phenomenon, a comparative table summary is presented in which the zones with a higher propagation risk can be identified, and the type of residence that functions better, in terms of the analyzed parameters during the COVID-19 crisis, can be assessed.

Limitations of the Study

For this analysis, generalizations have been made for each type of residence. These typological generalizations imply that each particular design can bring different and particular data that is worth evaluating independently. However, the presented methodology is clear and simple, which is why it is considered to be easily repeatable by any technician when comparing several projects.

Materials and Methods

Scope of the Study, Sample Selection, and Representativeness

According to the Kuratorium Deutsche Altershilfe, there are four types of generalized nursing homes in Europe classified as first-generation, second-generation, third-generation, and fourth-generation residences.

The first generation is a model developed between the 1940s and the 1960s, in which rooms are shared between two and six people. The bathrooms are centralized, and each person has 13.1 m^2 available. The second generation is characteristic of the 1960s and 1970s: In this generation, the common areas are centralized and are normally located on the ground floor or in the basement, and each person uses 28.5 m^2. The third generation was produced in the 1980s: In these, the shared and individual space is turned into a living space, rooms have their own bathrooms, and the common areas are decentralized and distributed on all floors in a way that each person uses 38.8 m^2. Finally, fourth-generation residences, constructed in the early 1990s, are composed of autonomous units. The centralized systems disappear, each unit has its own kitchen, and carers move to where the users are providing 40 m^2 per person (Montero, 2012).

Currently, in Spain, second- and third-generation residences coexist, and for a few years now, fourth-generation residential complexes have begun to be implemented, especially in Castilla León and the Basque Country (Jubilares, 2014). In Germany, some fifth-generation residences have been developed which are centered

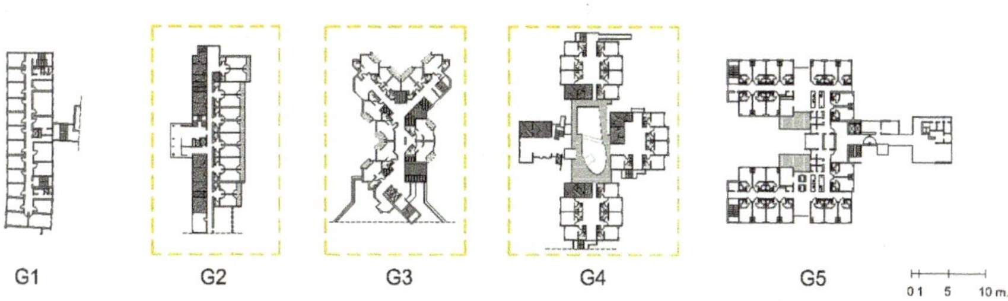

Fig. 12.1 The five generations of residences, indicating the three that will be studied in this text. (Own creation. Based on shown layouts in Michell-Auli and Sowinski (2012) 2020)

more around the person and where alternative forms of housing for the elderly can be found, such as protected and shared floors, or neighborhood projects that won't be considered for this article due to their typological variability. In focusing on the Spanish problem, this article will only analyze the three types of residences that occur in the region: second-, third-, and fourth-generation residences (Fig. 12.1).

Research Design

To select the indicators used in this article, the aspects that condition the spread of the virus were identified in the bibliography. The compilation of these aspects can be observed in Fig. 12.2 and contemplates the following factors: sectorization or isolation (appearing in 90.9% of localized texts); social distancing (86.4%); use of Personal Protective Equipment (PPE) (77.3%); density (59%); hand hygiene (54.5%); ventilation or open-air conditions (50%); general cleaning and disinfection procedures (50%); touching a surface or object that has the virus on it (50%); management of laundry, food service utensils, and medical waste (36.4%); information (36.4%); length of exposure (13.6%); contact tracing (13.6%); water hygiene (9.1%); urban air conditions (4.5%); and waste management (4.5%). From these factors, only those that are directly related to space construction were selected due to the typological and comparative nature of this analysis: sectorization or isolation, social distancing, density, ventilation or open-air conditions, information, water hygiene, and waste management. Because of the extension of this text, only the analysis of the four factors that have a higher rate of appearance in the bibliography is shown. It is also the reason why some repeated factors were eliminated, such as the adequate use of PPE or correct hand hygiene, among others, as these are aspects that can be solved with small but important actions that don't affect the space itself (Table 12.2).

The definition of the aspects that facilitate the spread of COVID-19, as well as how they condition residents' lives and how they will be measured in this investigation, is provided below. In all graphic analyses, traffic light colors (green, yellow, and red) will be used to distinguish the places with more risk (red), medium risk

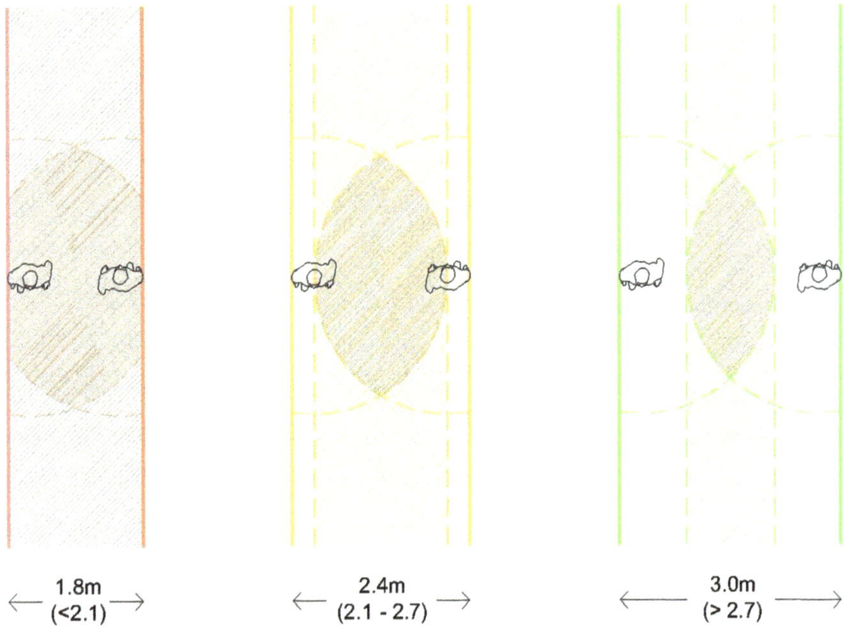

Fig. 12.2 The social distancing gradient used to zone the circulating area. (Own creation, 2020)

(yellow), and less risk (green) of virus spread. This method will be used to visualize the problem clearly and intuitively.

Isolation or *sectorization*, the most repeated aspect in the bibliography, is focused on the isolation between healthy, suspect, and sick residents. To understand this concept, it is important to distinguish between "quarantine" and "isolation". *Quarantine* "separates and restricts the movement of people who were exposed to a contagious disease to see if they become sick. These people may have been exposed to a disease and do not know it, or they may have the disease but do not show symptoms" (U.S. Department of Health & Human Services, 2020). *Isolation* "separates sick people with a contagious disease from people who are not sick" (U.S. Department of Health & Human Services, 2020). This analysis will highlight the possibility of making part of a building independent from the rest, whether vertically (by floors) or horizontally (wing or cluster of rooms). When representing this aspect, two types of floor analysis will be done. The first one will show if it is possible to define an isolation sector in the assessed type, and if the sector has an elevator and stairs, it will be indicated with green, and if it only has an elevator or stairs, it will be indicated with yellow. A greater possibility of creating different sectors on the floor means greater adaptability or transformability of the type against any circumstance, which is a positive quality when controlling COVID-19 in this type of infrastructure.

The second type of analysis focuses exclusively on the room area and indicates if a sick person can be isolated in his bedroom and if he has an independent

Table 12.2 Spread factors of COVID-19 in nursing homes according to the located bibliography and the appearance rate of the factors in it

Bibliography	Sectorization/ isolation	Social distancing	Personal protective equipment	Density	Hand hygiene	Ventilation/ open-air conditions	Cleaning/ disinfection procedures	Touching a surface that has the virus on it	Management of laundry and waste	Information	Length of exposure	Contact tracing	Water hygiene	Urban air conditions	Waste manage ment
CDC (2020h, How…)		•	•		•			•			•				
CDC (2020a, Infection Control…)	•	•	•	•	•	•	•	•	•	•					
Anderson et al. (2020)	•	•										•			
Fraser et al. (2004)	•											•			
Zhang et al. (2020)	•	•	•	•	•	•	•					•		•	
Murphy (2020)		•				•		•					•		•
Mass (2020b, Designing Spaces…)	•	•		•		•		•	•	•					
Salas and Zafra, (2020)	•	•	•	•		•		•			•				
Mass (2020d, Spatial…)	•	•	•	•	•	•	•	•	•	•					
Mass (2020a, Carceral…)	•	•	•	•	•	•	•	•	•	•					

(continued)

Table 12.2 (continued)

Bibliography	Sectorization/ isolation	Social distancing	Personal protective equipment	Density	Hand hygiene	Ventilation/ open-air conditions	Cleaning/ disinfection procedures	Touching a surface that has the virus on it	Management of laundry and waste	Information	Length of exposure	Contact tracing	Water hygiene	Urban air conditions	Waste manage ment
Mass (2020c, Rules…)	•	•	•			•	•	•		•			•		
Mass (2020, Redesigning…)	•		•	•		•	•	•	•	•					
Mass (2020b, Designing Senior…)	•	•	•	•	•	•	•	•	•	•					
Ministerio de Sanidad (2020)	•	•	•	•	•	•	•		•						
CDC (2020f, Responding…)	•	•	•		•		•	•							
CDC (2020d, Nursing)	•	•	•	•	•		•		•	•					
Center for Clinical Standards and Quality (2020)	•	•	•	•	•										
Gardner et al. (2020)	•	•		•	•										
McMichael et al. (2020)	•	•	•												
Kimball et al. (2020)	•		•								•				
Roxby et al. (2020)	•	•	•		•		•								
Aiello (2020)	•	•	•	•											
Representativeness rate of the factor	90.9	86.4	77.3	59.0	54.5	50.0	50.0	50.0	36.4	36.4	13.6	13.6	9.1	4.5	4.5

Own creation, 2020

•Represents that one of the main topics of the text is the one indicated in the column

bathroom in his room. In cases that both conditions occur, the room will appear green, otherwise it will appear red. From this mapping, a relation between the number of residents that can be accommodated in isolated rooms and the total number of residents will be established, transforming the data into a comparable rate.

Social distancing, also called *physical distancing*, is the second aspect with a higher appearance rate in the bibliography. According to the Centers for Disease Control and Prevention, *social distancing* means "keeping a safe space between yourself and other people who are not from your household" (CDC, 2020g, Social…). "Spread happens when an infected person coughs, sneezes, or talks, and droplets from their mouth or nose are launched into the air and land in the mouths or noses of people nearby" (CDC, 2020g, Social…). To practice social or physical distancing, residents must stay at least 6 ft (about 1.82 m or 2 arms' length) from other people in both indoor and outdoor spaces. These conditions restrict the use of common areas, especially circulating areas, and extremely restrict external visits, primarily from family. For social distancing representation, two analyses will be conducted. The first, focused on circulating areas, will show movement zones in which the social distance is less than 1.8 m (with a high spread probability) in red, areas that have between 2.1 and 2.7 m in yellow, and areas in which people can be separated by over 2.7 m, where the spread is less likely, in green (Fig. 12.2). From this analysis, the relation of the square meters of each spread zone and the total surface of the common areas of each floor is obtained, thus generating a rate that will be used to compare each case.

The second analysis of social distancing is focused on the rooms and living areas assessment, indicating the areas in which a physical distance of at least 1.8 m can be achieved while at rest. For the analysis of this aspect, all possible occupations for each space are drawn on each type of area, and the most suitable situation is chosen. Once this layout is charted, 1.8-m safety circles are overlaid, drawing in green those areas in which circles are not overlaid and in red those where they intersect, creating an unsafe area, like the one presented in Fig. 12.3. To quantify this parameter, a relation between the number of intersected circles and the number of total safety circles on the floor is created, obtaining a percentage value.

The third aspect that conditions COVID-19 spread is density. This refers to the average number of residents in an area in relation to a surface unit. In this case, a greater number of residents means a greater concentration and more exposure to the virus. Therefore, a greater density will imply a greater risk of infection. This aspect directly affects the communal life developed in common areas, especially in programmed social activities like group therapy or recreational activities. When representing density, common areas will be marked out on the floor, measuring its square meters and relating these with the number of residents per floor to make a comparable indicator.

The last indicator assessed in this text is ventilation. *Ventilation* "provides outdoor air into a building or a room and distributes air within the building. The purpose of ventilation in buildings is to provide healthy air for breathing by diluting pollutants originating in the building with clean air, and by providing an airflow rate to change this air at a given rate" (Atkinson et al., 2009). In the case of airborne diseases, the existence of adequate and natural ventilation that offers almost

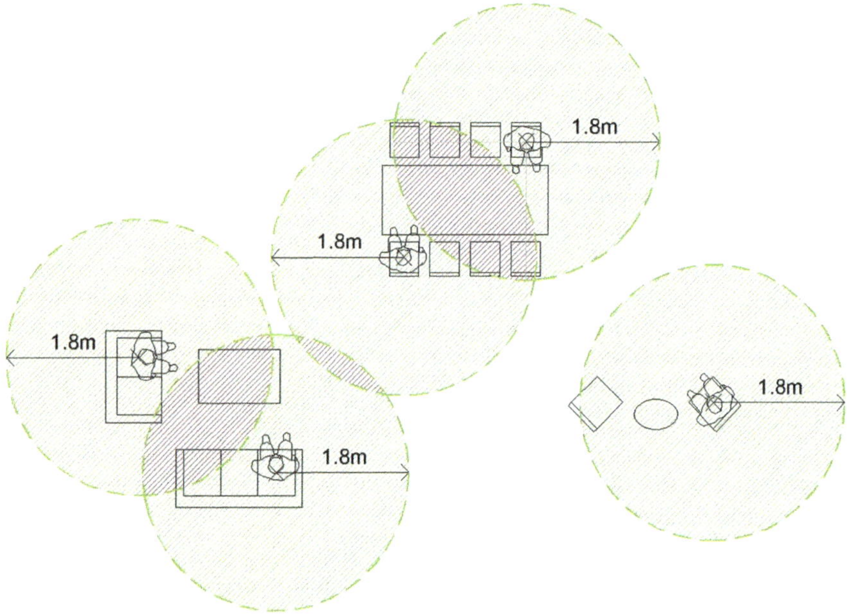

Fig. 12.3 Social distancing (6 ft radius) is used to zone the safe living spaces. (Own creation, 2020)

open-air conditions is necessary to reduce the risk of infection to the maximum level. This aspect conditions all the indoor collective activities.

For the analysis, only natural ventilation is assessed, which is the one that "uses natural forces to introduce and distribute outdoor air into or out of a building. These natural forces can be wind pressures or pressures generated by the density difference between indoor and outdoor air" (Atkinson et al., 2009). To clarify the complexity of this phenomenon, three indicators will be used. The first will evaluate the number of open-air areas per resident, which will be drawn, calculated, and divided by the number of residents per floor. The areas will be defined as exterior areas (used by only one resident), shared exterior areas (shared by one or two residents), and common exterior areas (shared by all residents on the floor).

Secondly, the air distribution or airflow pattern will be drawn in the rooms. This pattern analyzes if "the external air should be delivered to each part of the space in an efficient manner and the airborne pollutants generated in each part of the space should also be removed in an efficient manner" (Atkinson et al., 2009). In this pattern, natural ventilation that is crossed and effective will be marked with green, and when it is not, it will be marked with red. To obtain this data in a percentage value, the number of rooms with proper ventilation and the total number of rooms will be related.

Finally, to evaluate the ventilation area of each room, the area in square meters of windows or doors that allow ventilation is calculated with the help of the axonometric drawing.

Results, Recommendations, and Discussion

Having defined the aspects of this study (Table 12.3), each representative floor for each generation of residences was analyzed (Fig. 12.4). Subsequently, some recommendations for each case were developed, supported by the "Interim Infection Prevention and Control Recommendations for Healthcare Personnel During the Coronavirus Disease 2019 (COVID-19) Pandemic" from CDC (2020c). After this, the indicators were related through a table (Table 12.4) to be compared. The latter was done to identify the type that is relatively effective with respect to each assessed factor to minimize COVID-19 infections.

Isolation—Number of Possible Sectorizations

In this isolation analysis (Fig. 12.4), according to the number of possible sectorizations, three different behaviors can be observed for each type of residence. In the case of the second generation, the communication centers are located in the center of the floor, thus there is only one way of segregating the floor from these. In the third generation, the centers are located at the ends of the floor. This provides greater flexibility as rooms can be added in one sector or another, according to convenience. As for the fourth generation, thanks to its clustered architecture with independent stairs, each cluster can be easily isolated. However, in the case of needing an elevator, access can get complicated. It should be noted that in this case, if infection occurs inside a cluster, the subdivision would become more complicated due to a single access.

RECOMMENDATIONS: In the three studied cases, a lack of a wandering zone for patients with a neurocognitive disorder is observed. These spaces are needed in the three isolation sectors (healthy, suspects and infected) because of the unpredictability of these residents' movements. The existence of an exclusive zone for healthcare personnel (entry, storage to keep their objects and PPE separate, restroom, break room, and work area) separated from residents to minimize overlaps and touchpoints is recommended. It is imperative to create cleanable and disinfectable buffers to go from one sector to another.

Table 12.3 Summary table of analyzed aspects, indicators used, and its measure units

Aspect	Indicator	Units
Isolation	Number of possible sectorizations	#
	Isolated bedrooms ratio	%
Social distancing	Social distancing gradient in circulation areas	%
	Social distancing gradient in living areas	%
Density	Density	m^2/px
Ventilation	Open-air conditions area per resident	m^2/px
	Air distribution pattern	%
	Ventilation surface per room	m^2

Own creation, 2020

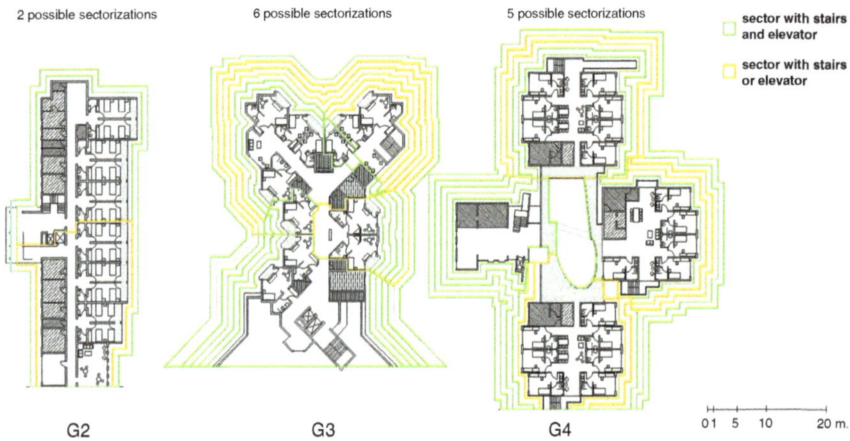

Fig. 12.4 Isolation analysis. Number of possible sectorizations in each of the three types of residences selected—second generation, third generation, and fourth generation. (Own creation, 2020)

Table 12.4 Comparative table of the analyzed indicators in each type of nursing home generation

Aspect	Indicator	Units	G2	G3	G4
Isolation	Number of possible sectorizations	#	2	6	5
	Isolated bedrooms ratio	%	0	100	100
Social distancing	Gradient in circulation areas (<2.1 m)	%	35.90	30.65	36.10
	Gradient in circulation areas (>3.0 m)	%	46.33	53.15	61.10
	Social distancing gradient in living areas	%	51.7	6.3	17.1
Density	Density	m²/px	9.40	19.20	25.38
Ventilation	Open-air conditions area per resident (individual exterior area)	m²/px	0.0	3.05	0.0
	Open-Air conditions area per resident (shared exterior area)	m²/px	1.99	0.0	0.0
	Open-air conditions area per resident (common exterior area)	m²/px	0.0	0.0	6.14
	Air distribution pattern	%			100%
	Ventilation surface per room	m²	6.8	3.2	0.5

Best practices number (summation of the previous ones)	#	2	5	5
Worst practices number (summation of the previous ones)	#	5	0	2

Own creation, 2020

Isolation—Isolated Bedrooms Ratio

Regarding the Isolated Bedrooms Ratio (Fig. 12.5), the behavior of the second-generation type should be noted as it is characterized by its shared bedrooms. Because of this, the only bedrooms that could be isolated would be the ones from the third and fourth generations because, besides being single-bedrooms, they have an independent bathroom.

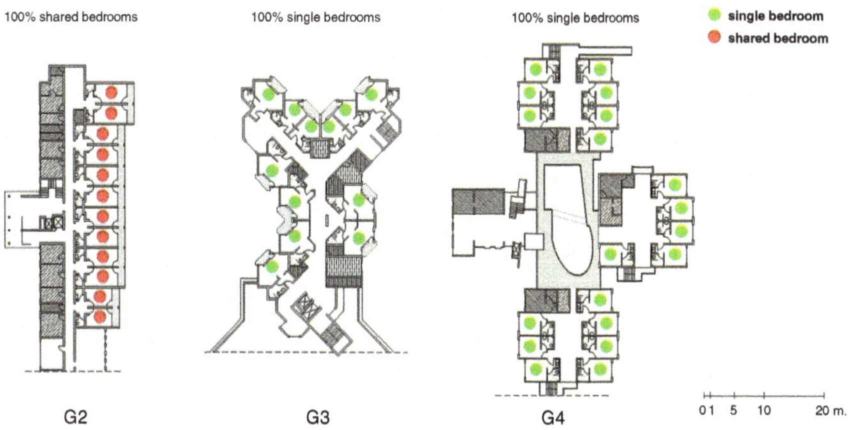

Fig. 12.5 Isolation analysis. Isolated bedrooms ratio in each of the three types of residence selected. (Own creation, 2020)

RECOMMENDATIONS: If there is no single room available, only exposed residents sharing a room should be allowed (CDC, 2020c, Interim…).

Social Distancing Gradient in Circulation Areas

When analyzing social distancing in circulation areas (Fig. 12.6), the three floors that have areas in which safe distancing cannot be respected can be observed.

The second-generation floor has a hallway narrow enough to facilitate the spread of the virus. While the third-generation floor has bags that broaden the hallway and can be used for people to wait and avoid encountering others in the narrower zones. The fourth-generation floor has clusters in which an adequate safe distancing can be achieved, except in the bedrooms. Once outside the clusters, however, the stairs and the hallways are too narrow and don't allow safe circulation.

RECOMMENDATIONS: For this aspect, it is imperative to design flows for infection control, reduce the number of people wandering, and enhance virtual contact when possible. If hallways cannot be broadened, the use of physical barriers can help reduce the spread. Another option is making one-way hallways if circulation allows it, i.e., corridors that have elevator cores at each end can become unidirectional.

Social Distancing Gradient in Living Areas

In the social distancing analysis for living areas (Fig. 12.7), the reduced physical distancing of the second-generation bedrooms stands out as these are shared, which

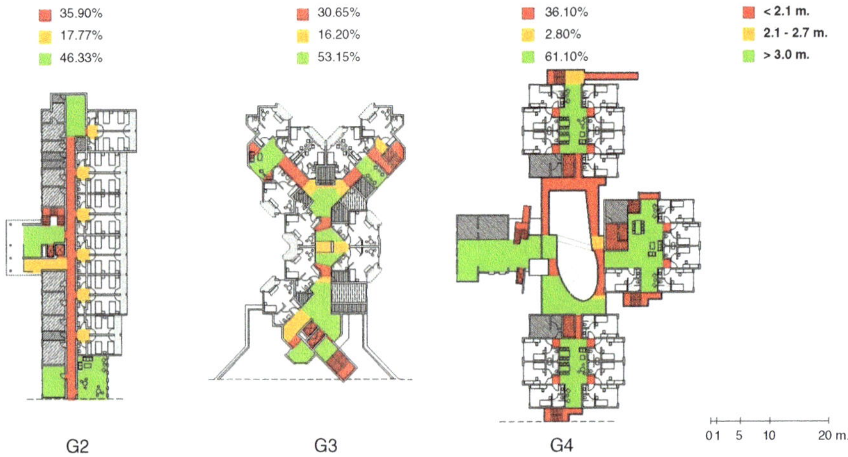

Fig. 12.6 Social distancing analysis. The gradient in circular areas in each of the three types of residences selected. (Own creation, 2020)

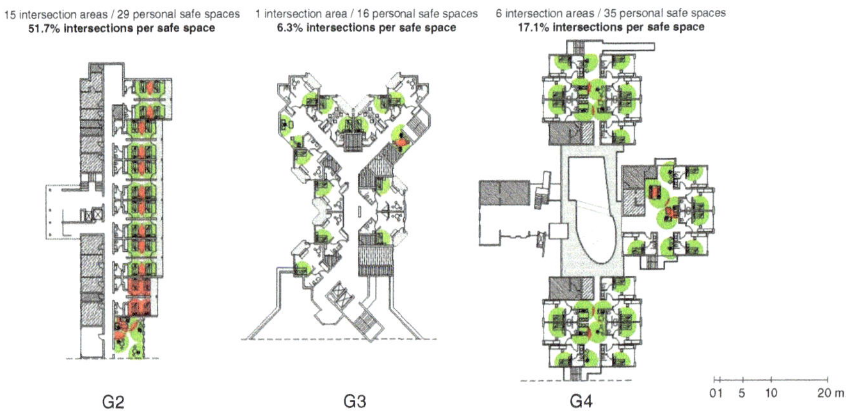

Fig. 12.7 Social distancing analysis. The gradient in living areas in each of the three types of residences selected. (Own creation, 2020)

does not happen in the other generation residences because they have single bedrooms. Regarding common living areas, the three generations possess waiting rooms that, due to their reduced size, expose residents to excessive contact. It should be noted that, while the intersections of the second-generation floor mainly occur in the bedrooms, in the other two cases, these are present in the common areas.

RECOMMENDATIONS: Rearrange spaces to ensure a safe distance between people. Use furniture that can be appropriately spaced for social distancing and easily sanitized. Create physical barriers between people, i.e., partitions between beds.

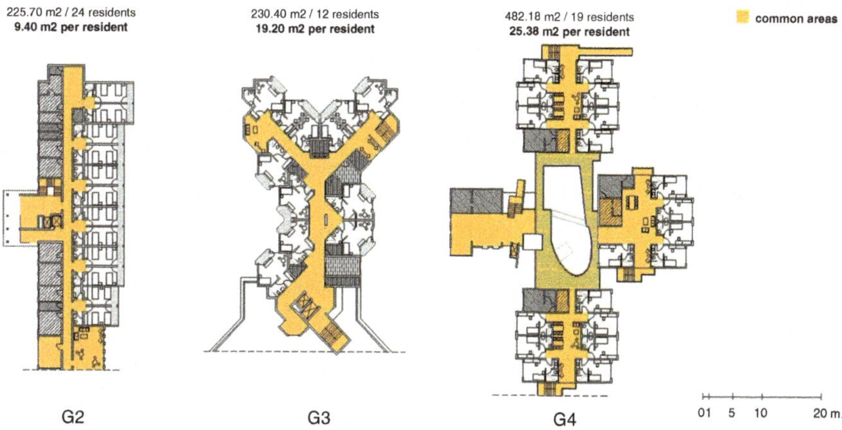

Fig. 12.8 Density analysis in each of the three types of residences selected. (Own creation, 2020)

Density

Concerning density, there is a substantial difference between the three cases, with the amount of common area per resident increasing exponentially in each generation, and this area duplicates or even triplicates from the second to the fourth generation (see Fig. 12.8).

RECOMMENDATIONS: Limit visitors to the facility to those essential for the patient's physical or emotional well-being and care. Schedule appointments to limit the number of patients in waiting rooms. Implement virtual methods for group healthcare activities. Implement systems for timed usage of outdoor space.

Ventilation—Open-Air Conditions Area per Resident

In the open-air conditions—area per resident analysis (Fig. 12.9), it can be observed that, with time, the area per resident almost duplicates and that each type specializes in a different exterior area without offering others. This lack of diversity reduces space flexibility, and it is imperative to have individual and common areas to be able to safely execute all daily activities.

RECOMMENDATIONS: If climate permits, keep residents outdoors most of the time. Providing access to the outdoors on each floor helps residents access nature, fresh air, and sunlight without having to take the elevator or stairs. Establishing protocols on times of use can help mitigate overcrowding. Claim additional outdoor space as programmed space and reassess the use of open bay recovery areas.

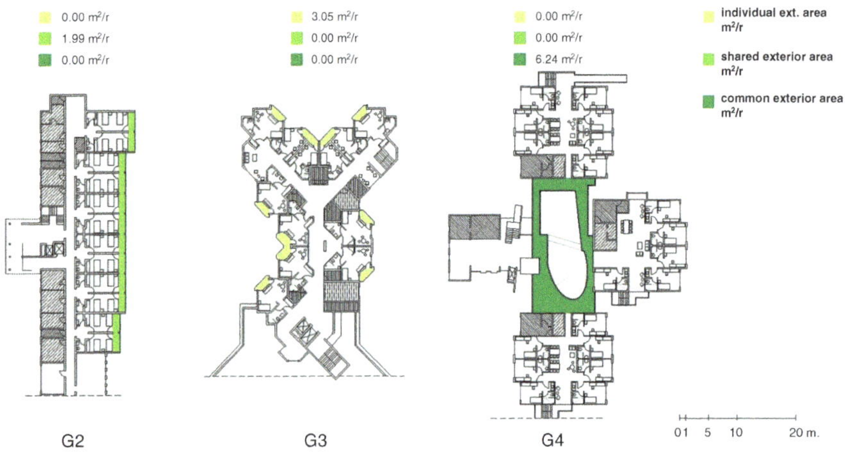

Fig. 12.9 Ventilation analysis. Open-air conditions—area per resident in each of the three types of residences selected. (Own creation, 2020)

Ventilation—Air Distribution Pattern

After assessing the air distribution pattern (Fig. 12.10), it is observed that the fourth-generation floor is the only one with 100% of residents getting effective crossed ventilation. In the third generation, crossed ventilation is produced between bedrooms and common areas. While in the third and fourth generations, crossed ventilation occurs from bedroom to bedroom. The fact that air goes through two bedrooms implies that both residents agree on opening doors and windows to ventilate the area. In this case, due to the path length, it is assumed that there is no infection exposure.

RECOMMENDATIONS: Avoid recirculation of air. Contaminated air can be diluted by adding fresh outside air via open windows, balconies, or doors. Develop innovative ventilation strategies. Consider the addition of portable solutions to augment air quality in areas when permanent air-handling systems are not a feasible option. Introduce air-purifying plants.

Ventilation—Ventilation Surface per Room

In the ventilation surface per room analysis (Fig. 12.11), it is observed that, although the surface of natural light (windows and doors) is steady in the four generations, it is reduced significantly with time. When relating this parameter with the air distribution pattern, it is understood that there is a bigger ventilation area when it is more difficult to obtain crossed ventilation to compensate for airflow.

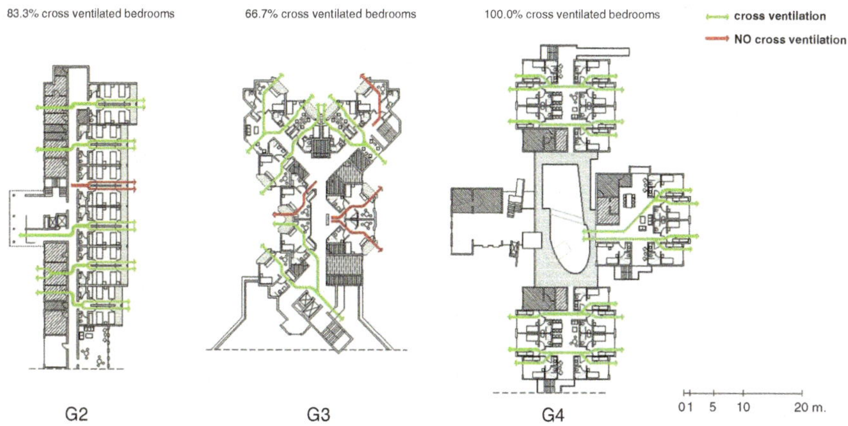

Fig. 12.10 Ventilation analysis. Air distribution pattern in each of the three types of residences selected. (Own creation, 2020)

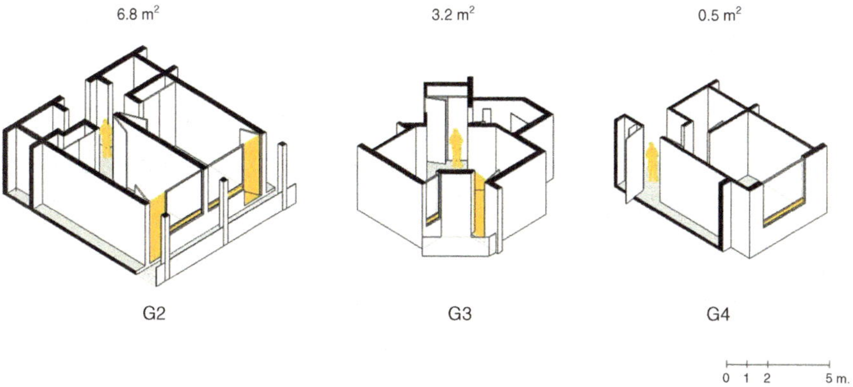

Fig. 12.11 Ventilation analysis. Ventilation surface per room in each of the three types of residences selected. (Own creation, 2020)

RECOMMENDATIONS: Optimize air-handling systems (directionality, filtration, exchange rate, proper installation, and up-to-date maintenance). Apply air cleansing strategies such as Germicidal Ultraviolet air disinfection units or air filters. Ensure operable portions are at appropriate and accessible heights for operation by those with mobility limitations.

After evaluating the four aspects (isolation, social distancing, density, and ventilation) in each nursing home generation, it is observed that none of the cases are optimal in avoiding the spread of COVID-19. As shown in Table 12.4, the second generation is hit the hardest as it offers isolation, social distancing, and density problems, while the fourth generation also presents isolation and social distancing problems. The third generation presents the same amount of successful strategies as the fourth generation but does not possess the negative aspects as the other two types of residence.

Conclusions

The layout design, the elevation configuration or its section relationship, an adequate election of type, and the correct space design have the power of damaging or keeping residents safe. In this work, it has been proven that the different space configurations and their space syntax directly influence the chances of airborne disease spread, such as COVID-19, in nursing homes.

From the three assessed types of nursing homes, it has been observed that none of these are exemplary cases for significantly lowering COVID-19 spread based on their spatial structure. This disturbing data evinces that much is still to be done in these facilities in spatial terms. Although the third-generation layout is characterized as having the greatest number of positive aspects compared to the rest, it is considered important to follow the recommendations indicated above to improve the space. Furthermore, it is considered necessary to develop a strong infection prevention and control program, which affects space management and how we relate to it, to protect residents and healthcare personnel from COVID-19 infection. All of this without ignoring the general considerations for the design of this type of facility allow adequate development of residents' lives.

At the same time, the inclusion of this network of nursing homes as an integral part of the cities' development, through the formalization of programs that recognize and complement it, would encourage the elderly's autonomy by allowing them to expand their everyday activities. Also, it would help to increment the resilience capacities of the communities, preparing them for future adversities, such as the current COVID-19 pandemic. For this to happen, local administrations and city planners should consider the integration of these facilities and their users as an essential urban element, creating a city that benefits all of its community.

References

Abramsson, M., & Andersson, E. (2016). Changing preferences with ageing – Housing choices and housing plans of older people. *Housing, Theory and Society, 33*(2), 217–241. https://doi.org/10.1080/14036096.2015.1104385

Aiello, R. (2020, April 13). Nearly half of known COVID-19 deaths in Canada linked to long-term care homes: Tam. *CTV News*. https://www.ctvnews.ca/canada/nearly-half-of-known-covid-19-deaths-in-canada-linked-to-long-term-care-homes-tam-1.4893419. Accessed June 2020.

Anderson, R. M., Heesterbeek, H., Klinkenberg, D., & Hollingsworth, T. D. (2020). How will country-based mitigation measures influence the course of the COVID-19 epidemic? *The Lancet, 395*(21–27), 931–934. https://doi.org/10.1016/S0140-6736(20)30567-5

Atkinson, J., Chartier, Y., Pessoa-Silva, C. L., Jensen, P., Li, Y., & Seto, W. (2009). *Natural ventilation for infection control in health-care settings*. World Health Organization.

Bachega, H. (2020, April 30). Coronavirus: Inside story of Spain's care home tragedy. *BBC News*. https://www.bbc.com/news/world-europe-52188820. Accessed May 2020.

BBC Radio. (2020, May 4). *Spain's care home nightmare* [Radio broadcast]. https://www.bbc.co.uk/programmes/m000hpct. Accessed May 2020.

Carreño, B., & Allen, N. (2020). Lockdown: Nursing homes in Spain a vector for deadly coronavirus. Reuters. Retrieved from https://www.reuters.com/article/ushealth-coronavirus-spain-lockdown-ins/lockdown-nursing-homes-in-spain-a-vector-for-deadly-coronavirus-idUSKBN2190N1

Center for Clinical Standards and Quality/Quality, Safety & Oversight Group. (2020). *Nursing home reopening recommendations for state and local officials.* https://www.cms.gov/files/document/qso-20-30-nh.pdf. Accessed June 2020.

Centers for Disease Control and Prevention [CDC]. (2020a). *Infection control guidance.* Centers for Disease Control.

CDC. (2020b). *Infection prevention and control assessment tool for nursing homes preparing for COVID-19.* Centers for Disease Control.

CDC. (2020c). *Interim infection prevention and control recommendations for healthcare personnel during the coronavirus disease 2019 (COVID-19) pandemic.* Centers for Disease Control.

CDC. (2020d). *Nursing homes & long-term care facilities.* Centers for Disease Control.

CDC. (2020e). *Preparing for COVID-19 in nursing homes.* Centers for Disease Control.

CDC. (2020f). *Responding to coronavirus (COVID-19) in nursing homes.* Centers for Disease Control.

CDC. (2020g). *Social distancing. keep a safe distance to slow the spread.* Centers for Disease Control.

CDC. (2020h). *How COVID-19 spreads.* Centers for Disease Control.

Comas-Herrera, A., Zalakaín, J., Litwin, C., Hsu, A. T., Lemmon, E., Henderson, D., & Fernández, J. L., (2020). Mortality associated with COVID-19 outbreaks in care homes: early international evidence. *International long-term care policy network*, 2020.

Costa-Font, J., Elvira, D., & Mascarilla-Miró, O. (2009). 'Ageing in place'? Exploring elderly people's housing preferences in Spain. *Urban Studies, 46*(2), 295–316. https://doi.org/10.1177/0042098008099356

Giorgi, E. (2020). *The co-housing phenomenon. environmental alliance in times of changes.* Springer Nature. https://doi.org/10.1007/978-3-030-37097-8_2

Rodriguez Martinez, M. (2020, March 24). Coronavirus: Elderly found 'dead and abandoned' in Spanish nursing homes. *Euronews.* https://www.euronews.com/2020/03/24/coronavirus-elderly-found-dead-and-abandoned-in-spanish-nursing-homes. Accessed May 2020.

Florida, R. (2020, April 3). The geography of coronavirus. *City Lab.* https://www.citylab.com/equity/2020/04/coronavirus-spread-map-city-urban-density-suburbs-rural-data/609394/. Accessed May 2020.

Fraser, C., Riley, S., Anderson, R. M., & Ferguson, N. M. (2004). Factors that make an infectious disease outbreak controllable. *Proceedings of the National Academy of Sciences of the United States of America, 101*, 6146–6151. https://doi.org/10.1073/pnas.0307506101

García Rada, A. (2020). Covid-19: The precarious position of Spain's nursing homes. *BMJ, 369.* https://doi.org/10.1136/bmj.m1554

Gardner, W., States, D., & Bagley, N. (2020). The coronavirus and the risks to the elderly in long-term care. *Journal of Aging & Social Policy, 33*, 310–315. https://doi.org/10.1080/08959420.2020.1750543

Jubilares. (2014, September 11). *La quinta generación. Modelos residenciales para personas mayores* [The fifth generation. Residential models for elderly people]. https://blog.jubilares.es/2014/09/11/la-quinta-generacion-modelos-residenciales-para-personas-mayores/. Accessed May 2020.

Kim, J. Y., & Kim, Y. O. (2020). The association of spatial configuration with social network for elderly in social housing. *Indoor and Built Environment, 29*(3), 405–416. https://doi.org/10.1177/1420326X17732612

Kimball, A., Hatfield, K. M., Arons, M., James, A., Taylor, J., Spicer, K., Bardossy, A. C., Oakley, L. P., Tanwar, S., Chisty, Z., Bell, J. M., Methner, M., Harney, J., Jacobs, J. R., Carlson, C. M., McLaughlin, H. P., Stone, N., Clark, S., Brostrom-Smith, C., … Jernigan, J. A. (2020). Asymptomatic and presymptomatic SARS-COV-2 infections in residents of a long-term care skilled nursing facility – King County, Washington, March 2020. *Morbidity and Mortality Weekly Report, 69*(13), 377–381. https://doi.org/10.15585/MMWR.MM6913E1

Lee, J. K., Shin, J., & Lee, Y. (2020). Circulation analysis of design alternatives for elderly housing unit allocation using building information modelling-enabled indoor walkability index. *Indoor and Built Environment, 29*(3), 355–371. https://doi.org/10.1177/1420326X18763892

Luciano, A., Pascale, F., Polverino, F., & Pooley, A. (2020). Measuring age-friendly housing: A framework. *Sustainability, 12*(3), 848. https://doi.org/10.3390/su12030848

Malik, K., & Mikołajczak, E. (2019). Senior housing universal design as a development factor of sustainable-oriented economy. *Sustainability, 11*(24), 7093. https://doi.org/10.3390/su11247093

Magdziak, M. (2019). Flexibility and adaptability of the living space to the changing needs of residents. *IOP Conference Series: Materials Science and Engineering, 471*(7), 072011. https://doi.org/10.1088/1757-899X/471/7/072011

Marcos, J., & Sosa Troya, M. (2020, June 17). 15% of residents in Madrid care homes died during the coronavirus pandemic. *El País*. https://english.elpais.com/society/2020-06-17/15-of-residents-in-madrid-care-homes-died-during-the-coronavirus-pandemic.html. Accessed July 2020.

Mass Design Group. (2020). Redesigning Hospital Spaces on the Fly to Protect Healthcare Workers. The Role of Architecture in Fighting COVID-19. USA: MASS.

Mass Design Group. (2020a). Carceral environments and COVID-19. In *The role of architecture in fighting COVID-19*. MASS.

Mass Design Group. (2020b). Designing senior housing for safe interaction. In *The role of architecture in fighting COVID-19*. MASS.

Mass Design Group. (2020c). Rules of thumb for limiting contagion in makeshift facilities. In *The role of architecture in fighting COVID-19*. MASS.

Mass Design Group. (2020d). Spatial strategies for restaurants in response to COVID-19. In *The role of architecture in fighting COVID-19*. MASS.

McMichael, T. M., Clark, S., Pogosjans, S., Kay, M., Lewis, J., Baer, A., Kawakami, V., Lukoff, M. D., Ferro, J., Brostrom-Smith, C., Riedo, F. X., Russell, D., Hiatt, B., Montgomery, P., Rao, A. K., Currie, D. W., Chow, E. J., Tobolowsky, F., Bardossy, A. C., … Duchin, J. S. (2020). COVID-19 in a long-term care facility – King County, Washington, February 27–March 9, 2020. *Morbidity and Mortality Weekly Report, 69*(12), 339–342. https://doi.org/10.15585/MMWR.MM6912E1

Michell-Auli, P., & Sowinski, C. (2012). *Die 5. Generation: KDA-Quartiershäuser. Ansätze zur Neuausrichtung von Alten- und Pflegeheime* [The fifth generation: KDA neighborhood houses – Approaches to realigning old people and nursing homes]. Kuratorium Deutsche Altershilfe.

Ministerio de Sanidad. (2020). *Guía de prevención y control frente al COVID-19 en residencias de mayores y otros centros de servicios sociales de carácter residencial* [Prevention and control guidelines against COVID-19 in nursing homes and other residential social services centers]. Gobierno de España.

Mosquera, I., Machón, M., Vergara, I., Larrañaga, I., & Martín, U. (2020). Social inequalities in health among the elderly population: review of indicators used in Spain. *Gaceta Sanitaria, 34*(3), 297–304.

Montero, M. (2012). Innovaciones en residencias para personas en situación de dependencia: el caso Alemán [Innovations in residences for people in dependence situations: The German case]. In P. Rodriguez Rodriguez (Coord.), *Innovaciones en residencias para personas en situación de dependencia* (pp. 73–86). Fundación CASER para la dependencia. https://www.fundacionpilares.org/docs/INNOVRESIDARQUITECYMODELO.pdf

Murphy, M. (2020, April 6). The role of architecture in fighting a pandemic. *The Boston Globe*. https://massdesigngroup.org/sites/default/files/multiple-file/2020-04/The%20role%20of%20architecture%20in%20fighting%20a%20pandemic_MMurphy_The%20Boston%20Globe%2004062020_0.pdf. Accessed May 2020.

Oliveira, N. A., Souza, E. N., Brigola, A. G., Rossetti, E. S., Terassi, M., Moretti Luchesi, B., Inouye, K., & Iost Pavarini, S. C. (2019). Senior caregivers in different housing arrangements:

Comparison of health and care profiles. *Revista Gaúcha de Enfermagem, 40*, e20180225. https://doi.org/10.1590/1983-1447.2019.20180225

Osman, L. (2020, April 13). Long-term care deaths expected to rise as growth of total cases slows: Tam. *The National Post*. https://nationalpost.com/pmn/news-pmn/canada-news-pmn/long-term-care-home-deaths-expected-to-rise-tam. Accessed May 2020.

Ossokina, I. V., Arentze, T. A., van Gameren, D., & van den Heuvel, D. (2019). Best living concepts for elderly homeowners: Combining a stated choice experiment with architectural design. *Journal of Housing and the Built Environment, 35*, 847–865. https://doi.org/10.1007/s10901-019-09716-5

Pettigrew, S., Rai, R., Jongenelis, M. I., Jackson, B., Beck, B., & Newton, R. U. (2020). The potential importance of housing type for older people's physical activity levels. *Journal of Applied Gerontology, 39*(3), 285–291. https://doi.org/10.1177/0733464819840978

Rodríguez, O. (2015, October 5). *Residencias para personas mayores: tipos, objetivos, servicios y requisitos* [Residences for the elderly: Types, objectives, services, and requisites]. Más que Mayores. http://masquemayores.com/magazine/residencias-para-personas-mayores-tipos-objetivos-servicios-y-requisitos/. Accessed Aug 2020.

Roxby, A. C., Greninger, A. L., Hatfield, K. M., et al. (2020). Detection of SARS-CoV-2 among residents and staff members of an independent and assisted living community for older adults—Seattle, Washington, 2020. *Morbidity and Mortality Weekly Report, 69*, 416–418. https://doi.org/10.15585/mmwr.mm6914e2externalicon

Rusinovic, K., Bochove, M., & Sande, J. (2019). Senior co-housing in the Netherlands: Benefits and drawbacks for its residents. *International Journal of Environmental Research and Public Health, 16*(19), 3776. https://doi.org/10.3390/ijerph16193776

Salas, J., & Zafra, J. (2020). An analysis of three Covid-19 outbreaks: how they happened and how they can be avoided. El país. Science & Tech. Retrieved from https://english.elpais.com/spanish_news/2020-06-17/an-analysis-of-three-covid-19-outbreaks-how-they-happened-and-how-they-can-be-avoided.html

Serrano-Jiménez, A., Lizana, J., Molina-Huelva, M., & Barrios-Padura, Á. (2020). Indoor environmental quality in social housing with elderly occupants in Spain: Measurement results and retrofit opportunities. *Journal of Building Engineering, 30*, 101264. https://doi.org/10.1016/j.jobe.2020.101264

Steels, S. (2015). Key characteristics of age-friendly cities and communities: A review. *Cities, 47*, 45–52. https://doi.org/10.1016/j.cities.2015.02.004

TeleMadrid. (2020, June 9). *El drama de las residencias desata la lucha política con la vista en los tribunales* [The nursing homes drama unleashes the political struggle aiming towards the tribunals]. https://www.telemadrid.es/programas/telenoticias-1/drama-residencias-desata-politica-tribunales-2-2239296075%2D%2D20200609035512.html. Accessed July 2020.

U.S. Department of Health & Human Services. (2020, July 22). What is the difference between isolation and quarantine? *HHS.gov*. https://www.hhs.gov/answers/public-health-and-safety/what-is-the-difference-between-isolation-and-quarantine/index.html. Accessed Aug 2020.

Valdivia, B. (2017). Hacia un cambio de paradigma: La ciudad cuidadora [Towards a change of paradigm: The caring city]. *Barcelona Metròpolis, 104*. https://www.barcelona.cat/bcnmetropolis/2007-2017/es/dossier/cap-a-un-canvi-de-paradigma-la-ciutat-cuidadora/

Valdivia, B. (2018). Del urbanismo androcéntrico a la ciudad cuidadora [From androcentric urbanism to caring city]. *Hábitat y sociedad, 11*. https://doi.org/10.12795/HabitatySociedad.2018.i11.05

Yang, Z., & Fu, Y. (2019). Physical attributes of housing and elderly health: A new dynamic perspective. *International Journal of Environmental Research and Public Health, 16*(24), 4961. https://doi.org/10.3390/ijerph16244961

Yourish, K. (2020). One-third of all U.S. coronavirus deaths are nursing home residents or workers. *New York Times*. Accessed Nov 2020. https://www.nytimes.com/interactive/2020/05/09/us/coronavirus-cases-nursing-homes-us.html

Zhang, R., Li, Y., Zhang, A. L., Wang, Y., & Molina, M. J. (2020). Identifying airborne transmission as the dominant route for the spread of COVID-19. *Proceedings of the National Academy of Sciences, 117*(26), 14857–14863. https://doi.org/10.1073/pnas.2009637117

Part III
Uncertainties

Chapter 13
Cultural Tourism and the Economic Recovery of Cities Post COVID-19

Emanuele Giorgi, Francisco Valderrey, and Miguel A. Montoya

Introduction

The year 2020 was rapidly creating a divide between an older way of living and a new lifestyle, known by many as "the new normal," which is still to be defined. Few aspects of our lives have remained untouched by the pandemic. People across continents have been witnessing the unstoppable spread of the virus, looking at damage in faraway countries before being hit themselves in their own territory. The consequences have been devastating due to the loss of precious lives and the catastrophic damage to the economy of nations, organizations, and individuals. The cost is so massive that only the combined efforts of many people are necessary to bring recovery. Indeed, the world after COVID-19 requires a multidisciplinary effort to solve the economic crisis while laying the foundations for a new society. Cities need to be rebuilt, perhaps leading the efforts across different industries. Tourism is among those sectors of influence due to its proven capabilities to impact the economy (Creaco & Querini, 2003) while reshaping human dwellings and modifying the interaction between material resources, esthetic values, and the local well-being of visitors.

E. Giorgi (✉)
Tecnologico de Monterrey, School of Architecture, Art and Design, Chihuahua, Mexico
e-mail: egiorgi@tec.mx

F. Valderrey
Tecnologico de Monterrey, Monterrey, Mexico
e-mail: francisco.valderrey@tec.mx

M. A. Montoya
School of Architecture, Art and Design, Tecnológico de Monterrey, Guadalajara, Mexico
e-mail: mmontoya@tec.mx

© The Author(s), under exclusive license to Springer Nature Switzerland AG 2021
M. A. Montoya et al. (eds.), *COVID-19 and Cities*, The Urban Book Series,
https://doi.org/10.1007/978-3-030-84134-8_13

In this investigation, we look at the city from different angles, including human geography, architecture, and economics, hoping to identify those synergies that may contribute to economic recovery. Since these elements are universal, findings from a specific nation may also be valid in many others. Nevertheless, we focus on China due to the growing importance of its tourism industry and the unparalleled experience of that nation throughout the pandemic. China was the first country to deal with the spread of the virus, and its efforts gained recognition by the World Health Organization (WHO). Once the health issues caused by COVID-19 were under control, the country took significant steps to jump-start the economy, providing meaningful results (Leung et al., 2020).

As this chapter's purpose is pragmatic, we concentrate on the steps that cities of all sizes may take toward the incremental recovery of the economy and social life without losing sight of the environment. To that end, we provide specific examples of how cultural tourism may benefit cities through the work of human geographers, architects, and economists, along with experts from a variety of professions. We present four different projects, pointing at the significance of architectural interventions as a driving force for rebuilding a city's image with a cultural endowment. Thus, the selected projects belong to China, leveraging its economic recovery management and compliance with the Sustainable Development Goals (SDG) from the United Nations. Cultural tourism has indeed been a significant force in China for many years, with cutting-edge architectural projects transforming the identity of numerous cities in recent times.

We aim to identify the features of architectural interventions for promoting tourism in terms of location, design approach, functions, users, economic impact, and methods for hospitality. Those differences surface in the four cases selected: *Dongtan Low Carbon Agricultural Park* in Shanghai, the *Confucius Temple* in Nanjing, the *Ruralation Shenaoli Library* in Zhejiang, and the *Jianamani Visitor Center* in Tibet. Therefore, we attempt to answer our research question:

> What are the features of architectural interventions that may positively impact cultural tourism promotion as a tool for the recovery of cities after the COVID-19 pandemic?

We selected China for further inquiry due to recent advances in the field, the role of urban areas, the tourism sector dynamics, and the wide range of examples offered. We provide a brief account of significant changes related to these topics, such as the shift from rural to urban life, the rise of the middle class, the demand for tourist services, and its impact on urban areas, to provide a context for the selected cases. Those cases may look modest but are representative of trends developing in cities with a cultural endowment. After presenting the four projects before the pandemic, we look at the actions undertaken in addressing the effects of COVID-19. Finally, we share our view on cultural tourism's role in the recovery of cities in the conclusion. Indeed, we believe that tourism may pave the way for the economic recovery of many cities outside of China, specifically in Latin America.

The Promotion of Cultural Tourism and Its Importance to the Chinese Economy

The last decades have witnessed significant changes in China, often related to demographic factors, such as the migration of millions of people from the inner provinces into the affluent coastal areas. The phenomena did not happen overnight but were the result of the modernization of the agricultural system coupled with an aspiration to attain a more desirable urban lifestyle. Things changed for the worse as the emptied cities became part of a vicious cycle of poverty, unemployment, and despair. Furthermore, in rural areas, the aging population has become more evident despite the recent return of migrant workers to their villages (Krishna & Mahalinga, 2020). The trend of urbanization is familiar to many countries, with an increasing rate on all continents. Cities quickly attract people from the countryside, lured by employment opportunities and the promise of leaving poverty behind. According to U.N. statistics, China has a 60.8% urban rate, which is not impressive (Worldometer, 2020). The caveat is the historical shift from rural to urban; for instance, in 1953, less than 14% of people lived in cities, and the urban population's total size accounted for approximately 875 million people (Worldometer, 2020).

As a result of people's displacement from the countryside to urban areas, 850 million people living below the poverty line (World Bank, 2020) joined the middle classes. Before the economic reforms started by Den Xiao Ping during the 1980s, the Chinese population had one of the world's lowest per capita incomes. Nowadays, this figure has grown significantly, placing the nation among the middle-income countries. People enjoy a more comfortable lifestyle, and consumption keeps the economic engine running smoothly. The numbers of the new middle class are astonishing, as well as their expectations. Under the current geopolitical conditions and the commercial frictions with the United States, it seems that China will most probably move further in that direction, with purchases from urban middle classes replacing exports of manufacturing goods. The so-called "double circulation" strategy points at a dual supply chain, addressing the internal market separately from the export channels (Blanchette & Polk, 2020).

Internal migration and the new prosperity are tipping the scales in favor of cities. In fact, out of the largest 150 cities in the world, measured by population, 37 are in China, with 6 of those surpassing 10 million people and 10 towns among the top 33 (City Mayor Statistics, 2020). The country is transforming its economy from manufacturing to a service-driven society, fostering the rise of the middle classes. As happens in almost every corner of the world, the urban population's prosperity imposes a demand for better products and, fundamentally, new services, such as those associated with leisure and travel. Consequently, China has experienced an exponential expansion in the tourism industry over the last decade, growing more than five-fold between 2008 and 2019 (CEIC, 2020). Accordingly, tourism is a fundamental part of society and a significant source of revenue. Sustainable Development Plans provide further proof of the strategic importance of this industry. Indeed, the word "tourism" is mentioned 27 times in the 13th five-year plan for the economic and social development of the People's Republic of China (2016–2020), with a general connotation to sustainability (Giorgi et al., 2020).

Tourism is a high impact human phenomenon, with great potential to promote sustainable activities and relations among communities, people, and the environment. In this regard, two trends in China are worth a profound analysis: close proximity to nature and visiting cultural sites, which often leads to combined efforts through cultural tourism. As defined by the United Nations World Tourism Organization ([UNWTO], n.d., par. 4), cultural tourism is:

> A type of tourism activity in which the visitor's essential motivation is to learn, discover, experience, and consume the tangible and intangible cultural attractions/products in a tourism destination. These attractions/products relate to a set of distinctive material, intellectual, spiritual, and emotional features of a society that encompasses arts and architecture, historical and cultural heritage, culinary heritage, literature, music, creative industries, and the living cultures with their lifestyles, value systems, beliefs, and traditions.

Such a detailed definition by the UNWTO contains many elements, although only indirectly allows for the inclusion of landscape and nature. For Chinese tourists, such a distinction is hard to visualize. Nature, indeed, is part of the national endowment and identity. Therefore, according to the Chinese way, we blend the appreciation of landscapes with heritage in our discussion. The city of Chengdu provides an exemplary case to show visitor appeal when it combines all those elements into the tourist offer. The results of a multidisciplinary study conducted by Japanese and Chinese scholars measured satisfaction with the tourist experience of historical neighborhoods, showing that "tourist satisfaction lies not only in infrastructure, historical buildings, natural environments and other tangible resources, but is also closely related to intangible heritage, such as history and culture, and the overall atmosphere" (Liu et al., 2017). Lijiang's ancient city offers a more detailed example of how historical endowment may become an asset if properly managed. The administrators launched a cocreation model to benefit the ailing Naxi ethnic minority (McCartney & Chen, 2020). In both cases, authorities followed some of the authors' recommendations, such as balancing cultural preservation and the inhabitants' well-being, while securing an income stream for the local population. Thus, research may lead to the betterment of public policies in this field.

A common theme for discussion is transforming a city after a World Heritage City declaration by UNESCO. Towns that receive such high consideration need to deal with unexpected visitors that may jeopardize any effort to preserve the surroundings. An example is the inclusion of the Ancient City of Pingyao among UNESCO's exclusive list, which turned a living city into an open museum, with great disturbance to the traditional lifestyle. Many residents could not reap the benefits, suffering instead from the nuisance crowds, thus raising the question about "whose heritage" and "restoration for whom." Careful planning of the tourist offer may adequately address those issues (Wang, 2012).

Adding to the positive economic impact, urban planning and architectural intervention may bring forth other fundamental changes to the local population's well-being. In any event, it is paramount to understand the user of cultural tourist services, as much of the typologies depend on their behavior. Among the many cultural

Table 13.1 The Chinese market for cultural services segmentation

Segment	Share (%)	Behavior
Purposeful	46	"Learning about the other's culture or heritage is a major reason for visiting a destination, and this type of cultural tourist has a deep cultural experience."
Sightseeing	30	"Learning about the other's culture or heritage is a major reason for visiting a destination, but this type of tourist has a more shallow, entertainment-oriented experience."
Casual Cultural	15	"Cultural tourism reasons play a limited role in the decision to visit a destination, and this type of tourist engages with the destination in a shallow manner."
Incidental	5	"Tourism plays little or no meaningful role in the destination decision-making process, but the person will participate in cultural tourism activities, having a shallow experience while at the destination."
Serendipitous	4	"Cultural tourism plays little or no role in the decision to visit a destination, but while there, this type of cultural tourist visits cultural attractions and ends up having a profound experience."

Source: Adapted from McKercher (2002)

tourist typologies, McKercher (2002) designed the one that seems to fit Chinese tourists better and is widely used in Asia (Chen & Huang, 2018) (Table 13.1).

From the supply side, the Chinese government took major steps to promote tourist services before the pandemic, both directly and indirectly. Some examples are the colossal plans to modernize land transportation, the creation of new airports, and the development of high-speed trains coupled with proper lodging facilities. Those improvements opened the opportunity for leisure and traveling to millions of residents. On the demand side, the rise in disposable income for Chinese citizens is well known. As China took a decisive leap toward prosperity, a younger segment of the population joined the middle classes, requesting services of all kinds, including such experiences as traveling to cities with cultural amenities. After the COVID-19 crisis, authorities are taking action to satisfy those underlying demands by fostering internal tourism (Soo, 2020).

Contrary to most nations, China successfully reinvigorated most industries, including tourism. As shown by the World Travel and Tourism Council, the tourism sector accounted for US$ 8.9 trillion and 330 million jobs worldwide for the year 2019 when considering the direct, indirect, and induced impact (World Travel & Tourism Council, 2020). Despite the positive aspects of tourism, some externalities may balance out the gains if not adequately addressed. For instance, the COVID-19 pandemic has exacerbated the need to promote local tourism, especially in the hardest-hit nations. The result has been an increase in competition among countries with more severe unemployment and economic stagnation, which benefits no one (Gössling et al., 2020).

Methodology and Cases

We started this investigation by looking at different cultural tourism aspects contributing to the economic recovery of cities. A report from the Italian University of Pavia came to our attention, showing other areas of tourism research that could fit our preference. Researchers pointed out the increasing number of tourists willing to visit cities off the beaten track. Furthermore, they indicated the research gap in cultural products' offering with the fusion of culture and landscape (De Lotto et al., 2017). Although the topic is not new to the literature, few studies recognize the transcendency of cultural and tourist activities as vital in urban contexts. Table 13.2 includes areas where research is most needed. Out of the suggested research topics, we found it most attractive to analyze architectural heritage and its potential to redefine tourism's role as a contributor to economic recovery. However, the research also embraces all the other topics.

The results provide insights into economic impacts, cultural heritage preservation, the strengthening of communitarian participation, integration with the local social context, and environmental and biodiversity protection. The projects encompass a megalopolis like Shanghai, a large city, Nanjing, and two smaller towns in Zhejiang Province and the Tibet Autonomous Region. Although the chosen projects' disparities are evident, a common denominator is the reclaim of physical space which previously had a different intended purpose. The contributions from architects are clearly at hand, although other professionals' input is equally important, even if not so visible.

All cases target urban dwellings, looking at different scales of interventions. The first one, Confucius Temple, is a project in Nanjing. The temple is at the pinnacle of an effort to rebrand the ancient town under a new identity and to enhance sustainability. The second one, Dongtan Low Carbon Agricultural Park on Chongming Island, aims to provide recreational space to the Municipality of Shanghai. Although the project may look rural, it serves to extend the metropolis under an eco-friendly approach. The third one, Ruralation Shenaoli Library, represents the new response to the local community's upper-middle-class and economic benefits. The last one,

Table 13.2 Proposed research topics in tourism for sustainable economic recovery

Topic	Guidelines
Architectural heritage	Recognize new roles for the architectural heritage.
The environment	Identify new roles and functions for the environment.
Small-scale services	Foster tourist services with small-scale interventions.
Countryside vs. sea and mountains	Integrate rural tourism with traditional tourist areas.
Tourism and water	Promote the use of water resources for recreational purposes.
Tourism and infrastructure	Improve competitiveness.
Tourism in less favorable areas	Encourage sustainable activities in less favorable areas.

Source: De Lotto et al. (2017)

Jianamani Visitor Center, provides a more affordable option to those with modest means but who are full of enthusiasm for religious pilgrimage.

The methodology is qualitative due to the nature of the selected projects. The cases draw from the anthological analysis of detailed descriptions of the projects regarding architecture, environment, and community participation. The information came from local magazines, online publications, and descriptions provided by the authorities managing the sites. Additionally, experts provided reports to illustrate building materials, construction techniques, and the different cases' technical aspects. An analysis of available data allowed for matching the findings through a comparative study. Standard features included the economic impact, cultural heritage preservation, the strengthening of communitarian participation, the integration with the local social context, and environmental and biodiversity protection.

Confucius Temple, Nanjing: Historical Heritage

Many cities across the Chinese territory are endowed with well-preserved ancient temples, such as Beijing, Shanghai, Hangzhou, Chengdu, Chongqing, Jinan, and Qufu. Nonetheless, the Confucius Temple of Nanjing provides a different meaning to the quest for cultural syncretism. Even if the Confucius Temple has witnessed many changes and some degree of structural transformation, it is part of the Song Dynasty's preserved heritage, as well as more recent events, such as the Japanese invasion and the Nanjing Massacre before World War II. Different events led to the destruction and later reconstruction of the religious site.

The temple embraces Confucian rituals, thus showing the beliefs and values of contemporary China. The nation's economic rebirth is somehow associated with Confucian values, even though Confucianism was considered a significant factor for China's previous decadence (Lemus, 2014). The spiritual monument also delivers the motion of traditions, acting as the underlying forces holding together the People's Republic of China's different ethnical identities. At the core of such proposals lies a mix of religious formalities, museum service offerings, and a gathering place for locals and visitors. When used in line with tourist promotion, the temple acquires a significant role in the economic development of its city, Nanjing. Tourist revenues provide financial means to merchants, local artists, and those catering for visitors.

Dongtan Low Carbon Agricultural Park: Natural Heritage

Since the nineteenth century, Shanghai has been a cosmopolitan city. In contemporary times, it has become China's open door to the world, with a disposable income well above the national average. Shanghai is also a preferred choice for expatriates and, consequently, provides an ample range of amenities, modern infrastructure, and business opportunities that cannot be matched by any other province. Above all, the city offers a perfect example of the new prosperity for the urban Chinese middle classes.

Prosperity elicits the demand for a more sophisticated offering of tourist services targeting national and foreign visitors. As a response, Shanghai's offering has been extended to include iconic projects, such as Disneyland Park, along with several theme parks rivaling the American colossus. Unfortunately, along with progress came some negative externalities, including severe damage to the environment and the oppressive demand for public services. Furthermore, those projects have compromised the proper balance of open spaces to population density, common to the first-tier cities such as Beijing, Shanghai, Guangzhou, and Shenzhen, as well as second-tier cities, or those urban areas "comprised of a large scale within its province" (Zhang & Li, 2020, p. 1). Those problems become more intense in those cities where historical districts impose severe limitations on commercial expansion and sustainability plans.

The response from the Municipality came with the Dongtan Low Carbon Agricultural Park. Despite the most peculiar conditions, such as Chongming Island's isolation, there are hopes to replicate the model in alternative geographical settings throughout the nation. The initiative came from the Shanghai Industrial Investment Group Co Ltd. with the Shanghai Science and Technology Committee's supervision. The park's primary objective was to find a synergy between architectural intervention and urban planning to offer recreational space and activities while serving a dual purpose. On the one hand, the residents may reap the benefits of a cleaner environment. Simultaneously, the project helps to spark economic activities in the area of influence, primarily related to commerce and the hospitality services offered to visitors. Transportation is also part of the master plan, along with sustainable infrastructure, to secure economic growth. According to the architectural master plan, the main issues involved were: (1) Preventing single-use sprawling development patterns occurring within Shanghai; (2) Accommodating tourism; (3) Minimizing the introduction of over-scaled highways and car-oriented developments; (4) Keeping development in balance with nature; (5) Maintaining the farming industry on the island; and (6) Organizing compact transit-oriented settlement patterns to accommodate growth (SOM, 2014). Overall, the project strives for equilibrium between urban and rural areas, all within the city limits.

After several architectural and urbanistic interventions, the island offers a unique space for business development and protected areas. A whole set of green villages, wetlands, and habitats for endangered species thrive along sites devoted to aquaculture and business-minded activities. The project has demonstrated the feasibility of reclaiming land to open space suitable for commerce, organic farming, and ecotourism, while preserving natural landscape. Additionally, regional tourism has become a contributing factor to the local economy.

Ruralation Shenaoli Library: Community Heritage

The Ruralation Shenaoli Library project is part of the new tourist offering for the more affluent population. The project welcomes interaction between guests and the local community at different times and in different spaces. The library and the exhibition hall follow a criterion of authenticity, a recurring topic in contemporary urban-architectural design in China. The transcendency of the initiative goes beyond architecture into the issue of sustainability. The master project includes many references to the Sustainable Development Goals, mainly through: (1) the enhancement of cultural heritage, both in terms of typological design and in terms of techniques and materials conceived in stages of discussion between local architects and artisans; (2) the differentiation of recreational offers by the interaction between guests and the local community; and (3) urban integration with the existing architectural heritage (China Design Center [CDC], 2018). The library provides an example of urban implantations, with an attractive "aim to attract urban residents, carrying urban lifestyle and maintaining a village atmosphere at the same time" (Wu & Guan, 2016).

Jianamani Visitor Center: Spiritual Heritage

Jianamani Visitor Center is a project with considerable international success. Jianamani has a deep significance for the Yushu community and is one of the most sacred places for Buddhists and Buddhist pilgrimage. This project shows the interpenetration of faith, community membership, and the economic benefits to the tourism sector. The design strategies also demonstrate how the urban-architectural practice follows the governmental indications and the SDG guidelines in countless aspects. Among the most relevant are: (1) the use of local materials that can connect the landscape, with full respect to spiritual values for pilgrims; (2) a territorial arrangement that allows for the visual connection with landscape icons, relating the building to the landscape itself; (3) the provision of essential services to pilgrims and the offering of new spaces and services for local citizens; and (4) the revival of the tourism sector to foster job opportunities (TeamMinus, 2020). The architectural intervention on Jianamani provides a perfect example of an integral design, as the project started using debris and abandoned materials after a powerful earthquake. The residents had a voice in the different stages of the project, and they found a way to secure their income.

Architectural Intervention and Cultural Tourism

The cases previously illustrated share differences and similarities. However, they represent a common theme: the efforts to regain physical spaces, values, and cultural identity through architectural interventions, with a holistic vision that includes

Table 13.3 Case comparison

	Confucius temple	Low carbon agricultural park	Ruralation Shenaoli library	Jianamani visitor center
Scale of intervention	Urban	Urban	Architectural	Architectural
Scale of influence	National	Regional	Regional	National
Context	Urban context/historical and religious center	Forestry, productive countryside	Urban context/historical village	Semi-urban
Design approach	Urban regeneration of the historical center, preservation, and partial reconstruction	Regional masterplan based on the redesign and protection of the island's biodiversity	The architectural renewal of historical buildings and interactions with the community	Architectural design and relations with the cultural landscape, local material, and techniques
Functions	Hospitality, museum, cultural tourism, commerce	Cultural tourism: Divulgation, sensibilization	Hospitality, culture (shared with locals)	Hospitality, visitor center, services for the local community
Users (mainly)	National tourists who aim to rediscover the city's role in the nation's history	Residents in the Shanghai urban area to find connection with biodiversity	Middle-high class of regional tourists	National pilgrims and local community
Recovering from a previous condition	Regeneration of attractiveness	Re-establishing "natural" condition as touristic attractiveness	Re-establishing "cultural—architectural" condition as touristic attractiveness	Regeneration of religious—touristic attractiveness
Different pathways	Previously mainly religious, now mainly touristic	Many communities have been relocated	New activities (library)	Creation of a new building is necessary for contemporary tourism

urbanization plans, residents' well-being, and the resources needed for full preservation of those sites.

Table 13.3 summarizes those differences based on the scale of intervention, the scale of influence, context, design approach, functions, users, recovering to a previous condition, and different pathways. The last couple of elements are of paramount importance since the architectural intervention in all the four sites analyzed aims to provide added value to their cultural endowment. Architectural interventions may contribute to restoration and differentiation (Cvitković & Kline, 2017), thus fostering those cities' resilience in facing the COVID-19 pandemic. In the end, those architectural efforts are geared toward the rebranding of a city with a unique cultural offering.

All cases have broad geographical influence, either regional or national. The scale of intervention is mainly urban for the Confucius Temple and the Low Carbon Agricultural Park. The temple is part of the historic downtown in a large city, Nanjing, whereas the agricultural park is in China's most populated city, Shanghai. The other projects are more rural and involve much smaller towns. Nevertheless, the library and the visitor center are less commercial, addressing cultural values. Due to the size of the first two projects, both the temple and the agricultural park show the intervention of urban planners more than the last two projects. The architectural contribution is at the center of the initiative, but attention to social dimensions and local community empowerment is also an essential issue. The four sites target national tourists, although all destinations are also attractive to foreign visitors. Finally, the four sites went through a regeneration process intended to recover cultural identity and promote economic activities, although the Shenaoli Library provides entirely new activities, and the Low Carbon Agricultural Park carries out an economic overhaul of the local economy.

Despite the differences, all the projects have an impact on their cities and their residents. Based on expert's opinions and an existing literature review, we offer some comments about the projects' overall effects. The Confucius Temple has a high economic impact, mainly from tourist revenues, whereas the agricultural park has great potential to create all kinds of business opportunities. According to the Emerging City Market Report, this project has been a strategic intervention in the key area of "tourist attractions" for Nanjing (Euromonitor, 2016). The agricultural park has great potential to create business opportunities of all kinds, with an investment of around 66 billion yuan (US$9.7 billion) in infrastructure projects (Koumelis, 2019), while the average annual per capita income of a village increased from 1100 yuan in 1986 to 30,000 yuan in 2019 (Yi, 2020). The library provides social engagement and interaction between tourists and the local community, following the contemporary Chinese approach to sustainable tourism and community empowerment. The project reached international awareness through journals, magazines, and architectural exhibitions. The visitor center is a well-known attraction of the Tibetan Autonomous Region, attracting millions of visitors and generating 320,000 jobs in the surrounding area (Denyer, 2016). Cultural preservation is a common theme, except for the agricultural park, which has the greatest positive impact on the community. The results are identical for a comparison based on communitarian participation and slightly similar in terms of the attention to the social context. Finally, the agricultural park shows the greatest possible impact on the environment and biodiversity, followed by the visitor center, with little influence from the temple and the library.

These projects have the potential to contribute to the post-COVID-19 recovery. The Chinese tourism industry will be "significantly and permanently" affected by the outbreak (Hao et al., 2020), although 2020 may be a better year than initially expected. Preliminary figures point to an increase of domestic trips to 2.38 billion visits (Statista, 2020). During the first part of the year, government figures were for 637 million trips nationwide, with a related revenue of 466.56 billion yuan (Yan, 2020). For example, during the first day of the 2020 Dragon Boat Festival, over

17.27 million domestic tourist trips in China were registered by the Ministry of Culture Tourism, with 4.47 billion yuan in tourism income (CGTN, 2020). Another example comes from Nanjing, where the Confucius Temple represents the main tourist attraction, showing a remarkable recovery (China Daily, 2020). This resilience is even more evident for the Chongming Agricultural Park, whose touristic attraction (high-end hotels and resorts) showed an increase of 6% in 2020, as compared to the same period of 2019, due to the strategic daily proximity to Shanghai (Ruofan, 2020). Furthermore, Shenaoli Library and the Jianamani Visitor Center are exemplary for social and economic COVID-19 recovery.

From a broad perspective, we may draw some lessons from the Chinese experience. It is necessary to understand that strategic plans in that country will most probably turn into actions. Consequently, as large as the number of successful cases might be, the results of similar experiences may yield different results elsewhere. Additionally, centralized decision-making and the abundance of financial resources may be challenging for other nations to duplicate those actions as quickly. However, there is valuable learning for urban areas in other locations. Policymakers making decisions regarding cultural tourism promotion should have a strategic plan and build upon a complete SWOT (strengths, weaknesses, opportunities, and threats) analysis of their influence on the region. It is paramount to understand those factors that may influence a visitor's behavior. There are five factors: the socioeconomic and cultural profile, trip organization, activities carried out in the destination, expense, and overall satisfaction. Each of those factors includes several variables, e.g., in the case of the socioeconomic profile, there are age, gender, education, and disposable income (Sánchez & Montes, 2019). Among the many actions that policymakers may undertake, there are offline and online marketing activities, participation in trade fairs, and digital advertising campaigns (Vasiliadis & Komninou, 2019), coupled with affinity and experiential marketing when tourists arrive.

Public policies should target economic recovery, although a long-term vision should prevail. Sustainability is gaining acceptance among tourists of many nationalities. The benefits of culture, landscape, and heritage preservation go beyond the city's attractiveness for outsiders and permeate to many local inhabitants. As seen in the four cases presented, the population's well-being has much to do with proper urban planning and sustainability. Examples of appropriate management of cultural tourism destinations are not limited to China. In that regard, the United Nations shares a clear message regarding sustainability, which is by no means opposed to competitiveness and private intervention into the tourism sector (UNWTO, 2020). The OECD also calls for a coordinated approach to rebuilding tourist destinations, especially those of higher dependency on international travelers (OECD, 2020). Indeed, globalization has not eliminated profound cultural differences, especially between Western and Eastern nations (Montt & Rehner, 2012).

Conclusions

The findings presented in this document are significant *per se*, but may also provide a road map to the recovery of towns in other latitudes, especially in Latin America. Indeed, several countries from that region are in the most profound need of renewed economic growth. Cultural and sustainable tourism may provide an opportunity for those nations. The tourism sector has a significant impact on the economy, social phenomena, resource usage, and overall well-being. Additionally, it may turn into a driving force toward a full accomplishment of the SDGs' guidelines. There are significant differences between China and Latin America in terms of political, administrative, and economic structures. However, promoting alternative forms of tourism will open the door to new opportunities. As with China, most Latin American nations have cities full of cultural attractions, and the citizens of both continents are proud of their historical heritage.

In terms of specific recommendations to Latin American authorities, we can state the need for creating bonds with the community. Residents may be great promoters of their cultural amenities if adequately included in the municipal plans. Developers may be public or private actors but will need to make joint decisions regarding urban planning, financial resources, and the share of benefits to most community members. Research is also an important tool to get acquainted with prospects before choosing a tourist destination. The Chinese tourist is hugely active on social networks, and if Latin American promoters would consult Chinese-outbound tourists, they would know the importance of those visitors' preferred communication methods. There are many other issues to consider when addressing those tourists, such as the availability of electronic means of payment, food issues, and local guides with language capabilities. Chinese tourists represent the fastest-growing segment of the market by nationality, and they are quickly preparing themselves to visit different cultural destinations.

Previously, we shared some advice for Latin American cities with a cultural heritage and agreeable landscapes. Those suggestions sound reasonable in times of a global economic crisis, but it is paramount to understand the great opportunity for change that will arise after the pandemic. Revenues and financial resources will be most welcome by mayors and urban planners for their cities. Nevertheless, the most significant opportunity is the possibility of promoting positive changes for those living in urban areas. The reconstruction of cities does not imply huge investments, relocation of populations, or cyclopean urban works. It is as simple as correctly identifying the residents' needs and building their perceived image of the new city and cultural heritage. The promotion of the culturally rebranded city comes afterward. The cases under scrutiny share a common ground: Those sites may contribute to the rebranding of entire cities, even if only on an incremental basis, but without the commitment of massive resources, as happens with cultural mega-events (Jones, 2020). As in the case of many cities in Europe, rebranding cities through art and culture is possible, even with "tough cities" (Massi et al., 2019). The rebranding of cities is a shared effort from all the stakeholders of a city, where academia may play a leadership role, proposing specific plans that may guide everyone to a post-COVID-19 future of the community (Haywood, 2020).

This research focuses on the promotion of sustainable tourism activities that can improve urban resilience. COVID-19 placed city life under considerable stress, but the pandemic came with a call for rethinking our cities. As happened to individuals and organizations hard hit by the spread of the new virus, administrators of cities of any size need to look for new proposals. In urban areas with a cultural endowment, there are important lessons to be learned. First of all, it is imperative to reclaim the historical value of abandoned sites, mainly through a multidisciplinary approach where architects work hand in hand with economists, astute businesspeople, urban planners, and public policymakers. Second, efforts geared to tourism promotion should emphasize a city brand's uniqueness, targeting segments where cultural appreciation is sought after, rather than competing for low pricing. Third, there is a need to investigate alternative proposals that have proven successful in other places. Yes, the cases described depict the Chinese reality, but could be considered valuable starting points to build proposals better suited to Latin America's local conditions. Finally, there is a need for the inclusion of local communities as promoters of tourism programs, after all, city dwellers are the most interested people in the sustainable development of the areas where they live.

We live in difficult times, and policymakers must be decisive to support those actions that would position culturally endowed cities to attract foreign tourists. Those visitors may provide the necessary resources for re-establishing activities leading to full economic recovery. Few positive things may come out of the pandemic, but at least one is the opportunity for a fresh start. Latin American cities have been waiting for such a moment to arrive.

References

Blanchette, J., & Polk, A. (2020, August 24). *Dual circulation and China's new hedged integration strategy*. Center for Strategic and International Studies. https://www.csis.org/analysis/dual-circulation-and-chinas-new-hedged-integration-strategy. Accessed 10 Oct 2020.

CEIC. (2020). *China tourism industry overview*. https://www.ceicdata.com/en/china/tourism-industry-overview. Accessed 1 June 2020.

CGTN. (2020, June 26). *17 million domestic tourist trips recorded on 1st day of Dragon Boat Festival*. https://news.cgtn.com/news/2020-06-26/17-million-domestic-tourists-recorded-on-first-day-of-holiday-RDdfz7qZmU/index.html. Accessed 10 Oct 2020.

Chen, G., & Huang, S. (2018). Understanding Chinese cultural tourists: Typology and profile. *Journal of Travel & Tourism Marketing, 35*(2), 162–177.

China Daily. (2020, May 6). *Top 10 cities by economic recovery after COVID-19. China Daily*. https://www.chinadaily.com.cn/a/202006/05/WS5ed97840a310a8b24115af8a_1.html. Accessed 10 Oct 2020.

China Design Center [CDC]. (2018, May 25). *Ruralation Shenaoli Library, Tonglu*. https://www.chinadesigncentre.com/works/ruralation-shenaoli-library-tonglu.html. Accessed 14 Aug 2020.

City Mayor Statistics. (2020). *Largest cities in the world: Cities 151 to 300*. http://www.citymayors.com/statistics/largest-cities-population-250.html. Accessed 12 Aug 2020.

Creaco, S., & Querini, G. (2003). *The role of tourism in sustainable economic development* [Conference Paper]. 43rd Congress of the European Regional Science Association: "Peripheries, Centres, and Spatial Development in the New Europe", 27–30 August 2003, Jyväskylä, Finland.

Cvitković, S., & Kline, M. (2017). Skopje: Rebranding the Capital City through Architecture and Monuments to Remake the Nation Brand. *Sociologija i prostor/Sociology & Space, 55*(1).

De Lotto, R., Cattaneo, T., Giorgi, E., & Venco, E. (2017). Coherences and differences among E.U., U.S., and PRC. Approaches for rural-urban development: Interscalar and interdisciplinary analysis. *Sustainability, 9*(4), 537.

Denyer, S. (2016, October 6). China's Tibet tourism statistics just don't add up. *The Washington Post.* https://www.washingtonpost.com/news/worldviews/wp/2016/10/06/tibettourism/. Accessed 10 Oct 2020.

Euromonitor (2016, November). *City Profiling study of China. Nanjing City.* https://www.euromonitor.com/cities. Accessed 7 July 2020.

Giorgi, E., Cattaneo, T., Ni, M., & Enríquez, R. (2020). Sustainability and effectiveness of Chinese outline for national tourism and leisure. *Sustainability, 12*, 1161.

Gössling, S., Scott, D., & Hall, M. (2020). Pandemics, tourism, and global change: A rapid assessment of COVID-19. *Journal of Sustainable Tourism, 29*(1), 1–20.

Hao, F., Xiao, Q., & Chon, K. (2020). COVID-19 and China's hotel industry: Impacts, a disaster management framework, and post-pandemic agenda. *International Journal of Hospitality Management, 90*, 102636.

Haywood, K. M. (2020). A post-COVID future: Tourism community re-imagined and enabled. *Tourism Geographies, 22*(3), 599–609.

Jones, Z. M. (2020). *Cultural mega-events: Opportunities and risks for heritage cities*. Routledge.

Koumelis, T. (2019, May 13). Chongming Island, a paradise of sports and nature. *Travel Daily News.* https://www.traveldailynews.asia/chongming-island-a-paradise-of-sports-and-nature. Accessed 10 Oct 2020.

Krishna, V. R., & Mahalinga, K. (2020). Covid-19 and returning migrants to villages: States responses and responsibility. *Education, 53*(32.4), 13–18.

Lemus, D. R. (2014). Confucianismo como humanidad: claves para complementar la modernidad [Confucianism as humanity: Keys to complement modernity]. *México y la Cuenca del Pacífico, 3*(9), 77–104.

Leung, N., Ngai, J., Seong, J., & Woetzel, J. (2020, May 6). Fast forward to China. *McKinsey.* https://www.mckinsey.com/featured-insights/asia-pacific/fast-forward-china-how-covid-19-is-accelerating-five-key-trends-shaping-the-chinese-economy. Accessed 19 July 2020.

Liu, Y., Ning, S., Oyama, I., & Li, L. (2017). Study informing policy on Chinese ancient town tourism based on a tourist satisfaction survey: A case study in the city of Chengdu. *Sustainability, 9*(7), 1087.

Massi, M., Piancatelli, C., & Pancheri, S. (2019). Culture and the city: Rebranding "Tough cities" through arts and culture–the case of Matera 2019. In *Positioning and branding tourism destinations for global competitiveness* (pp. 100–123). IGI Global.

McCartney, G., & Chen, Y. (2020). Co-creation tourism in an ancient Chinese town. *Journal of China Tourism Research, 16*(2), 159–182.

McKercher, B. (2002). Towards a classification of cultural tourists. *International Journal of Tourism Research, 4*(1), 29–38.

Montt, M., & Rehner, J. (2012). "Distancia cultural" entre América Latina y Asia. Reflexiones sobre el uso y utilidad de dimensiones culturales ["Cultural Distance" between Latin America and Asia. Reflections about the Use and Utility of Cultural Dimensions]. *Documentos de Trabajo en Estudios Asiáticos, 8.* https://estudiosasiaticos.uc.cl/publicaciones/dt/DT08_Maria_Montt_y_Joahnnes_Rehner_Cultura_America_Latina_Asia.pdf. Accessed 19 July 2020.

Organisation for Economic Co-operation and Development. (2020, June 2). *Tourism policy responses to the coronavirus (COVID-19).* https://www.oecd.org/coronavirus/policy-responses/tourism-policy-responses-to-the-coronavirus-covid-19-6466aa20. Accessed 29 Aug 2020.

Ruofan, W. (2020, September 24). Chongming attracts more tourists this year. *Shine*. https://www.shine.cn/news/metro/2009246754/. Accessed 10 Oct 2020.

Sánchez, M. D., & Montes, J. L. (2019). Dimensions of the Spanish cultural tourist: Definition of a behavior model. *ESIC Market. Economic & Business Journal, 50*(2).

SOM. (2014). *Skidmore, Owings & Merrill, Seagull Island Masterplan*. https://www.som.com/projects/seagull_island_master_plan. Accessed 21 July 2020.

Soo, Z. (2020, October 1). Virus has Chinese tourists heading for domestic destinations. *A.P. News*. https://apnews.com/article/virus-outbreak-travel-hong-kong-holidays-china-04a9409e2c1fe0d1b947a8de39297f46. Accessed 5 Oct 2020.

Statista. (2020). *The tourism industry in China – Statistics & facts*. https://www.statista.com/topics/1210/tourism-industry-in-china/. Accessed 10 Oct 2020.

TeamMinus Office. (2020). *Jianamani Visitor Center*. http://teamminus.com/. Accessed 27 Aug 2020.

United Nations World Tourism Organization [UNWTO]. (n.d.). *Tourism and culture*. https://www.unwto.org/tourism-and-culture. Accessed 14 July 2020.

UNWTO. (2020). *Tourism and the Sustainable Development Goals – Journey to 2030*. UNWTO.

Vasiliadis, L., & Komninou, M. (2019). *Regional tourism promotion policies in Greece: The case of the region of Western Greece* (Conference Paper).

Wang, S. Y. (2012). From a living city to a World Heritage City: Authorized heritage conservation and development and its impact on the local community. *International Development Planning Review, 34*(1).

World Bank. (2020). *China Overview*. https://www.worldbank.org/en/country/china/overview. Accessed 28 July 2020.

World Travel and Tourism Council [WTTC]. (2020). *Economic impact*. https://wttc.org/Research/Economic-Impact. Accessed 28 Aug 2020.

Worldometer. (2020). *China population*. https://www.worldometers.info/world-population/china-population/. Accessed 2 June 2020.

Wu, Z., & Guan, L. (2016). Urban implantation in rural China: Three representative works on rural construction in ancient villages, Zhejiang. In *Proceedings of the 11th international symposium on architectural interchanges in Asia (ISAIA 2016)*, Sendai, Japan (pp. 20–23).

Yan, Z. (2020, October 9). *China's Golden Week holiday, a driver for domestic growth, global recovery amid COVID-19. China.org.cn*. http://www.china.org.cn/world/Off_the_Wire/2020-10/09/content_76789447.htm. Accessed 10 Oct 2020.

Yi, X. (2020, August 7). Tourism changes a village's fortunes. *China Daily*. http://global.chinadaily.com.cn/a/202008/07/WS5f2c959ba31083481725ec22.html Accessed 10 Oct 2020.

Zhang, F., & Li, A. (2020). Housing sources of second-tier urban residents based on multivariate correspondence. *Advances in Civil Engineering, 2020*. https://doi.org/10.1155/2020/8435048

Chapter 14
City Governance and Resilience During the COVID-19 Emergency: A Case Study of Mexico City

Miguel Angel Gil Robles and Beatriz Alejandra Sanchez-Jimenez

Introduction

The city of Wuhan, China, experienced an outbreak of a new coronavirus disease labeled COVID-19. In about 40 days, the disease spread from one single city to at least 83 countries. However, the first sets of data showed that most infected individuals belonged to large urban centers (Richardson et al., 2020; Stier et al., 2020). As it became evident that cities are the main battlefield in the fight against COVID-19, the importance of how cities react to the disease rapidly gained attention (Daunizeau et al., 2020).

Understanding how cities react to the COVID-19 emergency has been analyzed from the medical (Sun et al., 2020), political, demographic (Dowd et al., 2020), and economic perspectives (Atkeson, 2020). However, these studies have not analyzed which sectors within the city have been accountable for their actions. Accountability plays a crucial role when analyzing how an organization reacts. When individuals and organizations are accountable for their actions, it is possible to assess their results and provide feedback and corrective action if necessary (Schedler, 1999). However, during a crisis such as the COVID-19 emergency, it becomes extremely challenging to assign accountability.

The purpose of this chapter is to analyze the case of Mexico City and its reaction to the COVID-19 emergency. Mexico City represents an excellent example of a large city, as in 2020, it ranked sixth in the world in terms of population and seventh (Citymayors, 2007) in terms of GDP. Moreover, while some other major cities in the

M. A. G. Robles (✉)
Jönköping International Business School, Jönköping University, Jönköping, Sweden
e-mail: miguel.gil@ju.se

B. A. Sanchez-Jimenez
Instituto Mexicano del Seguro Social, Centro Medico Nacional La Raza,
Mexico City, Mexico

© The Author(s), under exclusive license to Springer Nature Switzerland AG 2021

M. A. Montoya et al. (eds.), *COVID-19 and Cities*, The Urban Book Series,
https://doi.org/10.1007/978-3-030-84134-8_14

world have relative control of the situation, by July 2020, the state of emergency in Mexico City is still at its highest possible level.

To analyze city governance and resilience in the case of Mexico City during the COVID-19 emergency, the researchers used the Nobody Left Outside (NLO) framework proposed by Lazarus et al. (2020). Such a framework states that six dimensions are involved in the reaction of a city against a pandemic emergency. The six dimensions are leadership and governance, health workforce, health information systems, health products and technologies, financing, and system delivery. By analyzing each of the dimensions, the researchers were able to assign accountability and interpret its effect on how the city reacted to the emergency. To complete the case study, the researchers used public data from government, healthcare, and press organizations.

This paper has at least three contributions. First, it utilizes the NLO framework to assign accountability in a crisis such as the COVID-19 emergency. This analysis contributes to the body of literature in accounting, which focuses on accountability during periods of crisis (Hwang & Park, 2016; Schultze-Kraft & Morina, 2014). Second, this chapter intends to elaborate on the case of Mexico City so that other municipal policymakers can learn from this case (Reginato, 2010). Moreover, this chapter provides a profound analysis of how specific multilevel interactions between individuals and institutions allow change and generate city resilience in the medium and long term. Finally, the authors conclude by assessing the response of Mexico City during the COVID-19 emergency. Such an assessment should be taken into consideration when developing further policies regarding emergencies in Mexico City.

Literature Review

City governance is a concept broadly studied in the economics (Devas, 2001), politics (Beall et al., 2014), and management literature (Viale Pereira et al., 2017). Although there are different definitions for the concept of city governance, a generally accepted definition states that "*City governance can be defined as interaction and collaboration between different stakeholders in decision-making processes*" (Viale Pereira et al., 2017, p. 526). The current literature states that such interactions between different stakeholders in a city should be organized and efficient (Hill & Hupe, 2002; Piattoni, 2010). Thus, the objective of efficient city governance is to make decisions as quickly as possible, at the lowest possible cost, and with the best-expected outcome (Post, 1986).

However, achieving such objectives in practice is an overwhelming challenge. First, cities have limited financial resources (Taylor, 2007). Second, discussions between city stakeholders can be complex and take time to achieve a conclusion (Zito & Schout, 2009). To overcome such challenges, academics have proposed different theories of governance (see Bevir, 2013; Bingham et al., 2005). An important proposition, in terms of city governance, states that such a process must be completed through a multilevel structure (Kearns & Forrest, 2000). The authors argue that "*At the level of the city itself, space and society are becoming more fragmented and chaotic*" (Kearns & Forrest, p. 996). Such complexity forces city governments and organizations to create different levels to carry out discussions and make decisions. For instance, a city government could create an organization that takes care of security at the lowest level. This could, for instance, be police officers that would take care of low-impact disturbances, such as loud parties in a neighborhood or a street fight between drunken people (Harmes, 2019). However, the city government might also count on another organization to take care of more serious crimes, such as the investigation of a murder. The nature of such structures is what, in theory, is conceptualized as multilevel city governance.

Besides the short-term effect in city governance, city resilience is a topic of relevance in the current organizational literature (Spaans & Waterhout, 2017). City resilience implies that the changes and modifications to the system of governance have an impact in the long term, and that these changes provide a positive outcome to the members of the society (Falco, 2015). By combining the concept of multilevel governance and city resilience, it is possible to analyze, in a deeper manner, how interactions between individuals and institutions promote change and remain stable through time.

For multilevel city governance to be successful, each organization must be held accountable for specific tasks (Kersbergen & Waarden, 2004). Accountability in terms of city governance requires at least two mechanisms that would make it work: bylaws and systems (Benz, 2001). Bylaws are what set accountability in the first place. They must state in written form that an organization or even an individual is accountable for something. Additionally, in such bylaws, there must be stated consequences in the case that an organization or individual does not accomplish the stated objectives. Moreover, bylaws without systems might be useless. Systems are the procedures that organizations use to achieve the objectives stated in the bylaws. Systems must be coherent with the essence of bylaws. Thus, if bylaws and systems are in line, multilevel city governance can be successful and efficient.

Nevertheless, cities are suitable for contingencies that might affect how city governance is being performed (Moynihan, 2009). For instance, an earthquake would require quick adaptation and reaction from city governance bylaws and systems. Being able to maintain success and efficiency during a period of crisis is defined as city governance resilience (Thornton, 2009). Generally, bylaws should consider periods of crisis. Moreover, systems must adapt so as to react quickly during a crisis. In her study about Cape Town during a water crisis, Rodina (2019) found that systems reacted quickly to provide financial resources to key organizations in charge of water distribution. Thus, the city was able to make the required changes during a time of crisis. In another example, Thornton (2009) explained in her study of the SARS emergency in China that how the national healthcare system made adaptations in certain municipalities that allowed them to react quickly to the emergency. The author added that such adaptations were carried out in communication with the city governments.

Framework

As large-scale crises are unavoidable in any society, it becomes relevant to study how city governance can be resilient during a crisis. More specifically, health crises have been affecting societies throughout all the ages of civilization. Examples of such health crises are the black death, smallpox, and HIV pandemics. During such a crisis, city governments had to react quickly to alleviate the situation. More recently, the emergencies related to SARS, Ebola, and H1N1 have also put city governance resilience to the test. Academics have studied these emergencies and how city governance deals with these.

As a result of these studies, some theoretical frameworks have been elaborated to analyze each crisis management more coherently. One such framework is the Nobody Left Outside (NLO) framework. Such a framework intends to analyze the multilevel nature of city governance in the case of a crisis. The six dimensions are leadership and governance, health workforce, health information systems, health products and technologies, financing, and system delivery. This section of the paper explores the framework that will be used to make sense of the empirical findings from the case study.

Leadership and Governance

This dimension of the framework refers to how the city governance communicates with other governments, organizations, and citizens. Leadership and governance also refer to the capacity of the city government to communicate factual data to individuals. Without proper evidence, the message might not be received, or individuals might not be convinced that such a message is relevant during the time of crisis. Proper leadership and governance also mean that the city government can hear feedback from other governments, organizations, and citizens.

Health Workforce

During a health emergency, the health workforce is part of the system that should be able to adapt and react as quickly as possible. However, it might be impossible to adapt and react if the health workforce lacks training and resources. Thus, resilient city governance should consider emergency protocols that permit a quick reaction from the health workforce; otherwise, the health workforce might end up confused and without resources to deal with a health crisis.

Health Information Systems

When there is a crisis, information becomes the most valuable asset. It becomes critical to understanding the gravity of the situation and permits city governments to make better decisions. Thus, health information systems must be reliable and updated in real-time. Moreover, local health systems should be connected to larger healthcare systems, which can be national or even international. Without the proper information systems, decisions can be incorrect, leading to failure in city governance.

Medical Products and Technologies

Apart from a prepared and resourceful health workforce, it is also necessary to possess enough medical products and technologies. Such products and technologies are usually sourced from the private sector, which forces city governments to increase the speed at which they can negotiate with private third parties. The lack of medical products and technologies can lead to a shortage of medical supplies in hospitals, increasing the negative impact of the health crisis.

Financing

Managing a crisis is a costly operation. However, city governments need to think about how they are going to finance the costs. It can also be risky for a society when a city government increases its debt to dangerous levels to manage a health crisis. While managing the crisis might be the priority, financial stability is something that should not be forgotten about. Thus, the ability to manage the financial costs of a crisis is as important as managing health issues.

Service Delivery

Cities are complex and heterogeneous. This means that delivering healthcare services can be difficult. For instance, in some cities, there are marginalized regions where it becomes difficult to reach. Thus, city governance must also consider how to overcome such difficulties in order to provide health aid to every social group and individual in the city.

Case Study

The Mexican Institute of Social Security (Spanish: Instituto Mexicano del Seguro Social, IMSS) was founded in 1943 and is the largest social welfare institution in Latin America, attending 80 million people with an annual budget of 37 billion dollars. Financing for the institution came from three-party contributions: the government, the employer, and the employee. Since its foundation, IMSS has achieved remarkable medical success, such as the first kidney and heart transplants in Mexico in 1963 and 1988, respectively, a pediatric liver transplant in 1994, a successful intrauterine surgery, a successful thoracic–abdominal separation of conjoined twins in 2004, and a mechanical heart implant in 2012 (Gonzalez & Cuellar, 2015). Despite these accomplishments, IMSS has faced significant challenges, such as a double morbidity burden arising from its transition from an undeveloped to developed country, where infectious diseases and accidents that are common in developing countries continue to remain as the top causes of morbidity and mortality, but at the same time, an aging population with chronic and degenerative diseases continues to increase. There is also an outdated physical and financial resource management, designed 70 years ago, to meet the needs of the Mexican population of almost a century ago (Suarez et al., 2020).

In December 2019, the World Health Organization (WHO) was informed of a cluster of cases of severe pneumonia, of unknown cause, detected in Wuhan, China. A novel coronavirus (SARS coronavirus-2) was subsequently identified from patient samples. The WHO named this new illness "coronavirus disease 19" (COVID-19). The first case was reported in Mexico on February 27, 2020. On March 11, COVID-19 was declared a pandemic. By the end of August 2020, 64,158 deaths and 596,000 cases were reported in Mexico, and 844,000 deaths and more than 25 million cases worldwide (WHO, 2020).

Leadership and Governance

During March 2020, at the beginning of the pandemic, the Mexico City Government and the IMSS shared a joint message to the population. The message urged for calm and focused on social distancing (Rodríguez, 2020). As the crisis became more severe during April and May, the discourse from the Mexico City Government began to differ from the one from the IMSS and the federal government. For instance, during a conference on May 20th, Claudia Sheinbaum, the Governor of Mexico City, presented an emergency plan that aimed to provide local companies with financial aid and to establish rules to reopen some businesses in the city (Wong, 2020a, b). The financial aid strategy focused on loans and grants to businessmen, professionals, and the unemployed population. The city government claimed that the COVID-19 emergency was not only a health crisis, but also an economic one. Moreover, the strategy to reopen businesses focused on the use of masks and social distancing. The strategy intended to encourage as many people as possible to stay in their homes and slowly reactivate the economy. The Mexican City Government communicated on different occasions that the healthcare system situation was critical and the importance of being cautious.

During a conference on May 6th, Andres Manuel Lopez Obrador, President of Mexico, presented a plan which focused on financial aid for the elderly and students. Moreover, even as the President argued that the federal government did not have a structured plan to reopen businesses, he claimed instead that the emergency was being controlled and that shortly everything would return to normal (Estrada, 2020). Furthermore, the Mexican President has never worn a mask during his public appearances. The only exception was during his visit to President Donald Trump. During a conference, the Mexican President claimed that he will only wear a mask when the country eradicated corruption (Agren, 2020). In the case of IMSS, there were two main issues discussed during public conferences. First, the Head of IMSS, Zoe Robledo, presented a plan to provide Small and Medium Entreprises (SMEs) with loans of 1200 USD during the COVID-19 emergency, at an annual interest rate of 6.5% (Carbajal, 2020). The goal was to give 123,000 loans. Second, through advertisements and conferences, IMSS instructed the population about the benefits of social distancing. However, IMSS has rarely explained the status of the capacity of the healthcare system.

Health Workforce

The IMSS has 440,000 employees who are mostly healthcare personnel, including around 70,000 doctors and 100,000 nurses. During the COVID-19 pandemic, around 20,000 doctors were hired, yet the number of doctors per 10,000 citizens is only 1.46, which is far below the OECD average of 3.4. The health workforce is legally hired by the IMSS, so it is the organization accountable for preparing and managing the health workforce at the federal and local levels (Felix et al., 2020).

Health Information Systems

Regarding health information systems, the Mexico City Government, the federal government, and the IMSS shared certain data. For instance, the number of patients suffering from COVID-19 was shared in a national database (Gonzalez, 2020). Such standardization was required to keep track of the advances in the pandemic. In the end, all the information was kept by the federal government and then distributed to local governments.

As health information systems became standardized at the federal level, all government levels used the same information. This became useful in terms of reporting the number of cases and deaths to the population. For instance, during a conference on May 12, the President, Andres Manuel Lopez Obrador, and the Mexico City governor, Claudia Sheinbaum, reported the same data regarding the death of employees in the subway line of Mexico City (Morales et al., 2020). In general terms, the evidence shows that the health information systems were standardized and centralized at the federal level. Thus, there were no major disagreements, at least between Mexico City and the federal governments.

Medical Products and Technologies

Regarding medical products and technologies, the IMSS played a critical role during the early stages of the pandemic. The medical supplies used in public hospitals were acquired and delivered by the IMSS. The federal and local government did not play a major role in this process (Animal Politico, 2020a, b). Moreover, critical patients were treated using IMSS procedures and, in theory, these procedures were standardized, although in practice the procedures differed between hospitals. For instance, in some smaller hospitals, patients received different treatments because the hospital did not have the equipment stated on the standardized procedures.

Regarding medical products and technologies, the empirical evidence suggests that there was a major national effort by the IMSS to deliver the same standards in terms of healthcare. However, in practice, the outcome was not exactly the same as some smaller hospitals were not able to fulfill the requirements stated in such standards. Nevertheless, the role of the Mexico City Government and even the federal government was marginal, as the governments were not accountable for the distribution of medical products and technologies.

Financing

Financing during the COVID-19 emergency became a prime topic. While the Mexico City Government depends on the federal budget, the local government still has some degree to maneuver. During the early stages of the crisis, the Mexico City Government reacted with their budget and resources. Local hospitals required the acquisition of specific medical materials, most of which were provided by the local authorities and even patients and doctors (Corona, 2020). However, as the emergency became more severe, the Mexico City Government decided to contract debt to finance the aid for the crisis. However, according to some reports from the local government, the acquired debt does not put the financial stability of Mexico City at risk (Wong, 2020a, b).

According to federal bylaws, the federal government has the capacity and the obligation of financing the healthcare system in case of a national emergency (Cámara de Diputados del H. Congreso de la Unión, 2019). However, the federal government "*has resolved not to introduce any broad-based financial relief, tax reliefs, or stimulus measures*" (Martínez & Gonzales, 2020). The posture and discourse from the federal government are that increasing national debt is not necessary to manage the COVID-19 crisis. Moreover, the federal government has to reject additional financial resources to affected local governments such as Mexico City (Forbes, 2020). Furthermore, the federal government has not increased the budget to the IMSS, which has affected its operations, leading to protests from doctors and nurses (El Universal, 2020).

Service Delivery

Service delivery became especially relevant in the case of Mexico due to its increased levels in income inequality (Gutierrez & Bertozzi, 2020). In Mexico City, this has become even more problematic. For instance, in the case of poor areas of the city, the death rate of COVID-19 patients is higher than in richer areas (Peluffo & Viollaz, 2020). Moreover, a recent report claimed that 72% of the areas identified with the highest rates of mortality were those in zones of extreme poverty (Navarrete, 2020). Thus, the Mexico City Government has focused its attention on providing special aid to the poorest areas in the city. For instance, in an interview, Claudia Sheinbaum claimed that there were targeted campaigns to low-income zones in the city to urge the population to not leave their houses (Alejandra, 2020). Moreover, the Mexico City Government argued that there is an intense campaign to provide masks and antibacterial gel to the poorest members of the population.

While the federal government serves a larger population, there is no evidence of special efforts to redirect delivery services, in terms of healthcare, to the poorest areas in the country. Andres Manuel Lopez Obrador, President of Mexico, claimed that the federal strategy was to expand the already existent social programs which give a monthly payment of 200 USD to the elderly and students (Animal Politico, 2020a, b). However, such programs were not modified during the COVID-19 emergency. Besides this, the IMSS has not adopted new strategies to achieve proper distribution of medical supplies to the poorest areas of the country. There are reports of hospitals in the poorest regions of the city lacking medical supplies and personnel (Expansión, 2020).

Discussion

As already stated in the literature review section, city governance is a complex process of interaction and collaboration between the local government and different stakeholders. Moreover, being able to maintain success and efficiency in city governance during periods of crisis is conceptualized as governance resilience. This case study analyzes how the Mexico City Government exercises city governance and resilience during the COVID-19 emergency.

According to the theory of city governance and resilience, local governments should be able to manage an emergency through communication with other organizations and governments and by making decisions that are underpinned with bylaws and systems (Moynihan, 2009). However, in the study of COVID-19 in Mexico City, none of this took place. The main findings from this archival study are that there were huge differences between the stances taken by the Mexico City Government, the federal government, and the IMSS. On the one hand, the local government held a reactive stance on financial aid and healthcare assistance. On the other hand, the federal government and IMSS remained passive during the emergency. The previous phenomenon explains that the local government is accountable for different outcomes than the federal government and IMSS. First, during periods of crisis the communication between governments might not always be efficient. Thus, when the Mexico City Government saw an increase in the number of cases and a lack of response from the federal government, the local government decided to act on their own. Second, bylaws played a critical role in the way in which governments responded. As argued by Rodina (2019), bylaws permit or forbid local governments from making quick decisions. In the analyzed case, the Mexico City Government was able to acquire debt to provide financial aid to SMEs, professionals, and the unemployed population.

In terms of leadership and governance, while the local and federal governments started with a similar posture, this changed over time, when the Mexico City Government became more cautious and decided to implement an active strategy to promote social distancing. In opposition, the federal government did not become supportive of social distancing measures. Even the President did not wear a mask when he was doing public appearances. Such contradictions are not in line with what Moynihan (2009) suggests that city governance should be during a period of crisis. According to the author, during a crisis, local governments should act coherently with federal organizations, as it allows for quicker and more efficient responses. However, in the case of Mexico City, the contradictory reaction from the local government was influenced by the lack of response from the federal government. Moynihan (2009) did not consider that (federal) governments could neglect to communicate, leading to local governments having to decide strategies on their own. Regarding financing and service delivery, this case also found evidence contrasting with what is stated in the current literature, for instance, as stated by Kersbergen and Waarden (2004), city governance is a multilevel process through different organizations. Thus, in times of crisis, communication can be problematic, leading to misunderstanding. When misunderstandings occur, local governments might make decisions on their own, which would be underpinned in the existing bylaws. Thus, this paper found that the existence of bylaws that allowed local governments to increase their debt allowed for a quick reaction in terms of financing activities to control the pandemic. The findings from this paper urge scholars to incorporate the role of bylaws as a main factor that affects city governance and resilience in times of crisis.

Regarding the health workforce, health information systems, medical products, and technologies, the evidence suggests that the action between the local government and federal government was coherent. When analyzing the previous dimensions of the framework, it becomes evident that there could be better outcomes, in terms of efficiency and quickness, when the federal government takes the lead and communicates with the local government. As argued by Schedler (1999), communication is critical in terms of city governance and resilience, as it permits a quick reaction and exercises leadership. Moreover, when analyzing the interaction between the health workforce and all the systems and processes, it becomes evident that changes in institutions can remain over time (Falco, 2015). These changes can eventually be translated into city resilience, which is the outcome of a learning process experienced at the institutional level.

Conclusion

This paper has at least two major theoretical contributions. First, it criticizes the conceptualization of city governance and resilience of Moynihan (2009) by assuming that emergencies are handled through communication and bylaws. The evidence from this case study found that the Mexico City Government acted in opposition to the federal stance on multiple occasions, especially in terms of leadership and governance, financing, and service delivery (Lazarus et al., 2020). This paper calls for a reconceptualization of how governments communicate during times of emergency and how they deal with discrepancies. Second, this paper also highlights the importance of local governments during periods of crisis. As most of the current literature focuses on the leadership from the federal government (Kersbergen & Waarden, 2004), this paper urges for a better understanding of city governments and their leading role in city governance and resilience during a crisis.

A practical contribution of this paper aims for a better understanding of city governance and resilience by politicians and policymakers. This study highlights the positive and negative measures used during the COVID-19 crisis in terms of city governance and resilience. The findings from the case study should be acknowledged by politicians and policymakers around the world to prevent the replication of inadequate processes and replace them with positive strategies.

A major limitation of this study is that the COVID-19 pandemic has still not ended. Thus, the real outcomes of crisis management are impossible to document. A potential future study might consider the effect of the processes discussed in this paper when the COVID-19 crisis is over. Furthermore, another direction that this discussion might take is to do a comparative case study with other major cities in the world. For instance, the case of New York City (Wadhera et al., 2020) or Tokyo (Saito et al., 2020) is interesting, and such comparisons might be important for academics and practitioners.

References

Agren, D. (2020, July 31). Mexican president Amlo says he will wear a mask 'when there is no corruption'. *The Guardian*. https://www.theguardian.com/world/2020/jul/31/mexico-president-amlo-mask-coronavirus-corruption. Accessed Oct 2020.

Alejandra, E. (2020, May 28). 'Seguimos en alerta': Claudia Sheinbaum ['We're Still Alert': Claudia Sheinbaum]. *El Heraldo de México*. https://heraldodemexico.com.mx/cdmx/claudia-sheinbaum-refuerza-campana-quedate-en-casa-por-alta-tasa-de-contagios-y-casos-cdmx-coronavirus-covid-19/. Accessed Oct 2020.

Animal Político. (2020a, March 23). *Ayuda del gobierno solo a pobres, no habrá condonación a empresas por COVID-19: AMLO* [Government aid only for the poor, There won't be condonation for businesses due to COVID-19: AMLO]. https://www.animalpolitico.com/2020/03/ayuda-pobres-condonacion-empresas-covid-19-amlo/. Accessed Oct 2020.

Animal Político (2020b, April 1). *IMSS dará a pacientes medicinas para tres meses para que eviten ir a su clínica* [IMSS will give patients medicines for three months to prevent them from going to their clinic]. https://www.animalpolitico.com/2020/04/imss-surtir-receta-medicinas-tres-meses/. Accessed Oct 2020.

Atkeson, A. (2020). *What will be the economic impact of COVID-19 in the US? Rough estimates of disease scenarios* (Working Paper No. w26867). National Bureau of Economic Research.

Beall, J., Crankshaw, O., & Parnell, S. (2014). *Uniting a divided city: Governance and social exclusion in Johannesburg*. Routledge.

Benz, A. (2001). Restoring accountability in multilevel governance. *Governance and Democracy: Comparing National, European and Transnational Experiences*, 99–114.

Bevir, M. (2013). *A theory of governance*. University of California Press.

Bingham, L. B., Nabatchi, T., & O'leary, R. (2005). The new governance: Practices and processes for stakeholder and citizen participation in the work of government. *Public Administration Review, 65*(5), 547–558.

Cámara de Diputados del H. Congreso de la Unión. (2019). *Ley General de Salud* [General law of health]. http://www.diputados.gob.mx/LeyesBiblio/pdf_mov/Ley_General_de_Salud.pdf. Accessed Jan 2021.

Carbajal, B. (2020, May 10). IMSS dará créditos a trabajadores del hogar por 25 mil pesos [IMSS will give credits to home workers of 25 thousand pesos]. *La Jornada*. https://www.jornada.com.mx/ultimas/economia/2020/05/10/imss-dara-creditos-a-trabajadoras-del-hogar-hasta-por-25-mil-pesos-4666.html. Accessed Oct 2020.

Citymayors. (2007, March 11). *The 150 richest cities in the world by GDP in 2020*. http://www.citymayors.com/statistics/richest-cities-2020.html. Accessed Oct 2020.

Corona, S. (2020, March 29). Darán kits médicos a sospechosos y enfermos de Covid-19 [They'll give medical kits to Covid-19 suspected and sick people]. *El Universal*. https://www.eluniversal.com.mx/metropoli/cdmx/coronavirus-daran-kits-medicos-sospechosos-y-enfermos-de-covid-19. Accessed Oct 2020.

Daunizeau, J., Moran, R., Brochard, J., Mattout, J., Frackowiak, R., & Friston, K. (2020). Modelling lockdown-induced second COVID waves in France. *medRxiv*. https://doi.org/10.1101/2020.06.24.20139444

Devas, N. (2001). Does city governance matter for the urban poor? *International Planning Studies, 6*(4), 393–408.

Dowd, J. B., Andriano, L., Brazel, D. M., Rotondi, V., Block, P., Ding, X., … Mills, M. C. (2020). Demographic science aids in understanding the spread and fatality rates of COVID-19. *Proceedings of the National Academy of Sciences, 117*(18).

El Universal. (2020, July 1). *Protesta personal médico en estados por mejoras al presupuesto de salud* [Medical staff protests in states for improvements in the health budget]. https://www.eluniversal.com.mx/estados/protesta-personal-medico-en-estados-por-mejoras-al-presupuesto-de-salud. Accessed Oct 2020.

Estrada, F. (2020, April 5). Nula respuesta de AMLO a las peticiones de empresarios ante la crisis por Covid-19 [Null response from AMLO to the businesspeople's petitions against the Covid-19 crisis]. *Forbes*. https://www.forbes.com.mx/economia-finanzas-amlo-covid19-coronavirus-empresarios/. Accessed Oct 2020.

Expansión. (2020, April 27). *La CDMX vive jornada de protestas de médicos por insumos contra COVID-19*. https://politica.expansion.mx/mexico/2020/04/27/la-cdmx-vive-jornada-de-protestas-de-medicos-por-insumos-contra-coronavirus. Accessed Oct 2020.

Falco, G. J. (2015). City resilience through data analytics: A human-centric approach. *Procedia Engineering, 118*, 1008–1014.

Felix, V., Alcocer, S., & Soto, D. (2020). Dan su vida en batalla contra Covid [They give their lives in the battle against Covid]. *Grupo Reforma*. https://gruporeforma.reforma.com/interactivo/monterrey/sector_salud_covid_19/?md5=7a9e81ed1d1f5cb8ce7c6ac377e6ee8d. Accessed Oct 2020.

Forbes. (2020, August 9). *México tiene recursos para afrontar pandemia en 2020: AMLO* [Mexico has resources to confront the pandemic in 2020: AMLO]. https://www.forbes.com.mx/politica-mexico-recursos-afrontar-pandemia-2020-amlo/. Accessed Oct 2020.

Gonzalez, J., & Cuellar, R. (2015). The transformation of the Mexican Social Security Institute (IMSS): Progress and challenges. *Health Systems & Reform, 1*(3), 189–199.

Gonzalez, M. (2020, July 9). Coronavirus en México [Coronavirus in Mexico]. *BBC*. https://www.bbc.com/mundo/noticias-america-latina-53344337. Accessed Oct 2020.

Gutierrez, J. P., & Bertozzi, S. M. (2020). Non-communicable diseases and inequalities increase risk of death among COVID-19 patients in Mexico. *medRxiv*.

Harmes, A. (2019). *The politics of fiscal federalism: Neoliberalism versus social democracy in multilevel governance*. McGill-Queen's Press-MQUP.

Hill, M., & Hupe, P. (2002). *Implementing public policy: Governance in theory and in practice*. Sage.

Hwang, K., & Park, H. J. (2016). Dynamics of accountability in crisis management. *International Journal of Emergency Management, 12*(1), 95–112.

Kearns, A., & Forrest, R. (2000). Social cohesion and multilevel urban governance. *Urban Studies, 37*(5-6), 995–1017.

Kersbergen, K. V., & Waarden, F. V. (2004). 'Governance' as a bridge between disciplines: Cross-disciplinary inspiration regarding shifts in governance and problems of governability, accountability and legitimacy. *European Journal of Political Research, 43*(2), 143–171.

Lazarus, J. V., Binagwaho, A., El-Mohandes, A. A., Fielding, J. E., Larson, H. J., Plasència, A., … Ratzan, S. C. (2020). Keeping governments accountable: The COVID-19 assessment scorecard (COVID-SCORE). *Nature Medicine, 26*(7), 1005–1008.

Martinez, M., & Gonzales, R. (2020, June 8). Mexico stands alone in its tax relief response to COVID-19. *International Tax Review*. https://www.internationaltaxreview.com/article/b1lzjrk8hfk2fm/mexico-stands-alone-in-its-tax-relief-response-to-covid-19. Accessed Oct 2020.

Morales, A., Villa, P., & Miranda, P. (2020, May 12). Reconoce Sheinbaum fallecimiento de algunos trabajadores del metro por Covid-19 [Sheinbaum recognizes the death of some metro workers due to Covid-19]. *El Universal*. https://www.eluniversal.com.mx/nacion/la-mananera-de-amlo-reconocen-fallecimiento-de-trabajadores-del-metro. Accessed Oct 2020.

Moynihan, D. P. (2009). The network governance of crisis response: Case studies of incident command systems. *Journal of Public Administration Research and Theory, 19*(4), 895–915.

Navarrete, S. (2020, August 7). El 72% de colonias con más casos de COVID-19 en CDMX sufren marginación [72% of neighborhoods with the most COVID-19 cases in Mexico City suffer marginalization]. *Expansión*. https://politica.expansion.mx/cdmx/2020/08/22/44-colonias-de-cdmx-con-mas-casos-de-covid-19-sufren-marginacion. Accessed Oct 2020.

Peluffo, C., & Viollaz, M. (2020). *Intra-household insurance in the time of Covid-19: Lessons from Mexico*.

Piattoni, S. (2010). *The theory of multi-level governance: Conceptual, empirical, and normative challenges*. Oxford University Press.

Post, R. C. (1986). Between governance and management: The history and theory of the public forum. *UCLA Law Review, 34*, 1713.

Reginato, E. (2010). Accountability perspectives in Italian municipality accounting systems: The gap between regulations and practices. *Public Administration Quarterly*, 552–590.

Richardson, S., Hirsch, J. S., Narasimhan, M., Crawford, J. M., McGinn, T., Davidson, K. W., … Cookingham, J. (2020). Presenting characteristics, comorbidities, and outcomes among 5700 patients hospitalized with COVID-19 in the New York City area. *JAMA, 323*(20), 2052–2059.

Rodina, L. (2019). Water resilience lessons from Cape Town's water crisis. *Wiley Interdisciplinary Reviews: Water, 6*(6), e1376.

Rodríguez, F. (2020, March 17). La ciudad de México se prepara para la fase 2 del coronavirus [Mexico City gets ready for coronavirus' phase 2]. *Fashion Network*. https://mx.fashionnetwork.com/news/La-ciudad-de-mexico-se-prepara-para-la-fase-2-del-coronavirus,1197554.html. Accessed Oct 2020.

Saito, M., Adachi, E., Yamayoshi, S., Koga, M., Iwatsuki-Horimoto, K., Kawaoka, Y., & Yotsuyanagi, H. (2020). Gargle lavage as a safe and sensitive alternative to swab samples to diagnose COVID-19: A case report in Japan. *Clinical Infectious Diseases, 71*(15), 893–894.

Schedler, A. (1999). Conceptualizing accountability. In *The self-restraining state: Power and accountability in new democracies* (pp. 13–28). Lynne Rienner Publishers.

Schultze-Kraft, M., & Morina, E. (2014). Decentralisation and accountability in war-to-peace transitions: The case of Kosovo. *IDS Bulletin, 45*(5), 92–104.

Spaans, M., & Waterhout, B. (2017). Building up resilience in cities worldwide–Rotterdam as participant in the 100 Resilient Cities Programme. *Cities, 61*, 109–116.

Stier, A., Berman, M., & Bettencourt, L. (2020). COVID-19 attack rate increases with city size. *Mansueto Institute for Urban Innovation* (Research Paper Forthcoming).

Suárez, V., Suarez Quezada, M., Oros Ruiz, S., & Ronquillo De Jesús, E. (2020). Epidemiology of COVID-19 in Mexico: from the 27th of February to the 30th of April. *International Journal of Infectious Diseases, 104*, 572–579.

Sun, P., Lu, X., Xu, C., Sun, W., & Pan, B. (2020). Understanding of COVID-19 based on current evidence. *Journal of Medical Virology, 92*(6), 548–551.

Taylor, M. (2007). Community participation in the real world: Opportunities and pitfalls in new governance spaces. *Urban Studies, 44*(2), 297–317.

Thornton, P. M. (2009). Crisis and governance: SARS and the resilience of the Chinese body politic. *The China Journal, 61*, 23–48.

Viale Pereira, G., Cunha, M. A., Lampoltshammer, T. J., Parycek, P., & Testa, M. G. (2017). Increasing collaboration and participation in smart city governance: A cross-case analysis of smart city initiatives. *Information Technology for Development, 23*(3), 526–553.

Wadhera, R. K., Wadhera, P., Gaba, P., Figueroa, J. F., Maddox, K. E. J., Yeh, R. W., & Shen, C. (2020). Variation in COVID-19 hospitalizations and deaths across New York City boroughs. *Jama, 323*(21), 2192–2195.

Wong, P. (2020a, May 20). Los temas de Sheinbaum en conferencia por coronavirus del 20 de mayo [Sheinbaum's topics in conference due to coronavirus on May 20th]. *Milenio*. https://www.milenio.com/politica/comunidad/claudia-sheinbaum-coronavirus-cdmx-20-mayo. Accessed Oct 2020.

Wong, P. (2020b, June 16). Sheinbaum asegura que gobierno de CdMx tiene deuda controlada. *Milenio*. https://www.milenio.com/politica/cdmx-sheinbaum-dice-hay-endeudamiento-controlado. Accessed Oct 2020.

World Health Organization. (2020, July 17). *Country & technical guidance – Coronavirus disease (COVID-19)*. World Health Organization. https://www.who.int/emergencies/diseases/novel-coronavirus-2019/technical-guidance. Accessed Oct 2020.

Zito, A. R., & Schout, A. (2009). Learning theory reconsidered: EU integration theories and learning. *Journal of European Public Policy, 16*(8), 1103–1123.

Chapter 15
Building Strategies and Resilience in the Face of a Pandemic in Urban China and Brazil: COVID-19, Access to Water, and Inequality

Augusto F. J. Schmidt, Erick Tjong, Mariana Hase Ueta, Niklas W. Weins, and Roberto L. do Carmo

Introduction: COVID-19 Containment Strategies and Their Impacts on Unequal Societies

In early 2020, COVID-19 spread around the world, taking countries by surprise and demanding timely responses from governments in order to contain the effects of the pandemic. This crisis made it clear that, even though the entire world population was affected due to globalization, existing inequalities played an important role when one takes a closer look at the contagion and death rates in each region (Ahmed et al., 2020). Around the world, big cities tend to accumulate the highest number of cases, not only because of the high population density but also due to their place in the domestic and international transportation mobility networks, and especially due to existing inequalities in living conditions among people and neighborhoods. It is not surprising that spatialized and socioeconomic inequalities directly limit the response capacity to the pandemic in cities.

> The inequitable response to COVID-19 is already evident. Healthy life expectancy and mortality rates have historically been markedly disproportionate between the richest and poorest populations. The full effects of COVID-19 are yet to be seen, while the disease begins to spread across the most fragile settings, including conflict zones, prisons, and refugee camps. As the global economy plunges deeper into an economic crisis and government bailout programmes continue to prioritise industry, scarce resources and funding allocation decisions must aim to reduce inequities rather than exacerbate them. (Ahmed et al., 2020, p. 240)

A. F. J. Schmidt (✉) · M. Hase Ueta · N. W. Weins · R. L. do Carmo
University of Campinas, São Paulo, Brazil

E. Tjong
World Bank, Washington, DC, USA

© The Author(s), under exclusive license to Springer Nature Switzerland AG 2021

M. A. Montoya et al. (eds.), *COVID-19 and Cities*, The Urban Book Series,
https://doi.org/10.1007/978-3-030-84134-8_15

Inequalities often become most evident when it comes to accessing basic services. During the COVID-19 pandemic, this has been visible in that following the simplest of the World Health Organization's (WHO) guidelines, such as frequently washing hands with soap and water, has proven nearly impossible in some regions, in view of the lack of access to water (do Carmo & Teixeira, 2020). For instance, it is estimated that almost 40% of schools in Brazil do not have basic infrastructure allowing students to wash their hands.[1] In addition, the WHO's instruction to maintain social distancing has been made even more difficult to follow in crowded places that lack minimal sanitary infrastructure. This is notably the case in slums and socially vulnerable areas in major cities in Brazil and other countries in Latin America, which have no access to safe and clean water and sanitation services. As for the case of China, while it could be argued that China's densely populated coastal cities were mainly able to achieve lower contagion rates thanks to strict lockdown measures, we argue that the role of better sanitation systems cannot be understated.

It is likely that COVID-19 will not be the last pandemic of its kind (Marques, 2020). Authors such as Mike Davis (2005) were already foreseeing new and similar pandemics after the outbreak of Severe Acute Respiratory Syndrome (SARS) in 2003. It is thus imperative that governments build strategies to deal with this kind of emergency situation, and that cities invest in building resilience to avoid the spread of infections and protect their citizens. It is also essential for cities to have emergency plans prepared for when new epidemics hit, including not only immediate efforts such as lockdown strategies, but also economic relief efforts in the short- or long-term and other related policies that promote resilience, looking at alternatives like Nature-based Solutions (NbS) to improve urban infrastructure. Based on this premise, we carried out a study on the urban policies employed in both Brazil and China to contain and combat this pandemic, to verify what we can learn from the initial evolution of the epidemic in cities in the two largest countries in Latin America and East Asia.

Having a centralized strategy in place, that could coordinate actions in the provinces and cities, was crucial for the success of containing the spread of the virus in China. The lack of such prompt and coordinated action from the government at the national level, on the other hand, had disastrous effects in certain Latin American countries, including Brazil. Based on this observation, we proposed to carry out a study on the factors that negatively influence the spread of COVID-19 in Brazil, in order to discuss what the role of inequality is in the face of a pandemic in the Global South.

This study aims at contributing to our understanding of the relationship between cities and resilience in light of the COVID-19 pandemic, focusing on the role that long-term investment in infrastructure plays for improving urban resilience. This contribution proposes to explore key elements that can contribute to strengthening resilience in cities: investment in sanitary infrastructure and access to water;

[1] UNICEF, World Bank and Stockholm International Water Institute, 2020.

strategies to address the impacts of socioeconomic inequalities to a pandemic; and policies to prevent contagion, such as short-term quarantine measures and long-term urban planning practices. In the model used for our analysis, we also considered the impact that socioeconomic inequality can have in this emergency situation and included social aspects, such as literacy and income level. The paper is divided into four sections: The first covers a brief overview of the localized aspects of the current COVID-19 pandemic in China and Brazil; the second section explains the methodology employed for the quantitative analysis; the third section is dedicated to an analysis of the findings and results; and finally, the last section brings a discussion about the policy implications for each country.

The Local Spread of a Global Pandemic: The Cases of Brazil and China

Latin America and China were hit by the pandemic at different times. Unlike China, which had its first victim claimed in December 2019,[2] Latin America had more time to prepare government responses to combat the COVID-19 pandemic, as it reached the continent over two months later, at the end of February 2020.[3] Nevertheless, China had a more successful response to the first wave of contagion. As of April 2021, most countries across Latin America are still struggling to deal with the pandemic, dealing with second and third waves with continued high contagion and even higher death rates than in the first wave. Despite their differences, China and Latin America face similar challenges brought about particularly by urban inequality, which imposes additional constraints to the containment efforts. In both countries, the cases were concentrated in urban areas. The reason for that is not only the concentration of the population in the cities, but it is also due to the high level of urban connectivity across different regions, making them key places for spreading the virus.

A good indication to measure domestic interregional mobility would be by assessing overall passenger transport, including airborne travel as well as mobility by cars, buses, and trains. Even though it was not possible to obtain overall domestic passenger transport data for both countries, commercial flight movements can be used as a proxy. According to data from the June 2020 report of the International Air Transport Association (IATA, 2020), the pandemic caused a historically unprecedented drop in flight movements all around the world, with an average reduction of 86.5% (−96.8% on international, −67.6% domestic) of flown passenger kilometers. Thanks to the government's ready response, the recovery of domestic flights in

[2] WHO: Timeline of WHO's response to COVID-19. June 29, 2020. Statement. https://www.who.int/news-room/detail/29-06-2020-covidtimeline.

[3] Leoleli Schwartz: Brazil Confirms First Case of COVID-19 in Latin America. February 26, 2020. https://www.medscape.com/viewarticle/925806.

China was already possible in March, so that by June the country had the world's second lowest drop in flights compared to the previous year (second only to Russia, with a 35.5% drop). In comparison, Brazil's domestic flights saw a drop of 84.7% year on year. While the gradual restart in China since the low point in February was affected by the second wave of COVID-19 cases in June, the data indicated an upward trend in July 2020.

China's map of COVID-19 cases, besides Hubei (the province where the pandemic started), shows that the majority of cases are concentrated in the provinces in the coastal areas where the biggest cities are located. Zhang et al. (2020a, b) and Leung et al. (2020) also show that the spread of the virus from Wuhan to the other parts of the country was due to contact with infected people from Hubei province. Once the central government became aware of the importance of containing the virus, China was very fast in implementing localized control measures to enforce unprecedented neighborhood, or even city-wide, lockdowns and prevent contaminated patients from spreading it to different regions. The intensity of such measures varied according to the situation in each region, and they ranged from semi-lockdown up to exceptionally rare wartime policies (Leung et al., 2020).

The success of the Chinese response to the crisis was arguably not only the outcome of rapid and efficient government actions. The long-term investments in infrastructure made the cities more resilient to the pandemic and made it possible to have a successful lockdown policy. China has faced epidemics before, and in the 2003 SARS outbreak, despite political forces having caused a lack of transparency, the president at the time, Hu Jintao, aligned himself with the WHO and implemented several measures to contain the spread, investing about US$ 1 billion in the improvement of hospitals and public health services (Davis, 2005). A previous robust investment policy in water and sanitary infrastructure, such as the "toilet revolution" campaign, may have also contributed to improving the overall safety of the population (Cheng et al., 2018).

One of the difficulties that the most vulnerable part of the population faced when trying to follow the hygiene procedures to keep them safe was regarding water and sanitation. Although at a lower level and slower pace, access in Brazil has also improved over recent decades. Throughout a period of 25 years (1990–2015), access to sanitation saw a 25% increase in Brazil and a 60% increase in China.[4] In spite of the progress that has been made, lack of access to water and sanitation still poses health challenges in both cases: as of 2015, approximately one in five people in Brazil and one in four people in China still did not have access to improved sanitation facilities.[5]

[4] Our World in Data. Available at: https://ourworldindata.org/water-access.

[5] The share of the population with access to improved sanitation facilities was 82.8% in Brazil and 76.5% in China. Note: Improved sanitation facilities are designed to ensure hygienic separation of human excreta from human contact. Improved sanitation facilities include flush/pour flush (to piped sewer system, septic tank, pit latrine), ventilated improved pit (VIP) latrine, pit latrine with slab, and composting toilet. Source: Our World in Data. Available at: https://ourworldindata.org/sanitation.

Furthermore, access to water is insufficient in both countries. In China, as of 2015, around 65 million people (4.5% of the population) did not have access to improved drinking water sources; in Brazil, this affects around 4.2 million people or 2% of the population.[6] Even before the outbreak of the first cases of COVID-19, the insufficient access to water and sanitation represented a serious health challenge in both countries as a source of and aggravator of diseases. It is estimated that a total of 1.58 deaths per 100,000 people in Brazil were linked to unsafe water sources in 2017. This figure is 5 times higher than the estimates for China (0.32 sanitation-related deaths per 100,000) and around 30 times higher than the average estimates in the US and European countries (which are on average 0.02–0.05 deaths per 100,000 people).[7] As argued by the Inter-American Development Bank, rethinking infrastructure and investing in water, sanitation, energy, and transport will be vital for Brazil and other countries in the region to overcome not only the COVID-19 crisis, but also underlying problems of inequality, the health crisis, and low levels of economic growth (Cavallo et al., 2020).

Incidentally, Latin America's largest country is on the verge of adopting a new regulatory framework for water and sanitation services.[8] As this proposed water and sanitation reform has received several criticisms, in terms of deregulation and lack of incentives for the social and health aspects of private investments (Folha de São Paulo, 2020), a critical discussion about it could benefit from China's experience of ensuring a faster expansion of access to water and sanitation. The dialogue between China and Latin American countries like Brazil, on how to address inequality and provide sanitary infrastructure and access to water to all citizens, could contribute to the construction of a safer and more inclusive future for our cities. This dialogue has the potential of being instrumental for policies addressing inequalities and protecting people from future pandemics. Engaging in public–private partnerships requires caution as goals and accountability are not always well aligned among partners and profit priorities may conflict with achieving equity and social development (Stoler et al., 2021).

Furthermore, a dialogue about China's ever-advancing experiences of integrating NbS in urban planning to manage water in an integrated fashion, with other environmental and social concerns, promises advances in this direction. Decentralized techniques like NbS can supplement sanitation systems, not as a replacement, but increasing water safety and thus reducing scarcity. It has been observed that the centralized systems in water provision have been increasing its potential losses in efficiency (Schmidt, 2021). The particular configuration of urban water and

[6] Our World in Data. Available at: https://ourworldindata.org/water-access.

[7] Our World in Data. Available at: https://ourworldindata.org/water-access.

[8] On June 24, 2020, Bill No. 4,162/2019 was approved by the Brazilian Senate. It allows for the participation of private companies in sanitation services and establishes a one-year deadline for a mandatory procurement process in sanitation. Under this new framework, bidding agreements should promote the universalization of water and sanitation services, with the aim of expanding water services to 99% of the population and sanitation services to 90%. This bill is pending approval by the Executive branch.

sanitation systems is dated (Bell, 2012). High levels of urbanization have created large demands on water quantity and quality, as well as sanitation infrastructure, which has not kept pace with population growth and now requires large-scale investment (Hogan, 1993). The increased per capita consumption, higher than the urban population growth rate, is observed in many cities (Bell, 2012; do Carmo et al., 2014a).

The first cluster of cases of pneumonia that was later identified as the new coronavirus COVID-19 was reported in Wuhan on December 31st, 2019. It took 57 days for Brazil to register its first case of the same virus, on February 26th, 2020, which was brought in by a business traveler from Italy. Brazil became the first country in Latin America to confirm a COVID-19 patient, and as one of the countries with the greatest geographical distances from China, the time for instituting preventive and response measures was relatively long. Besides response time and capacity, the enabling or hindering of local conditions played a decisive role in the initial spread and (non)continuation of local infections. In this chapter, we argue that more analyses of local and systemic conditions can show factors that have had an impact on the spread of this new virus once it reached the region. The identification and analysis of such factors will be crucial to build better-suited public policies to deal with future pandemics.

Overview of the Methodology

Despite the common global experience of the pandemic as a unifying social experience, which can be exemplified by the often-cited observation that "the pandemic does not spare anyone" (see e.g., Lahiri-Dutt, 2020), we would like to question and reassess this simplistic assertion. The connection between contagion and inequality is not new, and it is known that pandemics, such as the Black Death in the fourteenth century, have hit the poorest and most vulnerable part of the population the hardest. The current COVID-19 crisis seems to occur in a similar manner, exposing existing inequalities (Davis, 2020). This article contributes to the debate on the role of inequality in the spread of pandemics by focusing on the access to water and sanitation infrastructure. These are, in turn, both a reflection of the spatialized and regional inequality within countries and cities, burdening communities and making them even more vulnerable to COVID-19 because they cannot follow the WHO hygiene guidelines.

This investigation was based on an initial analysis of city-level data on inequality, sociodemographic indicators, and water and sanitation infrastructure in Brazil, to verify their correlation with the COVID-19 propagation. The methodology applied in this study builds on interdisciplinary comparative studies on consumption, urban systems, and inequality in Brazil and China (do Carmo et al., 2014a; Hase Ueta et al., 2017). First, we investigated the sociodemographic indicators that correlated to the spread of COVID-19 around the country to identify which elements of inequality made the cities more vulnerable to the pandemic. Later, we focused on exploring the correlation between access to sanitation and the number and severity of COVID-19 cases. For this purpose, a preliminary analysis on the potential impacts of the availability and quality of water and sanitation services in Brazilian cities was carried out. A Weighted Least Squares Regression was executed using data on access to water from the Brazilian National Sanitation Information System (SNIS in Portuguese) and on the number of confirmed COVID-19 cases per municipality (from the Ministry of Health of Brazil).

Based on the assumption that this pandemic has interconnections similar to those formulated by Johansen and do Carmo (2015), considering the intersectionality (scientific research, public policies, education, etc.) of the dengue fever epidemic in Brazil, our regression model controlled for variables that would account for those different dimensions. Therefore, we considered the following variables (Fig. 15.1): average per capita water consumption; population density; hospital beds available (both as of December 2019 and additional beds as of June 2020); Human Development Index (HDI); population age; income per capita; income inequality (as measured by the Gini coefficient); life expectancy; literacy rate (as a proxy for education); and the level of adherence to self-quarantine measures (based on Google mobility data, evidencing the increase in smartphone users who stayed more at home compared to the period before the pandemic).

Finally, so as to avoid discrepancies caused by differences in the temporality of the pandemic in each city, the model included only the number of confirmed cases over the period of three months since the first case in each city. Cities with no cases for at least 3 months were excluded from the data sample. The total number of cases

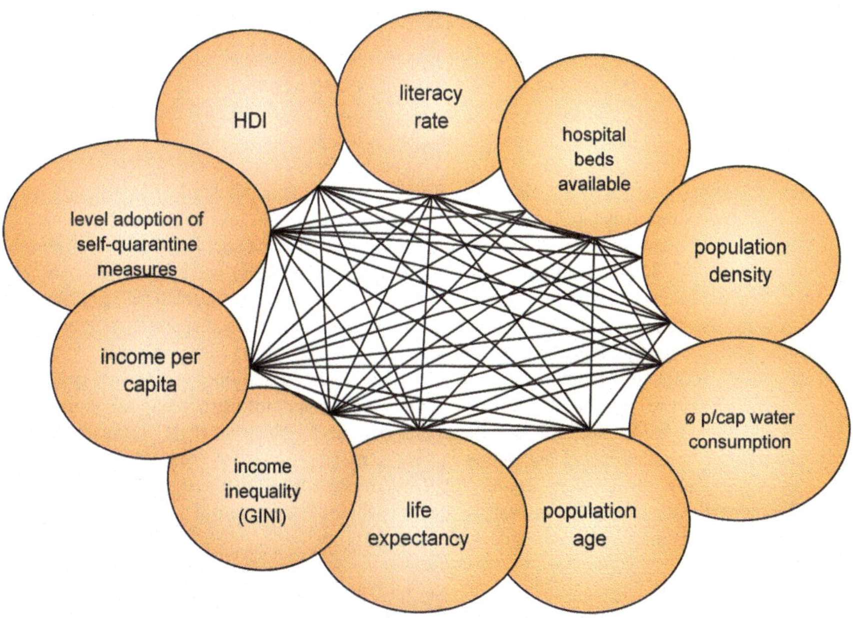

Fig. 15.1 Variables considered in the regression model for this study. (Elaborated by the authors)

(cities) considered in the model was 3265. The aim of this study was to contribute to the discussion and analysis of the public policies available for cities to combat this crisis and to be prepared for potential future crises. This study's findings, therefore, point out the importance of urban policies aimed at reducing inequalities, promoting education, and ensuring that social distancing policies can be followed.

Using Macroeconomic Data to Assess the Impacts of the Pandemic: Preliminary Findings

The results of this analysis point to a series of plausible interpretations. Although the results do not imply causality, it is relevant to note that, among all variables analyzed, income inequality was one of those most highly correlated with COVID-19 cases. An increase of 0.1 in the Gini coefficient corresponds to an increase of 44.5 cases (this would not be a minimal increase given that this coefficient ranges between 0 and 1). Income per capita also presented a correlation (−0.16 cases with an increase in wealth). The fact that inequality was demonstrated to be highly correlated with the pandemic can be explained by the importance of social issues in Brazil, from access to water and sanitation to healthcare options and living conditions. Income inequality unfolds itself in multiple forms of inequality, including an array of issues relating to gender, ethnicity, education, health, water and sanitation, consumption, mobility, housing conditions, safety, criminality, state neglect, and police violence (Hase Ueta et al., 2017). The high level of income inequality observed in Brazil, one of the world's most unequal societies, had a serious effect on the spread of the COVID-19 virus in the country. Racial, gender and regional components of income inequality have been playing a major role, as women, indigenous communities, and black people have been more severely affected by the pandemic:

> Furthermore, according to UN Women and the NGO Care, the pandemic affects men and women in different ways. (…) Women are overrepresented in informal settlements, which aggravates their lack of access to sanitation services and hygiene supplies (including menstrual hygiene). They depend more on public spaces to meet these needs, and there was a considerable increase in the records of domestic violence in Brazil, a situation aggravated by quarantine measures. In Brazil, indigenous communities are also especially vulnerable as they face more challenges in the access to water and sewage services: only one in three villages on indigenous lands has access to treated water. In addition, remote indigenous communities have limited access to hospitals and basic infrastructure. As a result, COVID-19's lethality rate among indigenous peoples is twice as high as the average national rate. Another important dimension is the racial dimension. Data collected in the city of São Paulo reveals that, among Brazilians infected by COVID-19, black people are 62% more likely to die of the disease than white people. The pandemic has therefore exacerbated pre-existing issues of exclusion and vulnerability.[9]

[9] UNICEF, World Bank and Stockholm International Water Institute, 2020.

In major urban centers such as São Paulo, Brasília, Manaus, and Fortaleza, which were among the first areas to be hit by the pandemic, considerable numbers of the low-income population live in socially and environmentally vulnerable areas (Fay, 2005). The relationship between income inequality and the availability of public services and infrastructure is crucial. Low-income neighborhoods are often neglected in cities throughout Brazil; at the same time, the country is plagued by persistent regional disparities. A recent study on access to water and sanitation found enormous differences between regions. For instance, the provision of sewage services is remarkably low in state capitals in the Amazon region, such as Manaus (where 12.5% of the urban population had access to sewage services as of 2018), Macapá (11.6%), Porto Velho (4%), and Belém (13.5%). In contrast, access to sewage services was nearly universal in most Southern and Southeastern state capital cities, reaching 99.9% in Curitiba, 96.3% in São Paulo, and 94.1% in Belo Horizonte (Trata Brasil, 2020).[10]

Income inequality has long been a serious problem in Brazilian cities, one that, not having been solved, was expected to create an additional challenge to the country's fight against the pandemic. People living in overcrowded housing, often without proper access to water and sanitation services, or even adequate healthcare facilities, are arguably more vulnerable to contagion and its consequences. For instance, in São Paulo, the city with the highest number of cases of COVID-19 at the time of writing, many vulnerable areas and low-income neighborhoods have been registering water shortages and outages.[11] Municipalities with less income inequality tend to offer better health and water services and better living conditions for their poorest citizens (Roaf et al., 2018).

It is also interesting that the literacy rate in the studied cities is significantly correlated with the number of cases; a 1% increase in the literacy rate corresponds to a decrease of 385 cases per 100,000 over the period analyzed by this study. This may point to the importance of education. Based on these findings, one could argue that more literate individuals will tend to have a higher capacity to respond more adequately to the crisis due to their access to written information. In this context, universalizing access to basic education in Brazil can be seen as an essential pillar of public policy in the country, one which remains incomplete despite the recent progress made. Between 2001 and 2012, the illiteracy rate among the population aged 15 and above dropped from 12.4% to 8.7%. At the same time, regional inequalities persist, also in the realm of education. Almost 20% of people in the Northeast region of the country remained unable to read as of 2012, while in the South region, 4.4% of people were illiterate in that period (Ministry of Education of Brazil, 2014).

---

[10] TrataBrasil. Planilha do Ranking, 2020. Available at: http://www.tratabrasil.org.br/images/estudos/itb/ranking_2020/Tabela_100_cidades_Ranking_Saneamento_4.pdf.

[11] As reported in local media, as of March 2020 water outages and shortages were taking place across low-income areas, affecting a total of 78 neighborhoods: https://g1.globo.com/sp/sao-paulo/noticia/2020/03/26/78-bairros-de-sp-reclamam-de-falhas-no-abastecimento-de-agua-em-tempos-de-coronavirus.ghtml.

Another finding that is worth mentioning is that self-quarantine measures are negatively correlated with the spread of the disease. According to the results of this study, a 1% increase in people staying at home (compared to the period immediately before the crisis) is correlated with a decrease of 420 cases per 100,000 in a city. This observation is an indication that further corroborates the quarantine and social distancing policies that have been advocated by international organizations, such as the WHO and the UN, since the outbreak of the pandemic, advice that unfortunately has been largely ignored by many in Brazil. Some extremist movements have been mirroring their counterparts in the United States, where right-wing activists also tend to minimize the dangers of the pandemic, or even deny its existence altogether. In this sense, continuous remarks and actions made by the President of Brazil, minimizing the risks and seriousness of the COVID-19 crisis, resisting social distancing recommendations, and claiming the economy would suffer less (Barberia & Gómez, 2020; Silva & Ventura, 2020), can only contribute to antisocial distancing sentiments, which in turn protract the quarantine measures and lower their effectiveness.

Even though there was a significant reduction in the number of flights in both China and Brazil, other means of transport were not considered in this study. In Brazil, the mobility infrastructure relies heavily on roads, even in the North Region where transport through rivers was the main factor shaping the occupation of the territories (do Carmo et al., 2014b). Those networks of mobility have had implications on the spread of previous epidemics, such as the Chikungunya, as the population moves through municipalities that connect different levels of mobility, both comprising interstate long-distance movements, intraurban migratory movements, and the daily commute (do Carmo et al., 2015).

Fortaleza et al. (2020) analyzed the expansion of the COVID-19 cases and mortality rates in the state of São Paulo. Their findings draw a conclusion similar to do Carmo et al. (2015) in the Chikungunya analysis, as they found two distinct patterns of epidemic spread of COVID-19 in the state: the spatial spread by contiguity into neighboring areas and metropolitan spaces; and the hierarchical spread through the degree of connectedness of smaller municipalities with their regional centers (Fortaleza et al., 2020).

For this reason, it is extremely important to consider intrametropolitan dynamics, as Fig. 15.2 shows, among the 40 cities where the confirmed cases grew the fastest during the initial period, only 4 are not part of a metropolitan region. By considering the "region of influence, i.e., the spatial reach of the commercial and service activities fixed therein" (Firkowski, 2012, p. 23), we can account for the metropolitan dynamic in Brazil. Commuter mobility expands those connections, increasing the flow and distances within the connected areas, and the movements that were more frequently of an intraurban scale start to take place in an interregional one (Cunha et al., 2018). In the state of São Paulo, for instance, there is already intense traffic and integration among the different metropolitan regions within the state.

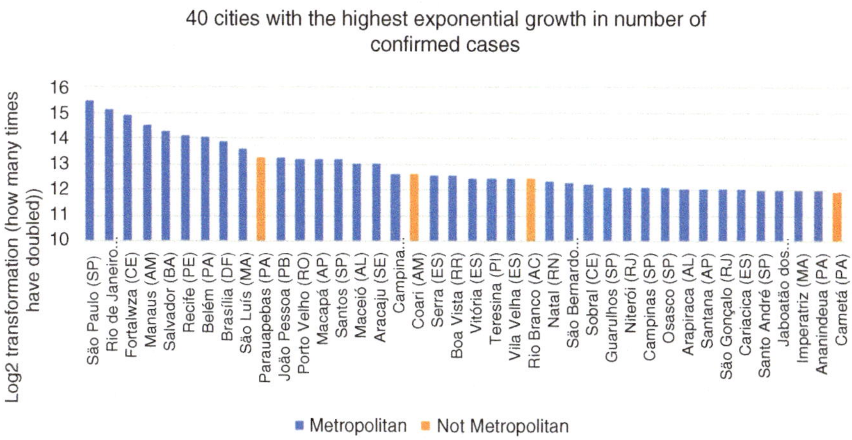

Fig. 15.2 Log_2 transformation of accumulated confirmed cases of the top 40 cities with highest exponential increase in COVID-19 confirmed cases in Brazil in June 2020. Cities that are part of a metropolitan region are marked in blue, and those that are not part of a metropolitan region are marked in orange. (Elaborated by the authors)

Discussing Policy Implications: No Simple Solutions for a Complex Problem

Conducting research on an ongoing pandemic is a highly challenging task, even more so, if the research should point to palatable policy solutions that can be approached through a small number of variables. This research emerged from continued interdisciplinary dialogues between demography, economics, sociology, and environmental studies on urban issues in Brazil and China, and thus has dealt with an array of methodologies, theoretical assumptions, and practical explanations for the issue studied.

One finding that we would like to highlight relates to the correlation of COVID-19 cases with lower literacy rates; it indicates that health issues alone cannot explain the difficulties of countries like Brazil to contain the pandemic. It therefore suggests that health can only be approached through complex and integrated considerations of other social variables. The importance of interdisciplinary studies becomes ever clearer as more scientific evidence is published, demonstrating that apparently unrelated issues add to a more complex understanding of virus propagation (such as the cases of do Carmo et al., 2015 and Roaf et al., 2018).

Access to water, sanitation, and hygiene are considered basic rights and responsibilities of the state and recognized as such by both China and Brazil as they are among the countries that voted in favor of a UN General Assembly Resolution on this topic in 2010.[12] The sudden wide recognition of coordinated state action in

[12] United Nations General Assembly Resolution No. GA/10967: Resolution Recognizing Access to Clean Water, Sanitation as Human Right. 28 July, 2010. The Resolution recorded 122 votes in

those fields during the pandemic has shown the necessity of continued and coordinated public policy action after decades of neoliberal policies that have weakened the crisis-response capacity of many countries (Goodwin, 2020). Especially in the process of reaching the 17 UN Sustainable Development Goals, it is of utmost importance to rethink the integration of social baseline policies (UN Department of Economic and Social Affairs [DESA], 2020). In this sense, it has been pointed out by some authors (Zhang et al., 2020a) that, in the case of China since the 1980s, there is a strong case for what has been termed a "return of the state" (Almond, 1988). The Chinese model, often termed as "state capitalism", does not come without criticism, but does present strength in crisis scenarios.[13] Brazil, on the other hand, has recently been moving toward a market-centered approach to economics, where the state retreats and shares a higher part of its roles with private firms. Specifically, in relation to access to water and sanitation, the level of success and effectiveness of the current government's strategy to achieve universal access through privatization of public services remains to be seen.

In Brazil, the lack of action from the federal government made local governments come up with their own diverse set of directives to deal with the specific challenges of each city during the pandemic. This has led to several problems as the population continued to move between jurisdictions and the different policies were oftentimes not coordinated. This may have contributed to the pandemic reaching all regions of the country, which in turn made regional inequalities in Brazil ever more evident, especially in the response capacities of the Northern and Northeastern regions. To address this issue, UNICEF, the World Bank, and the Stockholm International Water Institute pointed out that a more robust cooperation among the federal, state, and municipal governments, and among government sectors such as health and education, was necessary to provide the most efficient response to this crisis.[14]

Unfortunately, the response was the opposite. The political polarization around COVID-19 has led the federal government to keep as its agenda the constant undermining of the state governors who tried to impose stronger social distancing measures. It is difficult, though, to create a symmetry in this particular case, as the spectrum from right-center to left wing pleads for robust directives. The absence of a clear national strategy and the continuing denial of the healthcare emergency by the federal government further individualized the responsibility of citizens to keep themselves safe. That was clear as the president himself got involved in agglomerations, got himself and members of his staff infected, and even after this, constantly undermined the effectiveness of masks (Silva & Ventura, 2020). For this reason, it often came down to people's education to interpret the situation for themselves and

---

favor, none against, and 41 abstentions. Available at: https://www.un.org/press/en/2010/ga10967.doc.htm.

[13] The Economist. Xi Jinping is reinventing state capitalism. Don't underestimate it. Aug 13th, 2020. Available at: https://www.economist.com/leaders/2020/08/13/xi-jinping-is-reinventing-state-capitalism-dont-underestimate-it.

[14] UNICEF, World Bank and Stockholm International Water Institute, 2020.

their specific socioeconomic condition, to maintain self-isolation and follow WHO directives. This is in line with this study's findings on the correlation between literacy and inequality with COVID-19 cases in Brazil.

Conclusion: Fighting a Pandemic in the Context of Inequality

In the face of a pandemic, China and Brazil, as highly unequal societies, have to build strategies in order to reach the different parts of the country and address their needs. Once the decision to fight the pandemic was taken by the central government, China was very successful in its control measures by enforcing strict lockdowns and thus avoiding the spread of the virus by controlling the mobility of people in the contaminated areas. However, throughout this crisis and up to the time of writing, Brazil did not enforce similarly strict measures at the national level, and the pandemic spread all over the country. In this sense, as demonstrated in this preliminary analysis, inequality arguably played a decisive role regarding how the different states and cities in Brazil were able to deal with the crisis.

The present analysis brings together different elements to understand health and vulnerability as integrated with socioeconomic intersectionalities. In the context of an epidemic, we argue that not only fast containment strategies are important, but also long-term investment in access to water and sanitary infrastructure, which helps to build more resilient cities and allow them to be in a better position to fight new pandemics. Thus, it is important to consider the different spheres of politics, and the lack of coordination that made it more difficult to fight the pandemic in an efficient way in Brazil. The lack of action from the federal government forced state governments to take more action and assume greater responsibility regarding the crisis management of the pandemic. Furthermore, if the state and federal governments had been making stronger investments in sanitary infrastructure previously, a vulnerable population with universal access to water and sewage services would likely have had the means to follow basic WHO guidelines to decrease/lessen the spread of the disease. As the new sanitation law takes effect, the consequences are yet to materialize. As we see a global trend that cities around the world go back to nationalizing their water and sanitation services, liberal sectors claim that the goals are going to be stricter and better ensured. As mentioned before, Stole and collaborators (2021) have given attention to the priorities that the private sector has. The critics of the new law claim that profit might hinder investment and accentuate regional inequalities.

Another point worth mentioning is that during the pandemic, the federal government showed an inability to conduct its foreign affairs with countries such as China. This resulted in diplomatic tension and a missed opportunity to receive additional support in the form of health supplies and vaccines. It is considered that the unnecessary diplomatic crises created by Brazil's Minister of Foreign Affairs at the time, Mr. Ernesto Araújo, and the President's sons, who made systematic attacks against

China, have serious economic implications.[15] In the race to develop and provide vaccines against COVID-19, it became clear that Global South countries, such as China, India, and Russia, were moving fast: Among the 20 vaccines that had been approved or were being tested in the world at the time of the writing of this study, 6 are from China, 2 from Russia, and 2 from India (O Globo, 2021). Brazil announced only at the end of March 2021 that it had developed the first Brazilian vaccines and intended to start trials. The BRICS ties could have helped in the cooperation between these countries on vaccine matters. However, this was not a priority in the Bolsonaro government, which continued to show an anti-China position, as it was possible to see in the resistance to acquire the CoronaVac vaccine as well as racist and anti-Chinese remarks from the then Minister of Foreign Affairs. At the time of writing, recent signs are emerging, indicating a potential shift in the Brazilian government's attitude toward China. Mr. Ernesto Araújo was replaced in March 2021 in a movement considered by some to be as a result of pressure from Congress, worried about the commercial risks of the ongoing confrontation with China. The new head of the Ministry of Foreign Affairs, Mr. Carlos França, discussed cooperation in vaccine production in his first meeting with his Chinese counterpart, Mr. Wang Yi.[16]

The analysis of factors and issues related to access to water in Brazilian cities investigated in this research was not able to find a strong correlation between water consumption and COVID-19 cases in the country. This is potentially because it was only possible to identify city-wide data on water consumption, which did not indicate a statistical relation to COVID-19-related data and measures of quality of water provision and of sanitation infrastructure. We consider that the availability of such data would be highly beneficial for future studies. In fact, ensuring the availability of reliable and disaggregated data on hygiene and equitable access to water and sewage services in Brazil was one of the main recommendations of a technical note which was recently published on this matter by UNICEF, the World Bank, and the Stockholm International Water Institute.[17]

Nonetheless, the correlation shown by our model for the significance of literacy, inequality, and the reduction of intraurban movement due to adherence to self-quarantine measures indicates potentially effective policy recommendations, especially for the Brazilian case. It is important to consider that the ongoing pandemic is still unfolding and has possibly not even reached its peak in many countries of the

[15] GIELOW, IGOR. "Nova crise de Bolsonaro com a China ameaça superávit recorde com Pequim". FOLHA DE SÃO PAULO. November 25, 2020. Available at: https://www1.folha.uol.com.br/mundo/2020/11/nova-crise-de-bolsonaro-com-a-china-ameaca-superavit-recorde-com-pequim.shtml; SANCHES, MARINA. "Por que o Congresso quer demissão de Ernesto Araújo?". BBC. March 25, 2021. Available at: https://www.bbc.com/portuguese/brasil-56532188.

[16] Coletta, R. 2021. "Em 1ª conversa com ministro chinês, novo chanceler discute cooperação para insumos de vacina". Folha de São Paulo. April 10. https://www1.folha.uol.com.br/mundo/2021/04/em-1a-conversa-com-ministro-chines-novo-chanceler-discute-cooperacao-para-insumos-de-vacina.shtml; Coletta, R. and Uribe, G. "Ernesto Araújo deixa comando do Itamaraty após pressão do Congresso". Folha de Pernambuco. March 29, 2021. https://www.folhape.com.br/politica/ernesto-araujo-deixa-comando-do-itamaraty-apos-pressao-do-congresso/178033/.

[17] Ibidem.

Global South. At the time of writing this study, it is too early to draw more final conclusions on the impact of each variable to the spread of the disease. Based on the preliminary findings, this study points to the importance of taking into consideration a multilevel approach in designing public policies to prepare for pandemics and build urban resilience, one that considers inequalities, education, healthcare, access to water and sanitation, and urban and regional mobility, among other factors.

We propose that it is essential to raise the baseline water security so that citizens can benefit in periods of crisis and normality. Measures to complement the existing infrastructure could be, e.g., nature-based solutions for rainwater capturing and multipurpose use of green spaces, which could be one such integrated proposal. Future research on some of the incipient design proposals for Brazilian cities points in this direction, stressing social functions and connection to nature to promote education on ecosystems in cities. This kind of research can be used to increase coverage or provide safe and reliable water to more households. While such solutions can bring about long-term changes on the local level, the zoonotic origins of the pandemic have shown that a more immediate transformation of human ethics, as well as human–nature relations, is urgently necessary. Another crucial aspect is the multilevel integration of governance, both for ready responses to COVID-19 or for long-term water management.

Acknowledgments The findings, interpretations, and conclusions expressed in this work are entirely those of the authors and should not be attributed in any manner to the World Bank, its Board of Executive Directors, or the governments they represent.

References

Ahmed, F., Ahmed, N., Pissarides, C., & Stiglitz, J. (2020). Why inequality could spread COVID-19. *The Lancet Public Health, 5*(5), e240.

Almond, G. A. (1988). The return to the state. *American Political Science Review, 82*(3), 853–874.

Barberia, L. G., & Gómez, E. J. (2020). Political and institutional perils of Brazil's COVID-19 crisis. *The Lancet, 396*(10248), 367–368.

Bell, S. (2012). Urban water systems in transition. Emergence: Complexity and Organization, v. 14, n. 1, p. 45–58, 2012. https://www.proquest.com/scholarly-journals/urban-water-systems-transition/docview/1349940826/se-2?accountid=8113

Cavallo, E., Powell, A., & Serebrisky, T. (Eds.). (2020, July). From structures to services: The path to better infrastructure in Latin America and the Caribbean. *Inter-American Development Bank.* https://publications.iadb.org/publications/english/document/From-Structures-to-Services-The-Path-to-Better-Infrastructure-in-Latin-America-and-the-Caribbean.pdf. Accessed Oct 2020.

Cheng, S., Li, Z., Uddin, S. M. N., Mang, H.-P., Zhou, X., Zhang, J., Zheng, L., & Zhang, L. (2018). Toilet revolution in China. *Journal of Environmental Management, 216*, 347–356.

Cunha, J. M. P., Farias, L. A. C., Silva, K. A. A., & Silva, D. S. F. (2018). Síntese dos principais resultados e análise comparativa entre as nove RMs [Synthesis of the main results and comparative analysis between the nine RMs]. In J. M. P. Cunha (Org.), *Dinâmica demográfica e socioespacial no Brasil metropolitano*. EduFSCar.

Davis, M. (2005). *O monstro bate à nossa porta* [The monster knocks on our door]. Record.

Davis, M. (2020, March 20). The coronavirus crisis is a monster fueled by capitalism. *In These Times*. https://inthesetimes.com/article/coronavirus-crisis-capitalism-covid-19-monster-mike-davis. Accessed Oct 2020.

Do Carmo, R., Dagnino, R. S., & Caparroz, M. (2015). Modelagem de Expansão Hipotética do Chikungunya (MECHI) [Chikungunya hypothetical expansion modeling (MECHI)]. *Textos NEPO (UNICAMP), 72*, 60–80.

Do Carmo, R. L., Dagnino, R. S., El Saifi, S., Caparroz, M. B., & Craice, C. (2014a). Características demográficas e socioeconômicas de municípios do projeto URBIS Amazônia no Pará [Demographic and socioeconomic characteristics of municipalities in the URBIS Amazônia project in Pará]. *Núcleo de Estudos da População – NEPO/Unicamp, 68*(71).

Do Carmo, R. L., Dagnino, R., De, S., & Johansen, I. C. (2014b). Transição demográfica e transição do consumo urbano de água no Brasil [Demographic transition and urban water consumption transition in Brazil]. *Revista Brasileira de Estudos de População, 31*(1), 169–190. https://doi.org/10.1590/S0102-30982014000100010

Fay, M. (2005). *The urban poor in Latin America*. World Bank. http://siteresources.worldbank.org/INTLACREGTOPURBDEV/Home/20843636/UrbanPoorinLA.pdf. Accessed Oct 2020.

Firkowski, O. L. C. F. (2012). Por que as Regiões Metropolitanas no Brasil são Regiões mas não são Metropolitanas [Why metropolitan regions in Brazil are regions but not metropolitans]. *Revista Paranaense de Desenvolvimento, 122*, 19–38.

Folha de São Paulo. (2020, June 25). *Novo marco quer levar saneamento a todo o país até 2033* [New milestone wants to bring sanitation to the entire country by 2033]. https://www1.folha.uol.com.br/podcasts/2020/06/novo-marco-quer-levar-saneamento-a-todo-o-pais-ate-2033-ouca-podcast.shtml. Accessed Oct 2020.

Fortaleza, C. M. C. B., Guimarães, R. B., De Almeida, G. B., Pronunciate, M., & Ferreira, C. P. (2020). Taking the inner route: Spatial and demographic factors affecting vulnerability to COVID-19 among 604 cities from inner São Paulo State, Brazil. *Epidemiology and Infection, 148*, e118. https://doi.org/10.1017/S095026882000134X

Goodwin, M. (2020, May 12). COVID-19 will reshape our relationship with the state. Expert comment. *Chatham House*. https://www.chathamhouse.org/expert/comment/covid-19-will-reshape-our-relationship-state#. Accessed Oct 2020.

Hase Ueta, M. et al. (2018). China and Brazil: transitioning from the middle income trap to sustainable development? China: Fudan Latin America University Consortium (FLAUC), 2018. https://www.academia.edu/download/56081028/01_Inequality_middle-income_UETA_TJONG_WEINS_SCHMIDT.pdf

Hogan, D. J. (1993). Crescimento populacional e desenvolvimento sustentável [Population growth and sustainable development]. *Lua Nova: Revista de Cultura e Política, 31*, 57–78. https://doi.org/10.1590/S0102-64451993000300004

IATA. (2020, June). *Air passenger market analysis*. https://www.iata.org/en/iata-repository/publications/economic-reports/air-passenger-monthly-analysis%2D%2D-june-20202/. Accessed Oct 2020.

Johansen, I. C., & Carmo, R. L. (2015). A multicausalidade da dengue nos espaços urbanos brasileiros [The multi-causality of dengue in Brazilian urban spaces]. *Textos NEPO, 72*, 9–59. https://www.nepo.unicamp.br/publicacoes/textos_nepo/textos_nepo_72.pdf

Lahiri-dutt, K. (2020). Living in, and thinking about, the world in pandemic times. *Ecology, Economy and Society – The INSEE Journal, 3*(2), 1–3, 4. doi: https://doi.org/10.37773/ees.v3i2.283

Leung, K., Wu, J. T., Liu, D., & Leung, G. M. (2020). First-wave COVID-19 transmissibility and severity in China outside Hubei after control measures, and second-wave scenario planning: A modelling impact assessment. *The Lancet, 395*(10233), 1382–1393. https://doi.org/10.1016/S0140-6736(20)30746-7

Marques, L. Capitalismo e colapso ambiental. 3. ed. Campinas, SP: Editora da UNICAMP, 2018.

Ministry of Education of Brazil. (2014). *Report 'Educação Para Todos no Brasil 2000-2015'* [Report 'Education for all in Brazil 2000–2015']. http://portal.mec.gov.br/index.php?option=com_doc

man&view=download&alias=15774-ept-relatorio-06062014&Itemid=30192. Accessed Oct 2020.

O Globo. (2021, February 14). *O Brics e a barbárie global das vacinas* [Brics and the global barbarism of vaccines]. https://blogs.oglobo.globo.com/opiniao/post/o-brics-e-barbarie-global-das-vacinas.html. Accessed March 2021.

Roaf, V., De Albuquerque, C., & Heller, L. (2018). The human rights to water and sanitation: Challenges and implications for future priorities. In O. Cumming & T. Slaymaker (Eds.), *Equality in water and sanitation services* (pp. 26–45). Routledge.

Schmidt, A. F. J. (2021). *Transferring water and redistributing scarcity: A study of the São Paulo-Rio de Janeiro hydromegalopolis*. University of Campinas.

Schwartz, L. (2020). Brazil confirms first case of COVID-19 in Latin America. *Medscape*. https://www.medscape.com/viewarticle/925806

Da Silva, J. M., & de Lima Ventura, D. F. (2020). Between science and populism: The Brazilian response to COVID-19 from the perspective of the legal determinants of Global Health. *Revista de Direito Internacional, 2*(17). https://doi.org/10.5102/rdi.v17i2.6687

Stoler, J., Miller, J. D., Brewis, A., Freeman, M. C., Harris, L. M., Jepson, W., … Tutu, R. (2021). Household water insecurity will complicate the ongoing COVID-19 response: Evidence from 29 sites in 23 low- and middle-income countries. *International Journal of Hygiene and Environmental Health, 234*(January). https://doi.org/10.1016/j.ijheh.2021.113715

Teixeira, Maria do C. C., and A. R. P. Moreira. (2020). A construção do conhecimento agroecológico a partir da infância. Cadernos de Agroecologia, v. 15, n. 1, 2020. http://cadernos.aba-agroecologia.org.br/index.php/cadernos/article/view/6295

Trata Brasil. (2020). *Ranking do Saneamento 2020* [2020 Sanitation Ranking]. http://www.tratabrasil.org.br/images/estudos/itb/ranking_2020/Tabela_100_cidades_Ranking_Saneamento_4.pdf. Accessed Mar 2021.

UN Department of Economic and Social Affairs. (2020, May 15). *COVID-19: Reaffirming state-people governance relationships* (Policy Brief #75). https://www.un.org/development/desa/dpad/publication/un-desa-policy-brief-75-covid-19-reaffirming-state-people-governance-relationships/. Accessed Oct 2020.

UNICEF, World Bank, & Stockholm International Water Institute. (2020, August). *O papel fundamental do saneamento e da promoção da higiene na resposta à Covid-19 no Brasil* [The fundamental role of sanitation and hygiene promotion in the response to Covid-19 in Brazil]. http://documents1.worldbank.org/curated/en/998851596650728051/pdf/O-Papel-Fundamental-do-Saneamento-e-da-Promocao-da-Higiene-na-Resposta-a-Covid-19-no-Brasil.pdf. Accessed Oct 2020.

United Nations. (2010, July 28). *General Assembly Resolution No. GA/10967: Resolution recognizing access to clean water, sanitation as human right*. https://www.un.org/press/en/2010/ga10967.doc.htm. Accessed Oct 2020.

World Health Organization [WHO]. *WHO coronavirus disease (COVID-19) dashboard*. https://covid19.who.int/. Accessed 20 Oct 2020.

WHO. (2020). *Archived: WHO Timeline – COVID-19*. https://www.who.int/news-room/detail/27-04-2020-who-timeline%2D%2D-covid-19. Accessed 20 Oct 2020.

Zhang, S., Wang, Z., Chang, R., Wang, H., Xu, C., Yu, X., Tsamlag, L., Dong, Y., Wang, H., & Cai, Y. (2020a). COVID-19 containment: China provides important lessons for global response. *Frontiers of Medicine, 14*(2), 215–219. http://link.springer.com/10.1007/s11684-020-0766-9

Zhang, J., Litvinova, M., Wang, W., Wang, Y., Deng, X., Chen, X., Li, M., Zheng, W., Yi, L., Chen, X., Wu, Q., Liang, Y., Wang, X., Yang, J., Sun, K., Longini, I. M., Halloran, M. E., Wu, P., Cowling, B. J., … Yu, H. (2020b). Evolving epidemiology and transmission dynamics of coronavirus disease 2019 outside Hubei province, China: A descriptive and modelling study. *The Lancet Infectious Diseases, 20*(7), 793–802. https://linkinghub.elsevier.com/retrieve/pii/S1473309920302309

Chapter 16
Cities, COVID-19, and International Development Cooperation: Challenges and Opportunities

Carlos Cerda and Daniel Lemus-Delgado

Introduction

In the twenty-first century, cities are prominent players on the international scene. This situation is a result of a simultaneous process. On the one hand, it is clear from a historical perspective that cities, existing for more than 4000 years, have lived through waves of growth and expansion, participating in the process of contact between human groups and distant civilizations, giving way to the dynamics of the internationalization of cities (Clark, 2016). The last stage of this process has been evident since the second half of the twentieth century, when the processes of economic globalization and global production chains were underpinned by cities (Rennie-Short, 2004). On the other hand, the weakening of the modern nation-state in the face of the emergence of multiple transnational challenges has accelerated the process of decentralization in many countries, which has given cities a major role in the reconfiguration of the world.

At present, more than half the world's population is living in cities and that proportion is projected to rise to 60% by 2030; at the same time, cities and metropolitan areas are the heart of economic growth, contributing about 60% of the global gross domestic product (GDP) (United Nations, 2020a). This fact demonstrates the growing importance of cities as levers for development. For this reason, the United Nations, in the Sustainable Development Goals (SDGs), adopted a specific objective regarding the development of cities. So, objective 11 establishes that cities should be inclusive, safe, resilient, and sustainable. Although there is a specific objective for cities, there are many other goals in which cities play a fundamental role, such as climate action, reducing inequalities, promoting clean energy, and driving economic growth (United Nations, 2020b).

C. Cerda (✉) · D. Lemus-Delgado
School of Social Sciences and Government, Tecnológico de Monterrey, Guadalajara, Mexico
e-mail: carlos.cerda@tec.mx

© The Author(s), under exclusive license to Springer Nature Switzerland AG 2021

M. A. Montoya et al. (eds.), *COVID-19 and Cities*, The Urban Book Series,
https://doi.org/10.1007/978-3-030-84134-8_16

However, the emergence of COVID-19 has represented a major challenge for the multilateral international order and has led to a rethinking of the benefits of globalization. The outbreak accelerated tensions that were already present in our world and were already shaping a new generation of inequalities (United Nations Development Programme, 2020). Faced with the spread of the pandemic, states have acted unilaterally on more than a few occasions, closing their borders and adopting unilateral measures to contain the virus. The pandemic has generated a triple crisis: a health crisis, an economic crisis, and a political crisis. As noted by the United Nations, "The impact of COVID-19 will be most devastating in poor and densely populated urban areas, especially for the one billion people living in informal settlements and slums worldwide, where overcrowding also makes it difficult to follow recommended measures, such as social distancing and self-isolation" (United Nations, 2020b, par. 4). Despite the COVID-19 crisis deeply impacting the whole world, the worst effects of the disease are closely linked with urban areas, where death rates tend to be higher because of a complex combination of factors, including population density, national and international connectivity, and public health response (Dixon, 2020). Moreover, over 90% of COVID-19 cases are in urban areas (United Nations, 2021).

In March 2020, 2 weeks after the World Health Organization (WHO) declared a new pandemic, Eric Garcetti, Mayor of the City of Los Angeles, organized 45 mayors (who were part of C40 Cities[1]) from around the world to share their experiences on responding to COVID-19. So, they rapidly repurposed from their focus on tackling climate change to leverage their relationships, capacity, and expertise with cities to facilitate their leadership on the front lines of the response to COVID-19. In short, they rolled out a knowledge base, set up a recovery task force chaired by Mayor Beppe Sala of Milan, and signed up an influential set of global cities to make issues of equity and climate action central to the COVID-19 response and recovery (Pipa & Bouchet, 2020).

The emergence of the COVID-19 pandemic shows that cities have been challenged by unexpected crises, but at the same time, some cities can be a fundamental part of the solution; in the case of COVID-19, reacting faster than national governments to contain the spread of the virus, managing the donation of medical equipment and other supplies to combat the disease, and launching actions to mitigate the economic crisis and promote a speedy economic recovery through specific programs. The starting point of this article is that the COVID-19 pandemic is increasing the importance of cities in solving global problems. Due to the ineffectiveness or slowness in the response to the health crisis on the part of the nation-states, many cities have not only responded in an agile, flexible, and adequate manner, but have also woven international collaboration networks to share knowledge and give and receive international aid. We assume that this has been possible because, before the

[1] The network C40 represents more than 700 million citizens and one quarter of the global economy. Also, C40 Cities links 96 of the world's greatest cities to take bold climate action, leading the way toward a healthier and more sustainable future. The mayors of the C40 cities are committed to delivering on the most ambitious goals of the Paris Agreement at the local level (C40 Cities, 2020).

pandemic, there was already a trend toward the internationalization of cities. This process of internationalization has advanced over past decades, allowing cities to be a platform for International Development Cooperation (IDC). Thus, in the reconfiguration of the IDC regime, cities have become more important protagonists by the day. In this way, it is possible to affirm that the experiences accumulated during the pandemic, and the responses generated, will mean that cities will become more active actors in the IDC.

The main objective of this article is to reflect on the trajectory of cities as international actors and propose some recommendations on the way in which cities can increase their role as international actors in solving world problems. With the aim to analyze the significance of the responses of cities to the global health problem and its impact on the international regime of the IDC, this article is organized in four sections. First, we analyze the traditional role of the cities in the architecture of IDC with the intention of showing that cities are not newcomer actors on the international scene, since they embarked on an important path prior to the internationalization processes. In the second section, we discuss sustainable cities and communities as a specific goal of the SDGs as a result of the recognition of their value as an important actor in achieving many of the goals of sustainable development and the international actions that cities already carry out. Later, we analyze the impact of the COVID-19 pandemic on the SDGs and the SDG 11. Finally, we conclude with a series of recommendations on how cities can contribute to the development path from the new scenario caused by the pandemic, while assuming the importance of international cooperation as a tool to increase the capacity of cities to be resilient.

The Role of Cities in the Architecture of IDC

Cities as protagonists of international cooperation are not a new phenomenon. The initial international association of local authorities was founded in 1913 with the aim of exchanging information through a small number of direct city-to-city relations; however, it was in the aftermath of World War II, through the Sister Cities program, that direct connections between local authorities of two or more countries began to expand (Iocco, 2005). In this context, most of the early initiatives were among developed countries, but it was soon after that when the first links with developing countries began to be established (Iocco, 2005). Since 1950, more than 11,000 pairs of sister cities, in 159 countries, have entered into twinning agreements (Zelinsky, 1991). In recent times, the international connections of the cities have evolved from bilateral agreements to the creation of international networking. So, cities are progressively linking forces through transnational municipal networks and providing a platform for city-to-city learning. In this way, networks and cities have shown that, through network organizations, local policymakers aim to connect with peers from cities that face similar challenges (Haupt et al., 2020). At present, the idea of collaboration between cities has challenged the idea of the international network of cities with the aim of solving common problems such as climate change (Lee, 2013).

In the present situation, the emergence of global challenges reveals the weaknesses and fragility of states to solve these issues alone; other actors also claim leading roles, such as international organizations, transnational corporations, as well as cities (Martins Vaz & Reis, 2018). Even though the nation-state is still considered the main actor in the international scenario and holds the key responsibility for carrying out international cooperation, the current situation favors an increasing role for cities and their authorities in promoting development. So, the nature of local administration and local politics is rapidly and profoundly changing. As a consequence of the multifarious decentralization processes in most societies, a restructuring of the public sector is taking place, leading to a new interaction between the central and local governments, generating a rising involvement of the cities in activities of international cooperation with the aim to collaborate in the consecution of the SG (Bontenbal & van Lindert, 2006).

Since the beginning of the twenty-first century, Decentralized Development Cooperation (DDC) has been consolidated. This period has been characterized by the greatest quantitative growth, evolution of the institutional and normative framework, and doctrinal development (Iborra et al., 2013). City authorities have participated as important actors in cooperation, from the perspective of decentralized cooperation.[2] Although there is no single definition of DDC, there is a broad consensus that cities are participants in this cooperation model (OECD, 2018). So, there are points of convergence among these interpretations that suggest a common definition of DDC that includes the idea that the local governments are the lead actors, the sustainable local development is the main objective, and the nature of the activities carried out is exchanged and supported (Hafteck, 2003).

DDC between a Northern and a Southern municipality is known as city-to-city (C2C) cooperation. Among other characteristics, the activities have a relatively high level of involvement with the general public, generating specific projects that directly benefit particular target groups in the Southern sister city; the peer-to-peer approach, which means that professionals from the Northern and the Southern municipalities meet and exchange experiences, knowledge, and capacities; the mutual trust and reciprocity as well as the time frame implying a long-standing partner relationship that is increasingly deepened and extended over the years (Bontenbal & van Lindert, 2006).

[2] In a strict sense, centralized cooperation is the cooperation carried out by substate administrations (autonomous governments, councils, and municipalities). In a broad sense, this type of cooperation is a new in a strict sense, centralized cooperation is the cooperation carried out by substate administrations (autonomous governments, councils, and municipalities). In a broad sense, this type of cooperation is a new approach characterized by the decentralization of initiatives and new forms of relationships with the South, incorporating a wide range of novel civil society actors and generating greater participation by the actors from the developing countries in their development. These two approaches have in common its concern for the participation of new agents in development cooperation activity. We adopt the first approach to decentralized cooperation in the present article.

The importance of the role of local authorities in the IDC system was reinforced by two simultaneous phenomena. On the one hand, the crisis of the state that was reflected in the liberalization of the economies and the decentralization processes derived from the multiple waves of globalization. On the other hand, the increasing strength of participatory approaches, the drive for democratization, and the validity of human rights as a basis for the construction of society and the need to favor the local as a base for positive insertion in the process of globalization.

The concept of DDC is closely related to the idea of empowering civil society actors, giving them a more leading role in development (Bontenbal, 2009). For this reason, DDC strengthens the links between the city as the space in which cooperation practices take place and the city as a place for the formation of participatory, responsible, and even cosmopolitan citizens, who are interested not only in supporting the inhabitants of their cities, but the population of the whole world. From this perspective, although DDC includes a variety of actors, the modalities with which these agents interact are of greater importance. DDC aims to establish new forms of interrelation, where the public and private sectors, the economic, political, and social agents, and the organizations of the countries of the North with those of the South interact effectively to promote a more equitable development (OECD, 2018).

On the other hand, DDC does not pretend to be just another instrument to the means of aid that already exists. On the contrary, this is a different and new approach, complementary to the traditional forms of conceptualization and practices of cooperation. The three basic characteristics of this cooperation are institutional pluralism, participatory development, and decentralization, causing cities to play a vital role (Bontenbal, 2009). DDC generates valuable benefits to local governments, including staff capacity development, improved urban governance, internationalization of the city, business promotion, and a better understanding of diverse modes of contributing to facilitate better relationships with migrant communities (Ishinabe, 2010).

The most relevant feature of DDC is its greater proximity to citizens. Furthermore, decentralized cooperation, because it arises from cities, responds to the closest interests of citizens and has greater autonomy concerning the obligations and commitments of the nation-state for foreign policy. DDC allows local administrations to establish cooperation strategies focused on fulfilling the objective of the development of the poorest peoples and solidarity between peoples. The usual way of executing the budgets of DDC is through nongovernmental organizations. Furthermore, the vast majority of decentralized cooperation is done free of charge, with no burden on recipients.

DDC channels most of its programs through NGOs, allowing this cooperation to provide quality aid in terms of the search for sustainable human development, awareness of the population, and few ties to political or commercial interests. However, a frequent criticism is that this cooperation has an excessive atomization and dispersion in the destination of the resources that prevents results. Awareness of this risk has led to the creation of networks or groups between municipalities in various communities, forming what have been called “Cooperation Funds”. Its role has been very important in improving the quality of cooperation from municipalities, by allowing greater coordination of aid as well as more effective management. At present, the critical point is how DDC can be modified by the reality of a postpandemic world. In the next section, we analyze the necessity of re-thinking the role of cities and the achievements of the SDGs.

Sustainable Cities and Communities as a Specific SDG

At the end of 1961, the United Nations General Assembly adopted a resolution called "United Nations Development Decade", in which member states and their peoples would intensify their efforts to achieve a substantial increase in their rate of growth. By the end of the decade, the adoption of specific measures and the employment of new institutions of international cooperation for this purpose were realized. However, the quality of living for countless millions of people in developing countries was still pitifully low. In this context, the International Development Strategy for the Second United Nations for Development Decade was adopted. Progress was made, but not with optimal results, so that, in 1980, the Third Decade was proclaimed with its respective strategy.

For the United Nations, a Third Decade was necessary since "the limitations of a strategy, when conceived within the framework of the existing system of international economic relations, soon became obvious. Inequities and imbalances in these relations are widening the gap between developed and developing countries" (United Nations General Assembly, 1980). The beginning of this decade was also marked by a global recession in developed countries and an external debt crisis that significantly affected developing countries. Given the worsening conditions of development, it was decided to adopt a Fourth Decade, but there were already signs that it was necessary to modify the implementation in the face of a clearly discouraging performance. However, the strategy was adopted with the main goal of achieving accelerated development in developing countries and strengthening international cooperation.

Evidently, four consecutive decades were an indicator that the task was unfinished and the results unsatisfactory. This should not be conceived as failure, as the development issue is very complex and difficult to achieve, but it did show that the strategy was not functioning in its design and operation, so an inescapable and urgent change of approach was called for. In December 1998, the General Assembly decided to convene the so-called Millennium Summit to be held in September 2000, which would adopt the Millennium Declaration, later found in the document "Road map towards the implementation of the United Nations Millennium Declaration", resulting in eight concrete objectives and their respective tasks to be known as the Millennium Development Goals (MDGs), to be completed in the period 2000–2015. MDGs achieved global mobilization and are considered the most successful movement in history against poverty. The Secretary-General of the United Nations at the end of the MDGs period affirmed that "they had generated new and innovative partnerships, galvanized public opinion and showed the immense value of setting ambitious goals. By putting people and their immediate needs at the forefront, the MDGs reshaped decision-making in developed and developing countries alike" (United Nations, 2015).

However, the MDGs originated from a document adopted by the OECD Development Assistance Committee (DAC) in 1996 under the title *"Shaping the 21st Century: The Contribution of Development Co-operation*", which contains a set of international development goals formulated and adopted at the thematic meetings organized by the United Nations in previous years. It is clear that few actors participated in their redaction. During the United Nations Conference on Sustainable Development (Rio de Janeiro, 2012), it was negotiated to formulate Sustainable Development Goals (SDGs) to replace the MDGs (outcome document known as "The Future We Want"). A great effort was made that took into account several actors to appropriate SDGs in the international community. For example, the Secretary-General's initiatives, known as the "Panel of Eminent Persons" or "My World", the global survey to capture the opinion, priorities, and views of citizens, as well as the establishment of the Open Working Group to draft the SDGs, designed for 30 countries, which in the end had 70 participants because countries shared spaces.

Intergovernmental negotiations took place from January to July 2015, but also involving the so-called Major Groups,[3] one of which was the Local Authorities, including organizations representing subnational governments. On September 25, 2015, the 193 United Nations Member States unanimously adopted the document "Transforming Our World: The 2030 Agenda for Sustainable Development", containing 17 goals and 169 targets and the means of implementation. In addition to achieving recognition for the role to be played in the implementation of the 2030 Agenda, the Major Group lobbied to incorporate a specific SDG on cities and communities for sustainability, noting that an independent goal on sustainable urbanization would help mobilize subnational authorities considered as key partners in the implementation of SDGs (93 of the 169 targets involve regional and local governments), thus consolidating SDG 11, officially called "Making Cities and Human Settlements Inclusive, Safe, Resilient and Sustainable", in short, "Sustainable Cities and Communities". This SDG contains seven targets and three Implementation Medias.

It cannot be overlooked that the New Urban Agenda (adopted at the United Nations Conference on Housing and Sustainable Urban Development—Habitat III—held in Quito, Ecuador, on October 20, 2016) has incorporated the recognition of a correlation between good urbanization and development. The link between the New Urban Agenda and the 2030 Agenda is evident, particularly with Objective 11,

[3] Major Business and Industry Groups participated; Childhood and Youth; Farmers; Indigenous Peoples; Local Authorities; Non-Governmental Organizations; Science and Technology; Women; and Workers and Trade Unions. In addition, other interested groups, such as Educational and Academic Entities, were involved; Persons with Disabilities; Volunteer Groups; Elderly; and Global Networks.

and should therefore contribute to the implementation and localization[4] of the agenda.

The UN clarifies that the challenges cities face can be overcome in ways that allow them to continue to thrive and grow, while improving resource use and reducing pollution and poverty. At the same time, this goal has the expectation that in the future, cities will generate opportunities for all, gaining access to basic services, energy, housing, transportation, and more. The UN has defined 10 targets and 15 indicators for SDG 11, including safe and affordable housing, affordable and sustainable transport systems, inclusive and sustainable urbanization, protection for the world's cultural and natural heritage, a reduction in the adverse effects of natural disasters, a reduction in the environmental impacts of cities, and the provision of access to safe and inclusive green and public spaces, among others.

The Impact of the COVID-19 Pandemic on the SDGs and the Need to Accelerate the Achievement of the SDG 11

As it is in the public domain, on December 31, 2019, Wuhan, in Hubei Province, China, reported a group of pneumonia cases with unknown etiology. As early as January 9, 2020, the Chinese Center for Disease Control and Prevention identified a new coronavirus as the cause agent for this outbreak (PAHO, 2020). Coronavirus was officially called Severe Acute Respiratory Syndrome 2 Coronavirus (SARS-CoV-2), and the disease caused by it has been called COVID-19. On March 11, 2020, World Health Organization Director-General Dr. Tedros Adhanom Ghebreyesus announced that this outbreak could be characterized as a pandemic. This event, predicted by different scientific reports but ignored by politicians and society in general, represented an unexpected brake on progress regarding the accomplishment of the SDGs. However, this was not the first time that the development goals set by the international community were challenged by the outbreak of some surprising crisis.

In 2008, a significant global economic crisis erupted. In this context, the achievement of the MDGs was affected: "We are deeply concerned about the impact of the financial and economic crisis, the worst since the Great Depression. It has reversed development gains in many developing countries and threatens to seriously undermine the achievement of the Millennium Development Goals by 2015" (United Nations General Assembly, 2010, p. 22). History seems to have repeated itself with the SDGs, but the scale of the health and economic crises and their consequences are forecast far in excess of that of 2008. Just last September, the High-Level Political Forum on Sustainable Development, at its first session convened under the

[4] Localization is understood in the lexicon of the 2030 Agenda as the process that takes into account subnational contexts in the achievement of the 2030 Agenda, from the establishment of objectives and targets to the determination of means of implementation and the use of indicators to measure and monitor their progress.

auspices of the General Assembly (September 24 and 25, 2019), adopted a political statement entitled "Gearing up for a decade of action and delivery for sustainable development: political declaration of the Sustainable Development Goals Summit", in order to accelerate implementation work, using only almost a third of the original time to achieve it. In the same declaration, "a promise to make the next decade an action and dedication" was launched (United Nations General Assembly, 2019). The Secretary-General, as requested by the Political Declaration, called for a decade of worldwide action to achieve the SDGs by 2030, establishing their essential areas to drive his call: global action, local action, and people's action.

This concern had solid foundations. As previous experience shows, the effects on the growth of the world economy reduce the resources allocated to international aid. National governments prioritize programs for their citizens, and the economic crisis generated by COVID-19 was no small matter. Regarding the economy, 2019 was the worst year since 2009, with an economic growth rate of only 2.5%. By 2020, economic prospects were no better. Before the health crisis, a similar global growth was projected (CEPAL, 2020b). The crisis generated by the COVID-19 pandemic will have a visibly profound and negative effect on sustainable development efforts. A prolonged global economic slowdown will adversely affect the implementation of the 2030 Agenda for Sustainable Development (United Nations, 2020c). By July 2020, ECLAC changed its predictions and expected that the global economy would have its largest decline since World War II. So the gross domestic product (GDP) per capita would decline by 90% in most countries, in an unprecedented synchronous process. According to these projections, in 2020, global GDP would decrease by 5.2%. The fall would be 7.0% in developed economies and 1.6% in emerging economies (Comisión Económica para América Latina y el Caribe [CEPAL], 2020a). For Latin America and the Caribbean, ECLAC projects an average GDP drop of 9.1% in 2020, with decreases of 9.4% in South America, 8.4% in Central America and Mexico, and 7.9% in the Caribbean, not including Guyana, whose strong economic growth leads to a fall of 5.4% in the region (CEPAL, 2020b). Faced with this economic scenario (which could be further aggravated), accomplishment of SDGs can be threatened; Goal 11 is showing little progress and also has risks of slowdown and difficulties in achieving whole targets.

As the United Nations (2021) has noted, cities are a focal point for ideas, commerce, culture, science, and productivity, as well as social, human, and economic development. In consequence, in one way or another, the emergence of COVID-19 affected the life of cities in multiple ways, impacting present and future urban planning, transport systems, water, sanitation, waste management, disaster risk reduction, access to information, and education.

According to the Secretary-General's report on the progress of the SDGs 2019, on Goal 11 it states that "Substantial progress has been made in reducing the proportion of the global urban population living in slums, though more than 1 billion people continue to live in such situations. Urgent action is needed to reverse the current situation, which sees the vast majority of urban residents breathing poor-quality air and having limited access to transport and open public spaces. With the areas occupied by cities growing faster than their populations, there are profound repercussions for sustainability" (United Nations Secretary-General, 2019).

Meanwhile, the Bertelsmann Foundation and Bertelsmann Stiftung and Sustainable Development Solutions Network (2019) indicate that current assessments of SDG 11 show that, of the 193 countries in the United Nations membership, 43 have major challenges; 85 have significant challenges; 50 have challenges remaining; only 1 is considered as having achieved their goals, and 14 have no information available. In terms of trends, 4 countries show that their challenges are decreasing; 51 are stagnating; 56 are moderately improving; 16 are on track or maintaining SDG achievement; and 66 have no information available. Both reports show limited performance in achieving SDG 11.

The SDG 11 is key: meeting this goal or not can mean years of delay in achieving sustainable development for all people on the planet. The creation of a stand-alone goal on cities and urban development in the 2030 Agenda, that seeks to "make cities and human settlements inclusive, safe, resilient and sustainable", is a step to making cities a privileged place to realize multiple facets of development. The cities have a cross-cutting nature, impacting on several other Sustainable Development Goals, including SDGs 1, 6, 7, 8, 9, 12, 15, and 17, among others.

The COVID-19 outbreak unleashed a human development crisis. This crisis hit hard on all elements of human development: income—with the biggest contraction in economic activity since the Great Depression; health—the pandemic directly caused a death toll of over three million; education—with effective out-of-school rates, accounting for the inability to access the internet, affecting the quality of learning and increasing the school dropout rate. The Human Development Report elaborated by the United Nations Development Programme (2020, p. 3) warns that: "The pandemic was superimposed on unresolved tensions between people and technology, between people and the planet, between the haves and the have-nots".

Furthermore, the impact of COVID-19 taught us that the most devastating impact happened in poor and densely populated urban areas, especially for people living in informal settlements and favelas, where congestion also makes it difficult to follow recommended measures such as social distancing, frequent hand washing, and self-isolation for COVID-19 prevention.

Confronted with the greatest challenge that this generation has faced, cities are called to become a fundamental part of the solution. To face multiple problems generated or accelerated by the emergence of COVID-19, one of the three measures that the United Nations program proposes is to follow a coherent multidimensional approach. Since the crisis has multiple interconnected dimensions (health, economic, and several social aspects), a systemic approach is called for, rather than a sector-by-sector sequential approach. It is clear that cities are a privileged place for this to happen. The capacity of cities to weave horizontal and vertical cooperation networks, based on their previous experience of internationalization, is a fundamental tool that may allow progress to build a better quality of life in a postpandemic world. At the same time, the experience gained from the management of this pandemic, the international cooperation networks built from and for the cities, and the shared learning between the world's local governments will increase the resilience of cities and prepare us for the challenges of the future.

Conclusions: Rethinking the Role of Cities Not Only to Achieve the Sustainable Development Goals But Also to Build Resilient Cities

Cities can lead a new stage for development in a postpandemic world. Thus, from the analysis of historical trends in the internationalization of cities, it is possible to affirm that in recent decades cities have increased their capacities to interact internationally through collaboration networks on specific issues such as climate change and international security. In this way, cities have made considerable progress from establishing "sister cities" programs to consolidating solid networks where cities act in coordination to solve common problems together.

These networks of cities that existed prior to the pandemic were the first channel through which cities began to donate and receive international aid in the framework of the COVID-19 health emergency. In the context of the health crisis, the decision-making thought process of the local authorities, the decentralizations process experienced in multiple cities, as well as the previously established networks favored agile, precise, and concrete responses to health problems. However, we suggest that these responses have only been the first step and that after the pandemic, cities can become key actors in cooperation, not only as spaces where the achievements of many of the goals of the SDGs converge, but even more, as a robust platform for the IDC, complementing the activities of other actors in this international regime.

The importance of cities and the IDC was increasing during recent years, and the pandemic will strengthen this trend. At present, cities are a fundamental key to achieving SDGs. So, if we want to concretize a new phase of development characterized by the consecution of these goals, we need to recognize that cities are vital actors in the regime of IDC. Cities must generate initiatives to overcome the challenges, not only that the pandemic has caused, but also other longer-term challenges related to the well-being of the people who inhabit them, as well as other long-term problems. In this sense, cities must be consolidated as an indispensable platform for cooperation.

COVID-19 is an opportunity to see cities as a link in a strong chain for international cooperation. Cities must seek partners with whom to cooperate and solve a common problem. Therefore, it is necessary for cities to act more and more as part of networks, as networks neither discriminate nor establish hierarchical relationships. In the networks, all cities have something to contribute and something to learn. Thus, the consolidation of international networks aids in overcoming the North–South trends that were the dominant paradigm during the period in which the cooperation of cities was more bilateral through the initiatives of sister cities. The networks of cities are also a facet of the essential multilateralism needed to overcome the enormous challenges that humans face in the twenty-first century. In this sense, alliances are fundamental for the deepening of democratic life as mechanisms of political participation, and the citizens involved in the dynamics of the cities can be actors in a new phase of international cooperation.

At the same time, we must think of the territories of the cities as spaces that are crossed by transnational dynamics, such as capital, the progressive precariousness of working conditions, specific logistics of production and consumption, and cultural homogenization with the purpose of overcoming the vulnerability produced by these transnational dynamics in the territory. Cities should cultivate dynamics of proximity; the slowdown in the consumption of materials with short circuits, job creation based on value chains of proximity, presence, proximity; attempting to create housing markets, also generating proximity care spaces, with psycho-social and health home care for all the most vulnerable people. In addition, cities can be the platform for transforming the initiatives of collaboration, passing them from public–private partnerships into public–social or public–community partnerships.

Finally, the outbreak is an opportunity to improve cooperation practices that already existed. Specifically, regarding cooperation among cities, this kind of cooperation could be more selective in the networks, identifying the internal resources and capacities, providing a clear value about what and how each city, considering its reality, can support a common goal benefiting its citizens at the same time. Furthermore, cities should expand the diversity of their connections, inspiring a collective perspective rather than an institutional one. In this way, it will be more probable that in the next big challenge, like the COVID-19 pandemic, cities will not only be more resilient but better able to act together to overcome problems. In summary, the reflection on the relationship between cities and the achievement of the SDGs proves that, to the extent that cities are effective platforms for international cooperation, they increase their resilience due to finding agile ways to share knowledge and provide mutual aid, from donating specialized equipment to solve the crisis, to taking more collective actions beyond the narrow decision margins of nation states.

References

Bertelsmann Stiftung & Sustainable Development Solutions Network. (2019). *The sustainable development report 2019*. New York: Pica Publishing Ltd..

Bontenbal, M. (2009). *Cities as partners: The challenge to strengthen urban governance through North-South city partnerships*. Utrecht, the Netherlands: Eburon Academic Publishers.

Bontenbal, M., & van Lindert, P. (2006). Decentralized international cooperation: North-South municipal partnerships. In P. van Lindert, A. de Jong, G. Nijenhuis, & G. van Westen (Eds.), *Development Matters: Geographical studies on development processes and policies* (pp. 301–314). Utrecht, the Netherlands: Utrecht University.

C40 Cities. (2020). About Us. https://www.c40.org/about. Accessed Jan 2021.

Comisión Económica para América Latina y el Caribe [CEPAL]. (2020a). *Enfrentar los efectos cada vez mayores del COVID-19 Para una reactivación con igualdad: Nuevas proyecciones. Informe especial COVID-19 N° 5* [Facing the constantly increasing effects of COVID-19 for a reactivation with equality: New projections. Special report COVID-19 N°5]. Santiago: Naciones Unidas.

CEPAL. (2020b). *La agenda 2030 Para el Desarrollo Sostenible en el nuevo contexto mundial y regional: Escenarios y proyecciones en la presente crisis* [The 2030 agenda for sustainable development in the new global and regional context: Scenarios and projections in the current crisis]. Santiago: Naciones Unidas.

Clark, G. (2016). *Global cities: A Short history*. Washington, DC: Brookings Institution Press.
Dixon, T. (2020, June 8). What impacts are emerging from Covid-19 for urban futures? *CEBM;* Oxford University. https://www.cebm.net/covid-19/what-impacts-are-emerging-from-covid-19-for-urban-futures/. Accessed Aug 2020.
Hafteck, P. (2003). An introduction to decentralized cooperation: Definitions, origins and conceptual mapping. *Public Administration and Development, 23*, 333–345. https://doi.org/10.1002/pad.286.
Haupt, W., Chelleri, L., van Herk, S., & Zevenbergen, C. (2020). City-to-city learning within climate city networks: Definition, significance, and challenges from a global perspective. *International Journal of Urban Sustainable Development, 12*(2), 143–159. https://doi.org/10.1080/19463138.2019.1691007.
Iborra, J., Martínez, J. P., & Martínez, I. (2013). Spanish autonomous governments cooperation policies. In F. B. Dalmases & C. Coll (Eds.), *The debate on decentralized cooperation: Aid effectiveness after 2015* (pp. 25–47). Barcelona: CIDOB.
Iocco, M. (2005). *The international role of cities: Decentralized cooperation between domestic concerns and symbolic politics*. Doctoral dissertation, University of Siena. https://proyectoallas.net/wp-content/uploads/2018/01/The-international-role-of-cities-Decentralized-cooperation-between-domestic-concerns-and-symbolic-politics.pdf
Ishinabe, N. (2010). *Analysis of international city-to-city cooperation and intercity networks for Japanese national & local governments*. IGES Local Initiatives Discussion Paper. https://www.iges.or.jp/en/publication_documents/pub/discussionpaper/en/1837/iges_discussion_paper_local_initiatives_march_2010.pdf. Accessed Aug 2020.
Lee, T. (2013). Global cities and transnational climate change networks. *Global Environmental Politics, 13*(1), 108–127. https://doi.org/10.1162/GLEP_a_00156.
Martins Vaz, D., & Reis, L. (2018). From City-states to global cities: The role of cities in global governance. *JANUS.NET e-journal of International Relations, 8*(2), 13–28.
OECD. (2018). *Reshaping decentralised development co-operation: The key role of cities and regions for the 2030 agenda*. Paris: OECD Publishing.
Organisation for Economic Co-operation and Development [OECD]. (1996). *Shaping the 21st century: The contribution of development co-operation*. Paris: OECD Publishing.
Pan-American Health Organization [PAHO]. (2020). *Epidemiological Update. Novel coronavirus (2019-nCoV)*. Washington: PAHO.
Pipa, A. F., & Bouchet, M. (2020, August 6). *How to make the most of city diplomacy in the COVID-19 era*. Brookings. https://www.brookings.edu/blog/up-front/2020/08/06/how-to-make-the-most-of-city-diplomacy-in-the-covid-19-era/. Accessed Sept 2020.
Rennie-Short, J. (2004). *Global metropolitan: Globalizing cities in a capitalist world*. London: Routledge.
Secretary-General. (2019). *Report of the secretary-general on SDG Progress 2019* (Special Edn.). United Nations.
United Nations. (2015). *The millennium development goals report 2015*. New York: United Nations.
United Nations. (2020a). *United Nations Statistics, Goal 11*. https://unstats.un.org/sdgs/report/2019/goal-11/. Accessed Jan 2021.
United Nations. (2020b). *Goal 11: Make cities inclusive, safe, resilient and sustainable*. https://www.un.org/sustainabledevelopment/cities/. Accessed Jan 2021.
United Nations. (2020c). *Shared responsibility, global solidarity: Responding to the socio-economic impacts of COVID-19*. New York: United Nations.
United Nations (2021). *Overview: Make cities and human settlements inclusive, safe, resilient and sustainable*. https://sdgs.un.org/goals/goal11. Accessed Apr 2021.
United Nations Development Programme. (2020). *COVID-19 and human development: Assessing the crisis, envisioning the recovery*. The United Nations Development Program. http://hdr.undp.org/sites/default/files/covid-19_and_human_development_0.pdf. Accessed Jan 2021.

United Nations General Assembly. (1980, December 5). *Resolution 35/56, International Development Strategy for the Third United Nations Development Decade,* A/RES/35/56. https://undocs.org/en/A/RES/35/56. Accessed Aug 2020.

United Nations General Assembly. (2010, September 22). *Resolution 65/1, Keeping the promise: united to achieve the Millennium Development Goals,* A/RES/65/1. https://undocs.org/en/A/RES/65/1. Accessed Aug 2020.

United Nations General Assembly. (2019, September 9). *Resolution A/HLPF/2019/L.1, Political declaration of the high-level political forum on sustainable development convened under the auspices of the United Nations General Assembly.* A/HLPF/2019/L.1. https://undocs.org/en/A/HLPF/2019/l.1. Accessed Aug 2020.

Zelinsky, W. (1991). The twinning of the world: Sister cities in geographic and historical perspective. *Annals of the Association of American Geographers, 81*(1), 1–31. https://doi.org/10.1111/j.1467-8306.1991.tb01676.x.

Chapter 17
"Universities in Lockdown": The Impact of Reduced International Student Mobility Upon Cities in the Post-COVID-19 Era

Evgenia Likhovtseva

Introduction

Universities play a vital role in the economic development of every country. In many countries, universities have become key national centers of innovation, knowledge production, and human capital development. They have traditionally been leading focal points for the development of urban infrastructure, continually accumulating space for campuses, innovation parks, and science and humanities research hubs, together with residential complexes. To support such development, contemporary universities massively rely upon the presence of large numbers of international students and staff, as well as the cooperation of the wider global research community.

However, under the new conditions enforced by national governments to prevent the spread of COVID-19, universities have had to adapt to new realities. In particular, higher education institutions are now having to reorientate their learning practices from physical face-to-face interaction through group teaching in lecture halls and tutorial rooms, to online modes of teaching and learning. Since March 2020, higher education practitioners have tried to grapple with the evolving issues and challenges which present difficulties for the future of higher education. There is precious little research available which can provide an in-depth analysis on the current crisis; most available studies can only offer an opinion, or project a prognosis, upon the ever-changing situation facing higher education as a result of the pandemic.

As such, this chapter may be considered one of the first attempts to investigate how the circumstances of COVID-19, and its effects upon the activities of universities and other institutions of higher education, particularly those operating in urban areas, affect international student mobility, and how this, in turn, impacts on urban life and identity, along with the overall development of cities. Therefore, the aim of

E. Likhovtseva (✉)
Trinity College Dublin, Dublin, Ireland
e-mail: likhovte@tcd.ie

© The Author(s), under exclusive license to Springer Nature Switzerland AG 2021

M. A. Montoya et al. (eds.), *COVID-19 and Cities*, The Urban Book Series,
https://doi.org/10.1007/978-3-030-84134-8_17

the chapter is to examine how the relationship between universities and cities has been affected, adversely or otherwise, by the COVID-19 crisis. The chapter is comprised of three parts. The first outlines the interrelation between universities, cities and student mobility throughout history, and the effect that the latter has had upon the development of both universities and cities in the past. The second part examines the significant cultural influence that is brought to bear on cities and universities through internationalization, and the converse cultural capital that many cities, which lead as study abroad destinations, offer to international students. It also provides a reflection on how COVID-19 has altered this important commodity. The third section offers the reader a brief evaluation of the consequences of terminated student mobility, along with the measures that some national governments have enacted to overcome the restricted mobility of their students. However, it mostly provides a prognosis of the long-term impacts of COVID-19 upon both university life and city development.

The University, the City, and the Role of Student Mobility: From Medieval Times to the Contemporary Period

Cities and universities have always had a strong connection. Traditionally, cities and large urbanized towns have been seen as ideal locations, where civic institutions and developed urban spaces contributed a highly important component to the learning environment, especially those locations which represented the social, cultural, and ecological entity of the metropolis (Gruenewald, 2014). From the twelfth century, with European urbanization accelerating at a rapid pace, both universities and cities began to grow together. The university became part of the urban skyline, with its distinguishing architectural and symbolic features.

Urban spaces have attracted scholars to participate in public debates, while the city atmosphere itself enhanced the intellectual and social life of the city (Zerlang, 1997). While scholarly and student mobility is not a recent phenomenon, it is an extremely complex process, involving the intermingling of three variables. European scholarship inevitably benefited from the influx of foreigners: "academic pilgrimage" or "wandering scholars" was a form of collaboration within scholars' communities to help to explore and expand incomplete knowledge which was not available at a home university (de Ridder-Symoens, 1992; Leed, 1991).

Outside of Europe student mobility was also known. In fact, within the East Asian Confucian World, student mobility became more institutionalized than in Europe. Students from various parts of East Asia came to China in order to take their civil service examinations and to study the principles of the ancient Chinese bureaucratic system (Kim, 2009). Higher education systems became integrated into cities, creating those types of institutions which had relative ease of access and openness to people of various nations and social backgrounds (Hyde, 1991).

Therefore, by being located in cities, universities would be more open to a more diverse scholarly community than monastic institutions (Bender, 1991).

In preindustrial society, universities provided training in many key disciplines such as law, medicine, and theology, status professions which gave considerable power and prestige to their holders. The Renaissance brought about an orientation of university studies toward classical history and the empirical sciences, and consequently, new features of interaction between the university and the city began to take shape. New urban facilities, such as botanical gardens, libraries, and anatomical theatres, to name but a few, encapsulated the influence of the university upon urban public life (Bott, 2018).

Throughout the centuries of industrialization, new universities and technical high schools were established at the heart of industrial cities all over Europe in order to amalgamate scientific research with industrial production (Hall, 1997). Despite being motivated by exactly the same desire to travel in search of knowledge, student mobility became a central part of a far more complex process connected with both the industrial and scientific revolutions. Hammerstein points out that, in the case of the American universities, "scientific education and training in the United States was part of national prosperity and the country's international prestige" (Hammerstein, 2003, p. 640). Humboldt University, Berlin, Germany, became the model for the contemporary research university; amalgamated within its walls were the core academic freedoms in research, teaching, and the principles of self-administration. Located in the center of the city, Humboldt University became the basis for a distinctive "university district", which transformed the German capital into a "city for research, economics and the media" (Hu-Berlin, n.d., n.p). In the United States, the majority of universities are similarly located in city centers, with approximate connection to the urban facilities: MIT played an important role in the development of the electrical industry sector in the Greater Boston area throughout the 1880s, while the German Technische Hochschule had a similar role in Berlin (Hall, 1997).

In the decades which followed the end of the Second World War, a significantly increased student intake into higher education institutions led to an exponential expansion of the higher education sector, including measures to convert technical institutions into universities, which effectively doubled the size of the university sector.

By 1990, university education had become an industry, especially for those countries which held a world-class reputation for higher education. For the university towns of Oxford and Cambridge, the education industry has served as a primary source of income for centuries. This fact is no less valid for economic development today. Multinational corporations, such as Amazon and Apple, have recently expanded their headquarter operations to Cambridge in order to move into proximity with the University of Cambridge and its world-class research facilities. This relocation induced an important infrastructural development within the city, namely, the opening of a new railway station, Cambridge North (Ferguson, 2018). Therefore, education and learning, which have long been a highly noticeable characteristic of the city, continue to be essential functions in the development of its metropolitan areas (McFarlane, 2011).

Goddard and Vallance define the relationship between a city and a university as a unity of "interrelating physical, social, economic and cultural dimensions" (Goddard & Vallance, 2013, p.1). Campbell acknowledges that universities became entities that created jobs, built neighborhoods, and led to the development of goods and services even for city dwellers who did not relate to the academic profession (Campbell, 2005 as cited in Haar, 2011). Glasson states that universities are large organizations with a diverse labor force (Glasson, 2003). Universities are one of the biggest employment sectors for city inhabitants, alongside private companies, government departments, and cultural institutions. On the one hand, universities provide not only traditional academic and research employment, but also a variety of service-intensive jobs for administrative, technical, and support staff. One of the oldest universities in Europe, Trinity College Dublin, employed 2624 personnel during the 2016–2017 academic year (1264 academic and 1360 nonacademic), which is comparable to the number of employees in the largest industrial and consultancy firms in the Republic of Ireland (TCD, 2017). For a country with a population of 5 million, the Irish university sector has become a significant player in the Irish job market, contributing toward the wealth of the people and local economy. If we look at the profile of the United Kingdom, where the higher education sector currently occupies the position of the second largest in the world, universities support more than 940,000 jobs (3% of the total) and generate £95 billion for the country's economy (THE, 2017).

Today, every major city has a university; in most cases, urban development in these cities was induced by the internationalization and the massification of higher education. Universities are seen as a type of industry which produce "ready-to-go" candidates for the job market and accumulate knowledge for both public and private enterprises. Since the early 1990s, there has been a steady increase in the flow of scholarly students and highly skilled professionals from developing countries to the United States, Canada, the United Kingdom, and Australia. With a gradual reorientation of the international economy from industrial production to knowledge production, universities received major attention from governments and business communities. Universities became locations which attracted "knowledge workers" into a city; these would, in turn, contribute to the general development of the urban environment, transforming cities into knowledge-intense ecosystems (Power et al., 2010). Under these circumstances, the American higher education sector became an important channel for the U.S. private sector to recruit the most talented graduates. According to the McKinsey Global Institute, throughout the previous three decades, immigrants from developing countries "contributed an estimated 40 percent of labor growth in advanced economies: more of these workers have arrived with advanced skills" (Manyika et al., 2012). We must take from this statistic that this includes a considerable number of international students, which forms part of the processes of international student mobility.

However, following the impact of COVID-19 and the ensuing lockdown, modern universities have had to adapt to new conditions. University buildings have been shut down, students sent home, and teaching transferred to an online mode. The future of higher education, in its traditional sense, has become questionable for the first time in the modern era. The remainder of this chapter will, therefore, address each of these challenges and will speculate upon the potential solutions and opportunities that may be drawn from each challenge.

This study amounts to one of the first concerted efforts to understand the current climate for international student mobility and its impact upon the development of cities. The research was conducted using a qualitative research framework, incorporating a textual thematic analysis. The majority of the discussion around this issue is currently ongoing on online and social media platforms, inclusive of professional academic and nonacademic media. There is, understandably, little academic literature available on this topic. There were, therefore, two different modes of analysis: (i) an analysis of online material related to current COVID-19 international student mobility issues, and (ii) a systematic literature review of issues related to the impact of international student mobility on urban development.

Internationalization and the Cultural Impact Upon Cities

Nowadays, over 5.3 million people travel abroad to study, in comparison to the 2.1 million students who attended university outside their home country in 2001 (IIE, 2019). Before the COVID-19 crisis, student mobility patterns were well-established. Traditionally, the United States, the United Kingdom, and Australia have served as the most popular study destinations associated with world-class university education (IIE, 2019). In recent times, however, there have also been regional powers, such as China and Russia, which have emerged as top locations for higher education, attracting international students from neighboring countries. According to Project Atlas-2019, in Russia the majority of foreign students came from the former Soviet Republics of Kazakhstan, Tajikistan, and Uzbekistan, while in China, a majority pool of international students came from Pakistan, Thailand, and South Korea (IIE, 2019). COVID-19 brought about changes to established student mobility patterns, which I discuss in this section.

In the literature, a dominant framework in explaining the move of students abroad is the so-called "push-pull" factor. Altbach observes that "push" mobility is based on economic, political, or social conditions which influence the decision of a student to leave their country (Altbach, 2004). The "pull" factor, on the opposite side, is the attraction driven by opportunities available in a host country, including the opportunity to get a better quality of education and increasing the chances of getting a better job after graduation (Altbach, 2004; Chen, 2007). These socioeconomic and political factors are well-represented in the global university rankings, pushing the employability agenda as a key factor for graduates of good universities. Cities are also becoming a part of this agenda, represented by indicators as "good places to study".

However, international student surveys indicate that there are also many other underlying factors which define student motivation to study abroad: having fun, getting new life experiences, and travel are also important for students, as well as improving language skills, particularly in English (Llewellyn-Smith & McCabe, 2008; Lam et al., 2011). The idea of living through divergent cultural experiences connects with cosmopolitanism, which offers "contrasts rather than uniformity" (Hannerz, 1990, p. 239). Therefore, contemporary student mobility is hugely influenced by cultural globalization.

From the position of cultural globalization, contemporary academic and student mobility associates with the politics of recognition and identity politics (Gutmann, 2003; Taylor, 1992; Young, 1990). In particular, Taylor's "politics of equal respect" builds on mutual intercultural dialogue, where "the integrity of cultures has an important place" (Taylor, 1992, p.61). On the one hand, universities use this same idea to build a common educational space for local and international students: The English language becomes the modern language of education; the university curriculum becomes more adaptable for international students to prepare them for "global citizenship". Furthermore, those universities located in vibrant well-known cities attract more international students for the obvious fact that such institutions provide the additional variable of cultural capital, synchronizing with the pursuit of their own academic studies (QS, 2019). For instance, the old capitals of Europe, like Paris or London, have powerful cultural infrastructure represented by galleries, museums, and opera houses, which define a distinctive space, including the cultural quarters of cities and everyday urban surroundings (Savage et al., 2018). In Europe, in general, universities mobilize a city's cultural, linguistic, and historical potential in order to recruit international students. In the Catalan region of Spain, for example, the local authorities adopted the "tourist approach" for higher education institutions, which gives students additional experience in combining travel and study at the same time (Askehave, 2007).

On the other hand, international students themselves contribute new epistemologies through which to see the world, making universities and cities more culturally diverse places. University societies, for instance, organize culture nights, festivals, and food markets to promote the distinctive and varied cultures of international students beyond university walls. Within the United Kingdom alone, there are approximately 12 university-based Russian-speaking societies, promoting the Russian language and culture abroad, as well as building networking ties between Russian and foreign businesses. Agencies and cultural institutions, including well-established organizations such as Alliance Francaise, the British Council, and the Confucius Institutes, have vast representations in many cities across the globe. However, Ranson notes that cities are not homogenously internationalized, meaning that the majority of international activities, including cultural events and socialization, are concentrated in city centers (Ransom, 2018). As such, the presence of international students living in various locations of a city can help to demarginalize remote and impoverished neighborhoods located away from the city center.

Every year, international university rankings agencies, such as QS Best University Cities, publish the top cities as study destinations for international students, based on categories such as the global ranking of the city's universities, the student mix, the desirability of the city in terms of living standards, and, in particular, employment activity within the city, to name a few. In 2019, the top three cities in these rankings were London, Melbourne, and Tokyo, global cities which usually attract students who can afford to study abroad. Surrounding regional cities also serve the needs of the remainder of the international student population (QS, 2019).

However, the circumstances of the COVID-19 pandemic have radically changed this scenario, forcing national governments to rapidly seek alternatives; one example is Australia's New Colombo Plan. In the circumstances of the pandemic, the Australian response was notably strict; international students were encouraged to return to their home countries, especially those who were facing financial hardship (Ross, 2020). However, driven by the decline of international student intake for the 2020 academic year, this Australian government initiative allowed for a two-way exchange of international students between Australia and countries of the Indo-Pacific region. The New Colombo Plan also encourages Australian undergraduate students to become "ambassadors" in the Indo-Pacific region, travelling for study abroad and internship experience to build closer connections between their country and those of the region (Australian Government, n.d.). The geography of the region includes Nauru, New Guinea, and the Solomon Islands, which, by comparison, are far less visited places by students and tourists.

The crisis of COVID-19 has brought a shift in student mobility and enhanced already existing regional partnerships, making internationalization more localized; "regional" mobility is, for the moment, substituted for "global" mobility. Similar situations can be observed in global cities such as Shanghai, which is already perceived as a well-established study destination for Asian students. Shanghai builds its own image as a city with a "global vision", by "building international economic, financial, trade and shipping facilities, technology innovation centers and international cultural metropolis constructions" (Yueming, 2018, n.p.). Thus, Shanghai, a city considered as having the characteristics of being "open" and "similar to the West", can overtake the great majority of study destinations for international students coming to China (Ding, 2016, p. 328). In the perception of international students, other cities of China are still far from reaching the status of Shanghai. In this regard, COVID-19 can open a door to opportunities for Chinese cities to become more internationalized and more attractive in their strategy, both for foreign students from neighboring countries as well as Chinese students from wealthy backgrounds who traditionally go abroad to study in Western universities. There are new government initiatives, which concentrate on making cities more livable by introducing green spaces and ecological resilience to their urban planning, which are very important ranking criteria for study abroad destinations (Zhang et al., 2020).

A similar situation is occurring in Africa; the circumstances of the COVID-19 crisis can also improve inter-African mobility. Today, South Africa has the highest number of international students on the continent, with the majority coming from neighboring regions. Cape Town is considered the most international city in South Africa and is hailed by Price Waterhouse Coopers (PwC) as an "African city of opportunity" (PwC, 2020, p. 2). The city of Cape Town remains the top city, with the highest proportion of skilled jobs in SA (PwC, 2020). The impact of COVID-19 is now perceived as an opportunity for "reverse" brain-drain, getting back those professionals and students who returned from Europe and North America to their home cities in Africa during the time of the pandemic (Waruru, 2020). Such a turn of events can improve the capacity of emerging countries, such as South Africa, to use their own skilled human capital, not only to boost the development of the local economy, but also to become a bridge between western countries and their own.

However, among western countries, there were also "successful" examples of countries that proved capable of maintaining their numbers of international students. Swedish universities even experienced a 13% rise in the numbers of incoming foreign students (Erudera College News, 2020). This is explained by the strategy adopted by the Swedish government to bring measures which both minimized the severity of lockdown restrictions, while keeping measures to lower the number of COVID-19 cases. Bladh points out that "Swedish society has been open, with no strict lockdown", which is attractive for international students because it provides them with a sense of "stability" and "normality" (Erudera College News, 2020, n.p.). The Swedish course was in stark contrast to the majority of other western nations, which responded to the COVID-19 crisis with a combination of strict national self-isolation and metropolitan lockdown (Erudera College News, 2020, n.p.). It is widely acknowledged that international students are important, not only for the Swedish economy, but also for the local university environment, including the classroom dynamic and diversity among the student population (Myklebust, 2020).

International Students: The Financial and Infrastructural Impact on Cities

Campbell points out that a higher education institution "imports raw materials in the form of 18-year-old minds and bodies" who, after graduation, are able to go to the job market (Campbell, 2005, as cited in Haar, 2011, p.149). Barder et al. point out that the outputs of a university not only include degrees and research, but also contribute to the economy of a city or region (Barber et al., 2013). Thus, universities produce "ready-to-go" human capital necessary to supply both urban and national economies. However, alongside the traditional domestic stream of highly qualified workers, there is another: the stream of international graduates, many of whom have received their qualifications outside of their home countries. Therefore, Castles and Miller acknowledge that student mobility is equal to skilled immigration (Castles & Miller, 2003).

The international education sector contributes significant profits, not only to host countries, but to the cities themselves. Cities of global study destinations attract significant income from foreign students. This income is generated, not only from the payment of tuition fees, but also from rented accommodation and spending on general living expenses. For instance, the state of Queensland, Australia, generates approximately US$ 4 billion from international students alone, while London gets US$ 3.62 billion (Maslen, 2020; Universities UK, 2017). The Republic of Ireland has a significant income from foreign students, worth roughly €380 million annually to the Irish economy (O'Halloran, 2020). COVID-19 has, thus, significantly compromised the economy of the global university–city ecosystem in the following areas:

Reorienting University Courses Toward Online Learning

Online education is not a new occurrence. Since early 2010, online education has gained wide popularity among universities and private providers of online learning courses. For instance, Arizona State University and Florida State University doubled their online enrolment by almost 50% in the last decade (Brannen et al., 2020). However, the COVID-19 crisis has inevitably raised various problems with the approach to online learning, including those problems related to a reduction of tuition fees for obtaining a university degree.

The issue for international students arises around paying the same fees for online learning as for offline, taking into consideration that international student fees are normally higher than fees for local students. There are numerous magazine articles, qualitative interviews, and surveys indicating student opinion on the transformation of universities around e-learning. The general concerns are focused on the financial burden of tuition fees and living expenses, which are normally opportunity costs for most of the international students coming to a country to pursue a degree. For instance, an American student coming to Dublin, Ireland, is concerned about paying high tuition and accommodation fees to look at her computer screen from her Dublin room; a Chinese student may complain that, as a law student, classroom participation is key, and this simply cannot be substituted by an online course; for many other international students, especially those coming from Asian and African countries, problems may include "prejudice, xenophobia and racism" (Beckstein, 2020; O'Halloran, 2020; Zhang & Stucka, 2020).

As students voice the proposal of reductions in tuition fees, the universities are facing the reality that they require less expenses on maintaining buildings, paying staff, and engaging large numbers of students in classes (Brannen et al., 2020). However, while making sense from the position of students, this proposal invariably has an impact upon the general recruitment of international and local staff in universities. The recruitment patterns within universities were unstable even before the COVID-19 crisis arose. According to recent studies, in the United Kingdom, 54% of academic and 49% of teaching staff are hired on the basis of unsecured contracts (UCU, 2016). The majority of this type of academic personnel depend upon short-term funding and hourly paid contracts (UCU, 2016). Kings College London recently announced that 1000 contracts were under revision, the University of Liverpool put 600 jobs under review, and the University of Essex is also re-examining their finances for 300 posts (Grady, 2020). In short, universities will need less personnel for online teaching, and will lay off those not fortunate enough to secure a permanent contract, in order to maintain financial stability. Like international student mobility, academic internationalization will also change its patterns in accordance with ongoing economic trends.

Infrastructural Loss

In recent years, university campuses expanded their facilities beyond their university walls. The most important university-affiliated infrastructure is student accommodation. Faced with major shortages of residential accommodation, European cities have, until now, put in a lot of effort to sustain an inflow of international students. COVID-19 has impacted the rental market, driving students back to their home countries and parents' houses. Irish Universities accumulated significant income from renting accommodation to students. For instance, University College Dublin earned €28.6 million from their student housing rents in the 2018–2019 academic year (O'Halloran, 2020). In order to keep the economy going, the Irish government prioritized the development of student accommodation blocks for at least 9500 bedrooms over the period between 2017 and 2019, all built by private developers working alongside the universities (O'Halloran, 2020). In Newcastle, the newly built student-oriented city center apartment hall known as "the Met" faces a massive rental shortfall due to the withdrawal of foreign postgraduate students (McInnes, 2020). This is a noteworthy development since Newcastle is one of a number of cities in the United Kingdom where student accommodation is a profitable business. Similar occurrences have been noted in other countries which are leading student destinations; the student accommodation booking portal Student.com similarly summarized that bookings for Germany, the United States, and France had also fallen by 73% (Stacey, 2020). With a shortage of incoming international students, the rental market has had to readjust to new and challenging conditions. Moreover, other auxiliary enterprises, including student health services, stores, canteens, and transportation services, which generate income for the university business model and provide employment for city residents, will inevitably be similarly impacted (Kelly & Columbus, 2020).

COVID-19 has hit areas of university enterprise extremely harshly, providing uncertainty for the existence of face-to-face business (Kelly & Columbus, 2020). With the closure of universities and the redistribution of university space similar to business office infrastructure, the usage of these spaces becomes questionable, making university spaces available for meetings and socializing rather than for its primary purpose as a place for learning and study. Even if a vaccine is made available to every student in the near future, universities will utilize a mixed-learning mode more widely.

High-Skilled Human Capital and the Metropolitan Economy

The RSA City Growth Commission states that "money flows where ideas flow", arguing that international graduates provide cities with various entrepreneurial and business-like opportunities necessary for the "innovation ecosystems" of a city (The RSA City Growth Commission, 2014, pp. 7, 27). In 2014, the World Economic Forum similarly proposed a four-part taxonomy of city competitiveness. On the one hand, a city has to invest in hard connectivity—hard infrastructure in its different aspects. One the other hand, in order to support hard infrastructure, cities require another pillar—soft connectivity, understood as investments into the social capital of city development (World Economic Forum, 2014). Soft connectivity is formed via different aspects, including strengthening a city's education and training system (World Economic Forum, 2014). Ransom calls universities the "connective anchors" of a city, driving its local economy and social mobility, as well as providing a "window to the world" for a city (Ransom, 2015, p. 2). The educational level of expats indicates the ability of a city to attract and keep its intellectual capital. Therefore, cities with a high concentration of universities are important for a knowledge economy to maintain a consistently high standard in terms of the intellectual capital in a city. London, one of the most innovative cities in the world, has more than 60% of residents who are university graduates, while Cape Town has a mere 5.5% (PwC, 2020).

Alongside a university's reputation, one of the key factors behind the pursuit of study abroad is employability after graduation. Nearly 50% of international students from India travel abroad to pursue an education degree within STEM disciplines in the United States, the United Kingdom, and Germany (QS-IGAUGE, 2020). These top-three countries have accumulated a reputation of high potential for graduates to receive jobs in the technology sector, which contributes to the prosperity of the urban economy. If the United States and United Kingdom are the traditional study destinations for many groups of international students, Germany has become more attractive for its tech opportunities. German metropolitan regions have a very diverse range of specialization in information and communication technology (ICT) and STEM (Deloitte, 2017). Research shows that the job innovative sector creates five more jobs for every job available in other sectors of the same city (Deloitte, 2017). Munich is a key tech hub in Germany and has a GDP per capita similar to Stuttgart and Erlangen, while Berlin has the highest number of technology students in the country (Deloitte, 2017). Even tacit knowledge of being in a dynamic urban environment provides people with opportunities to build networks and contracts, whereas remote work and online education can take away from the intellectual capital of a city (Giles & Thomas, 2020).

Visa restrictions imposed by national governments is another reason for the inevitable decline of "intellectual migration". In June 2020, the U.S. Immigration and Customs Enforcement announced that the U.S. Department of State would not issue visas for the Fall semester, as all classes would take place fully online (U.S. Immigration and Customs Enforcement, 2020). Actions such as this will invariably reorient flows of international students between regions, and if the COVID-19 crisis causes a general shift to this tendency, this will contribute to a loss of talent within the advanced Western economies and mark an increase in cooperation among countries of the Global South (Brannen et al., 2020).

Conclusion

From even the briefest examination of the influence of COVID-19 upon international student migration, it becomes clear that several areas of urban and city development are immediately affected. First, COVID-19 has challenged the dominance of the traditional well-established study destinations of international students. Countries such as the United States, United Kingdom, and Australia question their ability to sustain a large international student intake for the academic year 2020/2021. Moreover, the stringent and uncertain circumstances of the COVID-19 pandemic and its fallout have caused international students to rethink their study choices abroad simply because it has put on hold global student mobility by restricting their physical movement.

New players in the "study destination" game, like Sweden and China, challenge American, Australian, and British dominance by giving international students more options during their study abroad period throughout the COVID-19 crisis. Sweden offers visiting students an excellent quality of education, a lively city environment, and a culture of toleration. Moreover, Sweden's response to the COVID-19 crisis was markedly different from the rest of the world. For instance, Swedish universities remain open and offer on-campus orientation weeks and classes for incoming first-year students, while transferring courses online for the older cohorts. This gives international students a sense of certainty, normality, and belonging, which has been absent over the previous months. China can also be considered as an exceptional case of a local power proving itself capable of attracting international students from the region. Chinese cities, especially the more international cosmopolitan hubs like Shanghai or Beijing, were well-placed to tackle the disease. This placed them in an excellent position to present themselves as "safe" places, while the rest of the world struggled with the pandemic.

Second, the crisis has potentially led to a general strengthening of national university sectors by bringing international students home to their own countries. This, in particular, may benefit the emerging economies of the Global South, by promoting regional student mobility and wider cooperation. In addition, any planned recovery stimuluses, which will inevitably be initiated once the pandemic has subsided, may give opportunities for cities to invest in new infrastructure, bounce back from the pandemic as better places to study and learn, and become more resilient to the impact of any future pandemics and health crises. Higher education institutions have already had to invest heavily in the development of their digital infrastructure, teacher training, student services, and robust IT support (Martin & Furiv, 2020). Recovery measures would invariably have to target student communities, and already a number of countries have outlined their plans in this respect. The COVID-19 recovery plan prepared by the region of Madrid will launch a program of scholarships for university students, as part of a grant of EUR nine million from the regional government and EUR three million from universities, and this will ensure that those most affected by the crisis can continue their studies at public universities (OECD, 2020). Likewise, research projects aimed at the treatment and diagnosis of COVID-19 will receive EUR eight million (OECD, 2020).

Third, COVID-19 has affected many other areas and sectors of metropolitan economies which are connected with the business of international education. Student-related businesses, such as language schools, catering, and student accommodation, now face a harsh winter. The crisis has provoked many universities to either update their resilience planning or to engage with this process for the first time. Resilience has become a major topic in the planning and design industry over the past decade, with nation states, cities, and entire regions facing an ever-growing threat of environmental and societal challenges, including natural disasters, sea level rise, climate change, terrorism, and financial insolvency. Universities are leading efforts in the sector, contributing research and problem-solving regarding resilience and sustainability in their broader communities. However, as campus planners work with higher education clients in the post-COVID-19 world, there is a growing responsibility for the leaders of higher education institutions to address their campus' own resilience. Therefore, campus master planning has long been identified as the "pinnacle opportunity to connect expert researchers with campus stewards and community leaders to engage in dialogue, identify priorities and advance resilience within their campus and community" (Storms et al., 2019, p. 187).

Fourth, in terms of helping to bolster the resilience of cities and their communities, the pandemic has shown how universities can be of service to urban communities in combating the pandemic, and providing mental health support, both during the pandemic and potentially for a long time after the crisis. In the case of Portugal, an innovative way of bringing, not only the university community, but also campus facilities, to bear in the fight against COVID-19, was shown in the city of Braga. The municipal authorities there created a public hot line to attend to questions related to COVID-19, while also creating a facility offering psychological support to citizens in partnership with the School of Health Sciences of the University of Minho. The municipality supported the University of Minho in the creation of a care center in the University Residence for people who are in nursing homes and similar facilities affected by cases of COVID-19 (OECD, 2020).

It is clear that the impact of COVID-19 is devastating for the agenda of the globalized world, an agenda upon which the Western model of university, tied up with the urban development of metropolitan areas, had become heavily dependent in recent years. Many leading international universities, including Oxford and Cambridge, have a major stake in the agenda of globalization and have a significant international student population. The consequential readjustments necessitated by the restrictions laid down by national governments to prevent a re-occurrence of pandemic conditions may prove disastrous for the global higher education sector as a whole. This, in turn, will invariably impact upon urban and city development.

This research can act as the commencement of a much wider analysis which both assesses the impact and reimagines the consequences of reduced international student mobility levels on cities around the world in the exceptional circumstances provoked by the COVID-19 crisis. The main limitation of this study is the obvious lack of academic research on this subject, to say nothing of the scattered nature of available data on the issue. However, in view of the challenges of the situation we are all living through at the time of writing, this research serves as an important note of introspection on what could be argued to be one of the most important and influential pillars of contemporary higher education, as well as a fundamental component in the development of cities.

References

Altbach, P. G. (2004). Higher education crosses borders: Can the United States remain the top destination for foreign students? *Change: The Magazine of Higher Learning, 36*(2), 18–25.

Askehave, I. (2007). The impact of marketization on higher education genres the international student prospectus as a case in point. *Discourse Studies, 9*(6), 723–742.

Barber, M., Donnelly, K & Rizvi, S. (2013). An avalanche is coming: Higher education and revolution ahead. Retrieved from: https://www.insidehighered.com/sites/default/server_files/files/FINAL%20Embargoed%20Avalanche%20Paper%20130306%20(1).pdf

Beckstein, A. (2020, July 24). *How are international students coping with the Covid-19 pandemic?* https://www.timeshighereducation.com/student/blogs/how-are-international-students-coping-covid-19-pandemic. Accessed Aug 2020.

Bender, T. (1991). Introduction. In T. Bender (Ed.), *The university and the city: From medieval origins to the present* (pp. 3–13). Oxford: Oxford University Press.

Bothwell, E. (2017). Universities 'generate £95 billion for UK economy'. Retrieved from: https://www.timeshighereducation.com/news/universities-generate-ps95-billion-uk-economy

Bott, H. (2018). City and university- an architect's notes on an intriguing spatial relationship. In P. Meusburger, M. Heffernan, & L. Suarsana (Eds.), *Geographies of the university* (pp. 375–439). Cham: Springer.

Brannen, S., Ahmed, H., & Newton, H. (2020). (Rep.). Covid-*19 reshapes the future*. Centre for Strategic and International Studies (CSIS), pp. 1–24.

Campbell, R. (2005, March 20). *Universities Are the New City Planners*. Boston Globe. https://www.newspapers.com/image/443623224/. Accessed Aug 2020.

Castles, S., & Miller, M. J. (2003). *The age of migration*. London: The Guildford Press.

Chen, L. H. (2007). Choosing Canadian graduate schools from afar: East Asian students' perspectives. *Higher Education, 54*(5), 759–780.

Ding, X. (2016). Exploring the experiences of international students in China. *Journal of Studies in International Education, 20*(4), 319–338. https://doi.org/10.1177/1028315316647164.

De Ridder-Symoens, H. (1992). A history of the university in Europe. Vol. I. Universities in the Middle Ages. Cambridge: Cambridge University Press.

Deloitte (2017). Germany's Digital Hubs: the Geography of the Tech Talents. Retrieved from: https://www2.deloitte.com/content/dam/Deloitte/de/Documents/Innovation/Digital-Hubs-Germany-Ranking-Deloitte-2018.pdf

Erudera College News. (2020, October 7). *Number of International Students at Swedish Universities Increases Despite COVID-19*. https://collegenews.org/number-of-international-students-at-swedish-universities-increases-despite-covid-19/. Accessed Nov 2020.

Ferguson, D. (2018). Cambridge tops the league … as Britain's most unequal city. Retrieved from: https://www.theguardian.com/uk-news/2018/feb/04/cambridge-most-unequal-city-population-divide-income-disparity

Giles, C., & Thomas, D. (2020, September 14). Cities count cost of lasting exodus from offices. *Financial Times*. https://www.ft.com/content/203cc83c-72b0-49c9-bea5-6fb38735a8fc. Accessed Aug 2020.

Glasson, J. (2003). The Widening Local and Regional Development Impacts of the Modern Universities - A Tale of Two Cities (and North-South Perspectives). *Local Economy, 18(1)*, 21–37. https://doi.org/10.1080/0269094032000073799

Goddard, J., & Vallance, P. (2013). *The university and the City*. London: Routledge.

Grady, J. (2020, July 28). Around 30,000 jobs may be on the line at universities. We have to fight back. *The Guardian*. https://www.theguardian.com/education/2020/jul/28/around-30000-jobs-may-be-on-the-line-at-universities-we-have-to-fight-back. Accessed Aug 2020.

Gruenewald, D. A.(2014). Place-Based Education: Grounding culturally responsive teaching in geographical diversity. In D. A. Gruenewald and G.A. Smith (Eds.), *Place-based education in the global age* (pp. 161-178). New York: Routledge

Gutmann, A. (2003). Identity in democracy. Princeton, N.J : Princeton University Press.

Haar, S. (2011). *The City as campus: Urbanism and higher education in Chicago*. Minneapolis: University of Minnesota Press.

Hall, P. (1997). The university and the city. *GeoJournal, 41*(4), 301–309.

Hammerstein, N. (2003). Relations with authority. In H. d. Ridder-Symoens (Ed.), *The history of the university in Europe: Universities in Early Modern Europe (1500–1800) (Vol. II)*, (pp. 631–671). Cambridge: Cambridge University Press.

Hannerz, U. (1990). Cosmopolitans and Locals in World Culture. *Theory, Culture & Society, 7(2–3)*, 237–251. https://doi.org/10.1177/026327690007002014

Hu-Berlin. (n.d.). *Humboldt-Universität zu Berlin: Education through learning and research*. https://www.hu-berlin.de/de/pr/medien/publikationen/pdf/humboldt-universitaet_en.pdf. Accessed Nov 2020.

Hyde, J. K. (1991). Universities and cities in medieval Italy. In T. Bender (Ed.), *The university and the city: From medieval origins to the present*. Oxford: Oxford University Press.

Institute of International Education (2019). A quick look at global mobility trends. Retrieved from: https://www.iie.org/Research-and-Insights/Project-Atlas/Explore-Data

Kelly, A. P., & Columbus, P. (2020). College in the Time of Coronavirus: Challenges Facing American Higher Education. *American Enterprise Institute Paper & Studies*. https://doi.org/10.2307/resrep25358.

Kim, T. (2009). Shifting patterns of transnational academic mobility: a comparative and historical approach. *Comparative Education, 45 (3)*, 387–403.

Lam, J. M. S., Ariffin, A. A. M., & Ahmad, A. H. (2011). Edutourism: Exploring the push-pull factors in selecting a university. *International Journal of Business and Society, 12*(1), 63–78.

Llewellyn-Smith, C., & McCabe, V. S. (2008). What is the attraction for exchange students: The host destination or host university? Empirical evidence from a study of an Australian university. *International Journal of Tourism Research, 10*(6), 593–607.

Leed, E. J. (1991). The mind of the traveler: From Gilgamesh to global tourism. New York, N.Y: Basic Books

Manyika et al. (2012). Manufacturing the future: The next era of global growth and innovation. Retrieved from: https://www.mckinsey.com/business-functions/operations/our-insights/the-future-of-manufacturing

Martin, M., & Furiv, U. (2020, December 12). COVID-19 tests the resilience of higher education. *University World News*. https://www.universityworldnews.com/post.php?story=20201211130427131. Accessed Jan 2021.

Maslen, G. (2020, August 13). Coronavirus: Impacts of school and university lockdowns. *University World News*. https://www.universityworldnews.com/post.php?story=2020081313184272. Accessed Nov 2020.

McInnes, K. (2020, October 13). Flats in prime Newcastle location are lying empty after pandemic causes student market to collapse. *Stoke-on-Trent News*. https://www.stokesentinel.co.uk/news/stoke-on-trent-news/flats-prime-newcastle-location-lying-4585856. Accessed December 2020.

McFarlane, C. (2011). The City as Assemblage: Dwelling and Urban Space. *Environment and Planning D: Society and Space, 29(4)*, 649–671. https://doi.org/10.1068/d4710
Myklebust, J.P. (2020). International student numbers up 13% despite COVID-19. Retrieved from: https://www.universityworldnews.com/post.php?story=20200930054856301
O'Halloran, B. (2020, August 13). Bord Pleanála gave approval for 9,500 student bedrooms. *The Irish Times*. https://www.irishtimes.com/business/construction/bord-pleanála-gave-approval-for-9-500-student-bedrooms-1.4276946. Accessed Nov 2020.
Organisation for Economic Co-operation and Development. (2020, July 23). *OECD policy responses to Coronavirus (COVID-19): Cities Policy Responses*. https://www.oecd.org/coronavirus/policy-responses/cities-policy-responses-fd1053ff/. Accessed Aug 2020.
Power, A., Ploger, J., & Winkler, A. (2010). *Phoenix cities: The fall and rise of great industrial cities*. Portland: The Policy Press.
Price Waterhouse Coopers [PwC]. (2020). *Cape Town: African City of Opportunity*. https://www.pwc.co.za/en/assets/pdf/cape-town-african-city-of-opportunity.pdf. Accessed Jan 2021.
QS-IGAUGE. (2020). *Indian Students' Mobility Report 2020: Impact of Covid-19 on Higher Education Choices*. https://www.igauge.in/news/2020/5/mobility-report-2020. Accessed Jan 2021.
QS (2019). QS Best Student Cities 2019. Retrieved from: https://www.qschina.cn/city-rankings/2019
Ransom, J. (2015). *Future of cities: Universities and cities*. Universities UK. https://assets.publishing.service.gov.uk/government/uploads/system/uploads/attachment_data/file/477295/future-cities-universities.pdf. Accessed Aug 2020.
Ransom, J. (2018). The city as a focus for university internationalisation: Four European examples. *Compare: A Journal of Comparative and International Education, 48*(4), 665–669.
Ross, J. (2020, April 3). 'Time to go home', Australian PM tells foreign students. *Times Higher Education*. https://www.timeshighereducation.com/news/time-go-home-australian-pm-tells-foreign-students. Accessed Aug 2020.
RSA City Growth Commission. (2014). *UniverCities: The Knowledge to Power UK Metros*. https://www.thersa.org/discover/publications-and-articles/reports/univercities-the-knowledge-to-power-uk-metros. Accessed Aug 2020.
Savage, M., Hanquinet, L., Cunningham, N., & Hjellbrekke, J. (2018). Emerging cultural capital in the city: Profiling London and Brussels. *International Journal of Urban and Regional Research, 42*(1), 138–149.
Stacey, V. (2020, October 9). Research shows where housing "fared best". *The Pie News*. https://thepienews.com/news/ireland-spain-and-uk-student-accommodation-fared-best-in-covid-19/. Accessed Dec 2020.
Storms, K., Simundza, D., Morgan, E., & Miller, S. (2019). Developing a resilience tool for higher education institutions. *Journal of Green Building, 14*(1), 187–197.
Taylor, P. (1992). Ethnic Group Data and Applications to Higher Education. *Higher Education Quarterly, 46 (4)*, 359–374. https://doi.org/10.1111/j.1468-2273.1992.tb01608.x
The Australian Government. (n.d.). *New Colombo Plan*. https://www.dfat.gov.au/people-to-people/new-colombo-plan/pages/new-colombo-plan. Accessed Dec 2020.
The U.S. Immigration and Customs Enforcement (2020). SEVP modifies temporary exemptions for nonimmigrant students taking online courses during fall 2020 semester. Retrieved from: https://www.ice.gov/news/releases/sevp-modifies-temporary-exemptions-nonimmigrant-students-taking-online-courses-during
Trinity College Dublin. (2017). *Profile 2016/2017*. https://hea.ie/assets/uploads/2017/04/TCD-Profile-2016.pdf. Accessed Aug 2020.
University and College Union [UCU]. (2016). *Precarious work in higher education: A snapshot of insecure contracts and institutional attitudes*. https://www.ucu.org.uk/media/7995/Precarious-work-in-higher-education-a-snapshot-of-insecure-contracts-and-institutional-attitudes-Apr-16/pdf/ucu_precariouscontract_hereport_apr16.pdf. Accessed Aug 2020.

Universities UK (2017). International Facts and Figures: Higher Education May 2017. Retrieved from: https://www.universitiesuk.ac.uk/sites/default/files/uploads/UUKi%20 reports/International_Facts_and_Figures_2017.pdf

Waruru, M. (2020, July 16). Internationalisation and COVID-19-challenges and lessons. University World News. https://www.universityworldnews.com/post.php?story=20200715110850412. Accessed Aug 2020.

World Economic Forum. (2014, August). *The Competitiveness of Cities*. http://www3.weforum.org/docs/GAC/2014/WEF_GAC_CompetitivenessOfCities_Report_2014.pdf. Accessed Aug 2020.

Young, I. M. (1990). Justice and the politics of difference. Princeton: Princeton University Press.

Yueming, R. (2018). The future of Shanghai as an international and Cosmopolitan City of culture. *The Asia Dialogue*. https://theasiadialogue.com/2018/07/09/the-future-of-shanghai-as-an-international-and-cosmopolitan-city-of-culture/. Accessed Aug 2020.

Zerlang, M. (1997). The university and the city. *GeoJournal, 43*(3), 241–246.

Zhang, D., & Stucka, M. (2020, August 19). COVID-19, visas, Trump: International students turning away from US colleges for lots of reasons. *USA Today*. https://eu.usatoday.com/story/news/education/2020/08/19/covid-college-fall-semester-2020-international-student-visa-donald-trump/5585675002/. Accessed Nov 2020.

Zhang, F., Chung, C. K. L., & Yin, Z. (2020). Green infrastructure for China's new urbanisation: A case study of greenway development in Maanshan. *Urban Studies, 57*(3), 508–524.

Chapter 18
Vulnerability After COVID-19 and the Response of a Developing City: The Case of Bogotá, Colombia

David Arboleda and Andrés Zambrano

COVID-19 has posed formidable challenges for societies. On the one hand, it has generated a health crisis that threatens to cause millions of deaths. On the other hand, it has produced an economic recession that is expected to be the worst in modern history, endangering the improvements in livability achieved in the last decades and deepening previous inequality. These challenges are even greater for developing economies since they have fewer resources to cope with the health and economic crisis. Efforts to improve their health system capacities and to support vulnerable households most affected by the slowdown would be restricted by their fiscal capacity and the evolution of the pandemic within their territories.

Most societies have relied on lockdowns to ease the speed of transmission of the disease and to better prepare their health systems for the contingency. Therefore, the mobility of most citizens was reduced to within the city where they live, even after easing the confinement, thus increasing the importance of the measures taken by local governments. While national governments have created large welfare programs to cope with the economic crisis, local governments have an opportunity to complement them and adjust such policies to their context. Moreover, local governments have the possibility to implement revolutionary policies that are harder to carry out at a national level and can improve their response to future crises. These measures become even more central when the local government of the capital of a country implements them, since they also serve as an example and set expectations for smaller municipalities.

The purpose of this chapter is to study the economic consequences of COVID-19 in the city of Bogotá, the capital of Colombia, and the responses taken by the local

D. Arboleda · A. Zambrano (✉)
Universidad de los Andes, Cundinamarca, Colombia
e-mail: de.arboleda@uniandes.edu.co; ja.zambrano@uniandes.edu.co

© The Author(s), under exclusive license to Springer Nature Switzerland AG 2021

M. A. Montoya et al. (eds.), *COVID-19 and Cities*, The Urban Book Series,
https://doi.org/10.1007/978-3-030-84134-8_18

government to address these impacts.[1] The pandemic has taken a large epidemiological toll on the city, forcing it into recurrent quarantines and restrictions that have significantly affected the economic outcomes. Unemployment has doubled, and the whole economy has experienced an unprecedented contraction, close to 8%.

The national government has reacted with a fiscal stimulus establishing transitory cash transfers to vulnerable households that complement and expand previously existing ones, as well as loans and employee subsidies to formal firms, among other policies. However, its response has not been sufficient for the magnitude of the crisis, leading poorest households to seek income in informal markets that are more prone to contagion. Bogotá has been able to counteract their response by further complementing those transfers to households that had not received any before, and in some cases increasing the size of the transfers to households that had received some. It has also developed a plan to provide incentives for informal firms to become formal. These ambitious programs will contribute to a stronger social safety net and, arguably, to greater productivity in the long run. Nevertheless, these measures are costly and harder to implement at a national level, thus their political support is more difficult. If these programs prove to be successful and sustainable in Bogotá, it will be easier to replicate them nationwide. Bogotá is funding them through debt, using its ample fiscal space generated in previous administrations, and although there was a heated debate in the local council, its implementation has been approved for the next few years. The inherited fiscal space has been key for improving the resilience of the city to the current large shock and should be preserved after the recovery of the economy to cope with future crises.

This chapter is organized as follows: In the first section, we provide a context on how Bogotá has fared over the last two decades in terms of socioeconomic indicators and the impact of the recent pandemic on these. The next section discusses the impact of COVID-19 on health outcomes, while the third section describes the fiscal stance of Bogotá. The fourth section will focus on the policies followed by the local government to cope with the crisis, and how they have interacted with the policies implemented at the national level. The final section gives conclusions.

Bogotá's Performance Over the Last Two Decades

Bogotá has 7.4 million inhabitants (10.2 million when considering the metropolitan area) (DANE, 2018) and is responsible for almost a quarter of Colombia's GDP (Cotelo, 2020). From 2006 to 2019, its local economy has grown at a general real annual rate of 3.87%, which has been remarkably steady throughout these years, indicating that the city has been characterized by a healthy and stable growth dynamic (Departamento Administrativo Nacional de Estadística [DANE], 2020).

[1] We restrict attention to the economic dimension, while omitting political considerations, which could take an entire book.

Table 18.1 GDP per capita (PPP) in 2019 for the main LAC cities

City	GDP per capita (PPP)
Ciudad de México	17,961.03
Santiago de Chile	34,030.18
Lima	21,351.97
Montevideo	23,584.15
Bogotá	22,879.94

Source: Own calculations based on World Bank (2020), INS (2020), INEGI (2020), INEI (2020)

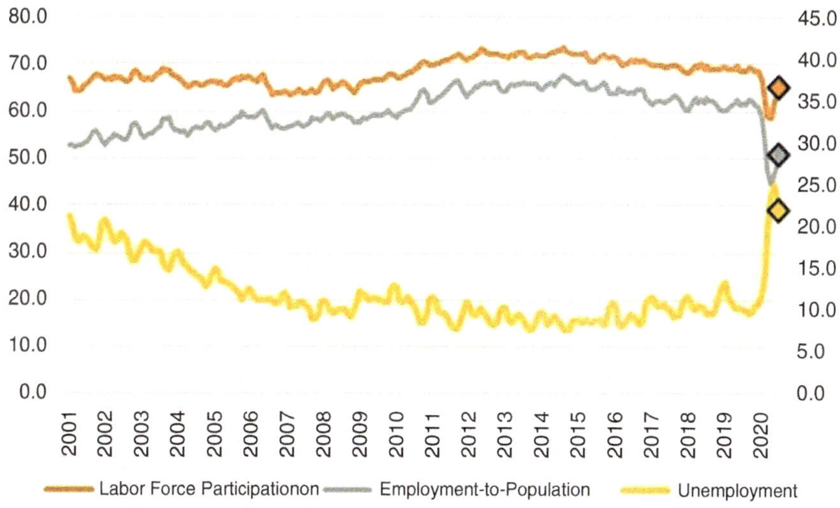

Fig. 18.1 Labor Market Indicators for Bogotá
Source: DANE (2020). Latest observation corresponds to the 2020 April–June trimester. Unemployment rate on secondary axis

For 2019, its per capita GPD (PPP) was 22,879. Table 18.1 shows a comparison with other major Latin American cities. Bogotá ranks over Lima and Ciudad de México, but below Montevideo and is considerably behind Santiago (World Bank, 2020). For 2020, initial forecasts predicted a 3.5% increment of the GDP. Data suggest that a considerable part of this growth would have derived from commerce, real estate, and financial activities. These sectors represent, on average, 19.7%, 13.5%, and 8.2% of the GDP and have grown at a rate of 3.08%, 2.7%, and 5.45%, respectively, since 2014. However, previous growth predictions now show a contraction of 8% due to the economic crisis arising from the pandemic itself and the measures taken to counteract it (Redaccion Bogotá, 2020). .

Regarding the labor market, Bogotá was also exhibiting a positive performance. Throughout the last two decades, unemployment showed an overall downward trend with a considerable flattening during recent years (see Fig. 18.1). At the beginning of the sampled period , the city's unemployment rate was over 30%, a clear repercussion of the 1999 financial crisis. Nonetheless, this number continually decreased until 2011, and the second-quarter unemployment rate has orbited toward 10% (with a mean value of 9.98%) ever since. Similarly, both the labor force participation rate and the employment to population ratio have been deemed stable, with an average of 68.5% and 60.5%, respectively. Nevertheless, the crisis unraveled by COVID-19 has triggered an unprecedented increase in unemployment. Data for the March–May trimester show a 7.3 p.p. increase in the unemployment rate, peaking to 19.2%, which implies a return to unemployment levels unseen since the beginning of the century. The workers most affected by the crisis were those that were salaried and the self-employed, accounting for nearly 288,400 of the 515,000 jobs lost. This negative effect has only deepened: The latest labor market report available by the time this chapter was written recorded a 23.6% unemployment rate and a sharp drop of both the Labor Force Participation and the Employment-to-Population ratio (DANE, 2020).

In terms of poverty and inequality, Bogotá's indicators evidence a stagnant behavior for the past 5 years (see Fig. 18.2). In 2002, the city's extreme monetary poverty rate was estimated at 7.2%. It then showed a decreasing trend until 2013 when it reached a minimum of 1.6%. Nonetheless, from this point forward, the extreme poverty rate has stalled and even increased slightly, resulting in a 2.5% rate in 2018. Furthermore, the multidimensional poverty rate presents an analogous pattern: In 2010, it was 12.1%, then continuously decreased to 4.7% in 2015, and remained approximately constant thereafter (SALUDATA, 2020).

Above all, Bogotá's accomplishments in alleviating poverty have resulted in a substantial recomposition of the population's distribution among the various social classes, as depicted in Fig. 18.3. Two facts stand out: On the one hand, the percentage of the population categorized as poor diminished notably, moving from 19.5%

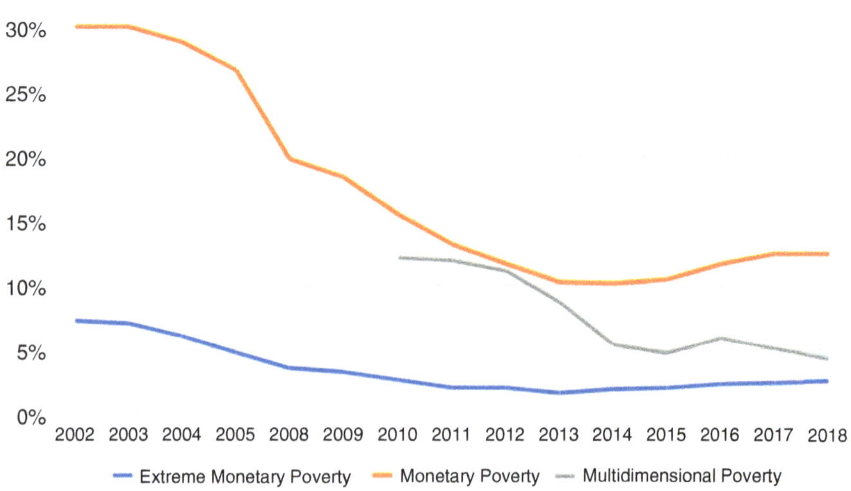

Fig. 18.2 Poverty Rates
Source: SALUDATA (2020)

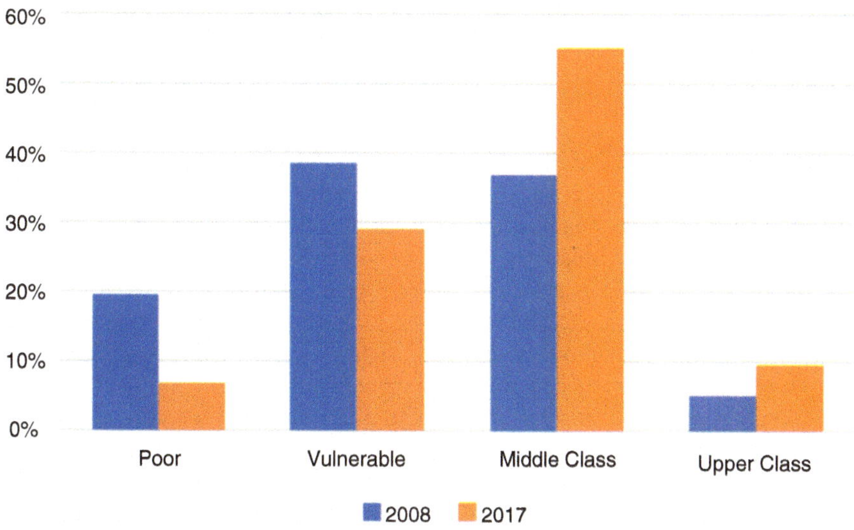

Fig. 18.3 Bogotá's Social Class Composition
Source: Puche & Villa (2018)

in 2008 to 6.7% in 2017. On the other hand, there has been a notable expansion of the middle-class population, which previously accounted for 37% of Bogotá's citizens, but by 2017 represented nearly 55%. However, a large proportion of the population remains vulnerable (29%), and the impact of a shock like COVID-19 threatens to make them fall into poverty (Puche & Villa, 2018). The policies implemented by the national and local government are key to preventing deterioration from previous social advances. In fact, the situation poses an opportunity to reform the social protection programs to better prepare for future crises.

In terms of inequality, the Gini coefficient has decreased from 0.572 in 2002 to a minimum of 0.497 in 2012. From then on, inequality remained rather invariant, with the Gini coefficient taking a value of 0.498 in 2018 (SALUDATA, 2020). The stagnation of these indicators reveals that both poverty and inequality are time-persistent phenomena that withstand key challenges to the city's economic progress.

In summary, the COVID-19 pandemic both jeopardizes the healthy economic behavior of the city in terms of growth and unemployment and threatens, due to its higher impact over the poor and vulnerable, to obliterate the progress obtained in matters of inequality and poverty reduction. Thus, given the insufficient progress in reducing inequality and poverty over recent years, it becomes of utmost importance to study the repercussions of the pandemic in terms of the living conditions of Bogotá's inhabitants, and understand the possible effects of the policies proposed to respond to the crisis.

The Health Panorama in Bogotá

On March 6th, 2020, a 19-year-old female was confirmed as the first case of COVID-19 in Bogotá and the nation. Thirteen days later, Bogotá's mayor, Claudia López, announced that the city would have a 3-day lockdown simulation to contain the virus' spread, but that ended up being extended until March 22nd when the Bogotá District, following the mandates of the national government, decreed 23 days of compulsory isolation (Alcaldía Mayor de Bogotá, 2020b). Only essential workers (those involved in medical, pharmaceutical and financial services, transportation, food production, etc.) were allowed to leave their homes. Although some modifications and relaxations have been introduced since then, several restrictions over mobility and working conditions remain active. As a result, the local economy has experienced a large negative shock, with a considerable proportion of the economic apparatus partially or entirely being put on hold. By the time of the first lockdown (March 19th), Bogotá reported a total of 55 confirmed cases, 2 deaths, and a 5-day moving average of 14 cases per day (INS, 2020).

Despite the quarantine measures, the disease continued to spread, and by the beginning of July 2020, the 5-day average daily variation of confirmed cases and deaths escalated to 1058 and 24, respectively. Accordingly, the accumulated number of cases went up to 36,532, with a total of 786 deaths and 13,484 recoveries, as reported on July 4th. Nearly a month later, the moving averages for cases and deaths were 3558 and 61, and the city reported a total of 106,168 cases. However, the marked augmentation of COVID-19 patients pictured on Fig. 18.4 does not provide conclusive evidence regarding the effectiveness of the quarantine. On the one hand, the larger number of cases reported is also partially due to a more aggressive testing policy. In only 2 months, the city multiplied its testing by a factor of 6, and in 3 months by a factor of 12, thus achieving an accumulated figure of close to 7200 processed tests per 100,000 people, and over 10,000 daily tests (INS, 2020). On the other hand, the quarantine measures have been progressively reduced, with the easing on June 14th, 2020, allowing 80% of the work force to move freely within the city, which corresponds with the biggest jump in the number of cases hitherto (Alcaldía Mayor de Bogotá, 2020a).

As exemplified by the increase in the availability of ICUs, the sharp rise in the number of cases posed a major challenge to the city's health system. On April 8th, 2020, the city possessed around 8 ICUs per 100,000 people. At the time, only 19.5% of these were in use. As the city prepared to face the peak of COVID-19 cases, the local government made big efforts to broaden its ICU stock, thereby reaching a level of 23 ICUs per 100,000 people by early July; notwithstanding, the attempts to guarantee a sufficient supply of intensive care units were proven dangerously scant at best. As pictured on Fig. 18.5, by July 5th, 83.5% of the COVID-19 ICUs were already in use; consequently, the city hall declared a red alert on the healthcare system, thus bestowing the control of all available ICUs, public and private, to district government. A subsequent strengthening of the isolation measures, in the form of localized quarantines, managed to slow down the progression of the occupation rate and stabilize it around 90%.

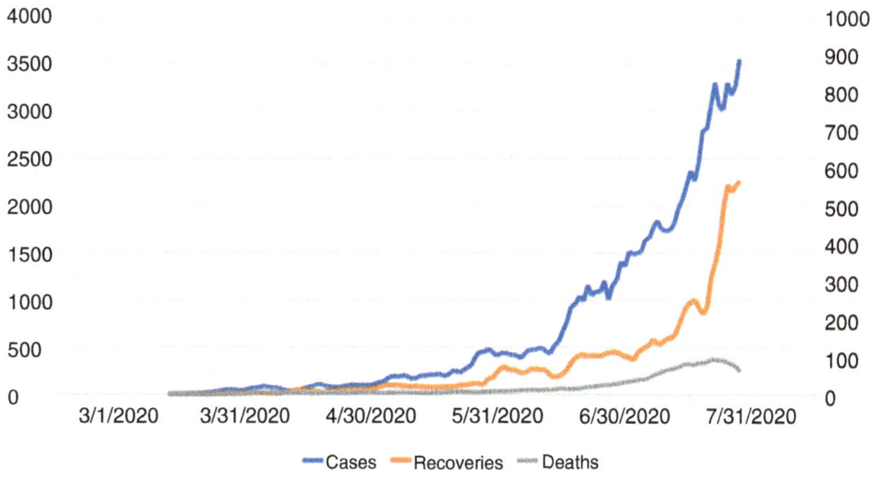

Fig. 18.4 Five-day Moving Average Daily Variation Indicators
Source: INS (2020). Deaths graphed on secondary axis

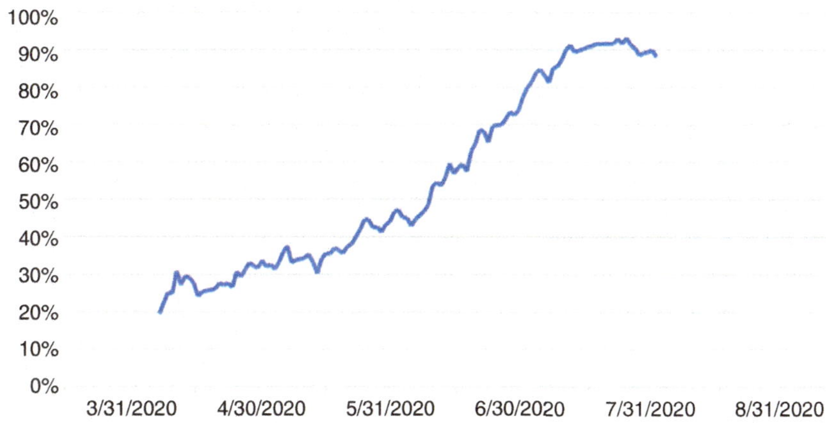

Fig. 18.5 COVID-19 ICUs Occupation (%)
Source: SALUDATA (2020)

Furthermore, the severity of COVID-19 cases has been heterogeneous among the socioeconomic strata. While the bottom three comprise 77% of Bogotá's households, they represent 94% of patients hospitalized due to complications, and 92% of the COVID-19 cases remitted to an ICU. Even more disquieting, 92% of the deceased individuals belonged to these lower strata, with the greater affectation posed on the stratum level 2 (48% of deaths, see Fig. 18.6). Such findings become even more alarming when considering that, within the bottom-half of the strata, the percentage of the population over 65 years old, that are considered to be particularly

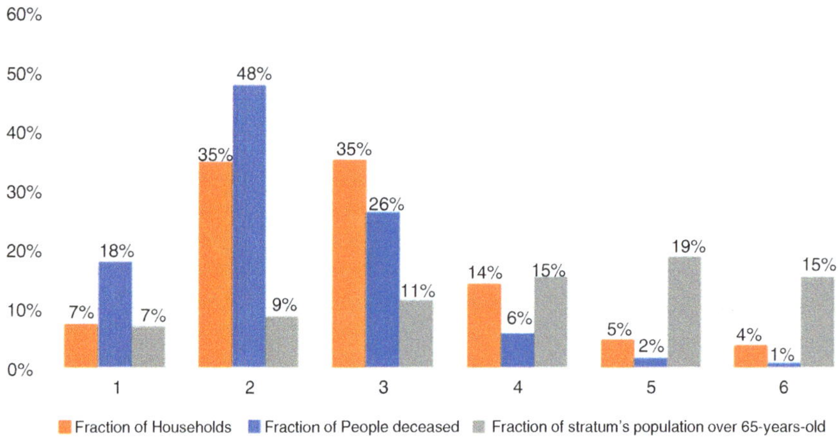

Fig. 18.6 Bogotá: Fraction of Households vs. Deceased people by stratum
Source: Grupo de Investigación en Macroeconomía (2020)

endangered by the virus, is systematically lower than that within the upper-half of the strata. Therefore, despite being compounded by a proportionally less risky population, strata 1, 2, and 3 seem to suffer more and have greater losses due to the virus. The explanation is threefold. First, poor households work in more informal jobs and have a greater need to work in the streets since they have less savings to help them comply with a quarantine. Second, they have fewer resources to spend when they fall ill and have less access to good quality healthcare. Third, these households believe less in the existence of the virus and do not perceive it to be as harmful as it is. Moreover, they think their neighbors share their beliefs (Grupo de Investigación en Macroeconomía, 2020).

The Fiscal Stance of Bogotá

In this section, we examine the fiscal space that Bogotá has to implement programs to alleviate the effects of the crisis. Since most of the social assistance policies are funded and implemented by Bogotá's Central Administration (BCA), the focus will be placed on the Central Administration's fiscal indicators.

To begin with, the Central Administration's income is considered. In 2018, the latest reported year, BCA's income was 7.26% of local GDP, which represents a 0.81 p.p. increase with respect to 2017. Additionally, Fig. 18.7 illustrates the composition of income, and its disaggregated components, as percentages of Bogotá's GDP since 2005. Some facts immediately stand out. First, most of the Central Administration's resources come from tax revenues, national transfers, and capital resources in that order. Nontax revenues and other types of transfers have relatively low relevance in the budget. Second, the overall income to GDP ratio has been

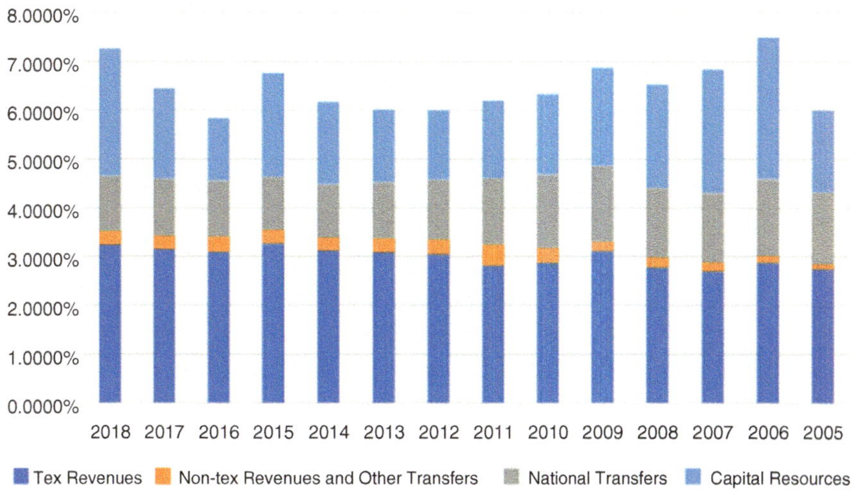

Fig. 18.7 Income Composition
Source: Contraloría de Bogotá (2020)

remarkably stable. It averaged 6.48%, and most of the observations fall considerably proximate from this mean. While most of the variability derives from capital resources and national transfers, tax revenues remain nearly constant at around 3% of the GDP. However, the pandemic has changed this panorama with initial estimates calculating that the current income will see a decrease of 38% and that the local government is expected to compensate with debt (Contraloría de Bogotá, 2020).

When it comes to expenditure, a different dynamic is observed. On the one hand, Fig. 18.8 shows that executed expenditure has been systematically lower than definitive expenditure, thus suggesting that the Central Administration strictly adheres to its planned budget and presents no tendency to over-expend. On the other hand, albeit until 2009, expenditure was calculated to be over 6% of the local GDP, in 2010 this percentage went down to 3.84% and did not recover afterward, even though, as previously discussed, income did not suffer great disturbances and only slightly decreased during the 2010–2013 period. From then on, expenditure averaged 4% of the GDP (ídem).

Disaggregated data corroborate that such a reduction in expenditure was mainly achieved through cut-offs on investments. While in 2009 investment represented circa 5.1% of Bogotá's GDP, in 2010, it was only 3%, and despite it having progressively increased in recent years, by 2018, it reached only 4% of the GDP. Simultaneously to the investment reduction, the Central Administration also lowered its functioning expenses and the amount spent on debt service. This behavior may be a sign of improved efficiency in expenditure. Certainly, as the sudden drop in expenditure was not accompanied by less income, the Central Administration managed to accumulate significant resources that allowed it to increment its surplus as a percentage of the GDP by a factor of 5. Before 2010, the Central Administration's

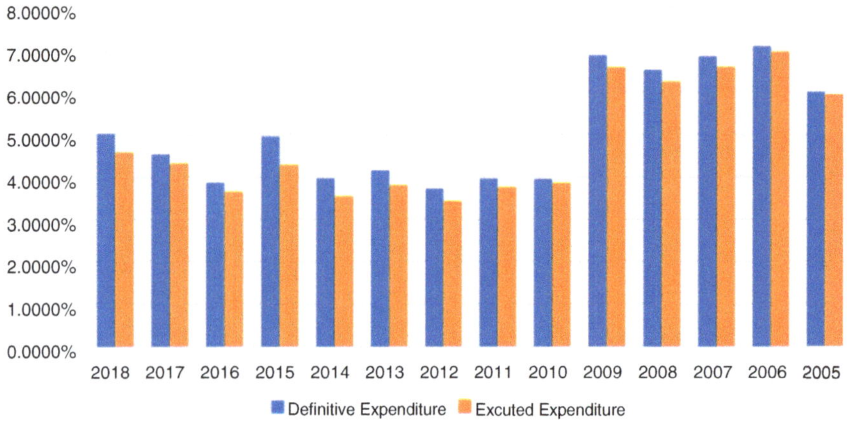

Fig. 18.8 Expenditure
Source: Contraloría de Bogotá (2020)

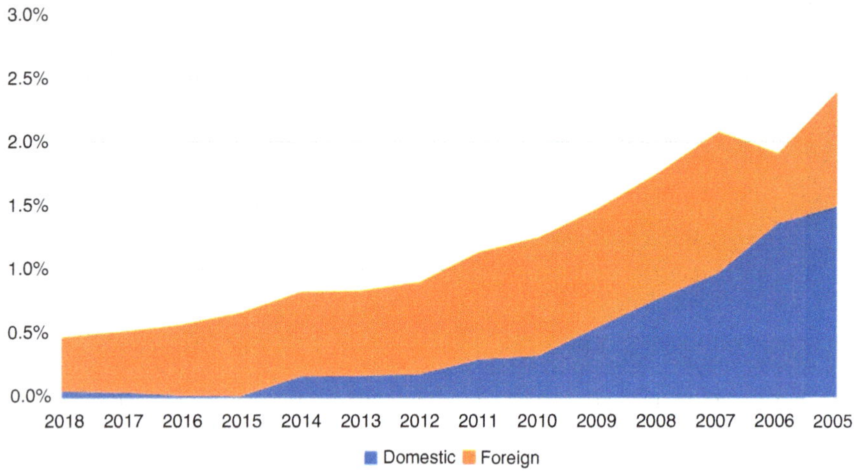

Fig. 18.9 Debt Composition
Source: Contraloría de Bogotá (2020)

surplus was less than 0.5% of the GDP. Nonetheless, the dynamics of income and expenditure described above resulted in a surplus equal to 2.5% of the GDP that has continued until recent years.

To conclude, it is important to examine the composition of the Central Administration's debt and its trends (Fig. 18.9). In 2005, total debt equaled somewhat less than 2.5% of the GDP, and close to two-thirds of that amount represented domestic debt. Nevertheless, the domestic portion of the debt decreased steadily and became virtually nil since 2015. Foreign debt, however, presented only a subtle reduction. By 2018, total debt, mainly compounded by foreign debt, was under 0.5% of the local GDP, meaning that the Central Administration is capable of fully paying its financial responsibilities and yet preserve a surplus. Thus, it seems that BCA's finances are healthy, sturdy, and bestow the district with an ample response margin in case of an economic emergency, such as the COVID-19 crisis, thus improving its resilience to adverse shocks.

The Implemented Policies

National Government Policies

The national government strategy to face the crisis has had to balance its policies to attend to both the health and economic costs of the pandemic: While the virus has taken approximately 10,000 lives, the shock to economic activity (due both to the pandemic and the measures undertaken to prevent the spread of the virus) lowered the growth forecast down to −7.8%. Therefore, once the initial lockdown was announced, the national government stepped up with a wide variety of economic measures to soften the impact of the quarantine on poor and vulnerable individuals, and formal businesses.[2]

Like most countries, Colombia confronted COVID-19 with a mix of contact tracing, health system reinforcement, greater testing capacity, and compulsory lockdowns. In the initial period after the introduction of the virus, lockdowns were viewed as appropriate to reduce the spread rate of the virus and provide the health system with sufficient time to prepare for the pandemic. For instance, the increase in ICU capacity allowed the national ICU occupancy rate to remain under 75%, even through the peak of the contagion. However, now that compliance with the quarantine has weakened significantly as the national government seems to repeatedly extend the lockdown, questions have arisen regarding the effectiveness of mandatory isolation and the pertinence of its rather early implementation. The largely informal population of the country lacks the means to remain in lockdown indefinitely. Moreover, were they to be allowed to resume work, the economic standstill still implies that their income would diminish substantially. Therefore, Colombia's national government was forced to accompany health-related policies with an extensive fiscal policy.

The flagship of the social assistance policies has been the Solidarity Income: a 160,000 pesos (around 40 US dollars) monthly transfer aimed at 3 million households that are not beneficiaries of other previously established social programs, such as Families in Action, Youth in Action, or "Colombia Mayor". The Solidarity Income was initiated in April 2020 and is expected to be extended to June 2021.

[2] For a complete revision of the measures taken by the national government, see Alvarez et al. (2020).

Table 18.2 National Government Social Programs

Program	Transfer	Beneficiaries	Total Cost in millions
Families in action	145,000	2,600,000	377,000
Youth in action	356,000	276,000	98,256
Colombia Mayor	80,000	1,700,000	136,000
Solidarity income	1,440,000	3,000,000	4,320,000
VAT return	75,000	1,000,000	75,000
Total			5,006,256

Source: Own calculations

Furthermore, for families that were included in the previously established social programs, the government stipulated a supplementary cycle of transfers, which required an additional expense of over 4.9 trillion pesos. Finally, the government also implemented a novel tax return program: a million of the most vulnerable households of the country, identified through the SISBEN and the databases of other social programs, would receive a transfer of 75,000 pesos every 2 months as a compensation for the burden imposed by the VAT (Value Added Tax). The value of resources designated for each program and the number of beneficiaries are summarized in Table 18.2. Other poverty alleviation policies include: direct subsidies to public services in rural areas and the opportunity for individuals cataloged as stratum 4 or less to defer public services payments at no cost; grace periods and renegotiations for loan payments for over 10.9 million debtors, with no interests charged for possible deferments; and baskets of goods donated to vulnerable communities.

Complementarily, the national government launched a series of financial aid programs directed to safeguard employment and protect vulnerable firms from bankruptcy. On the one hand, for firms that report a 20% or greater fall in income compared to 2019, the government agreed to grant a 220,000 pesos contribution (a fourth of the minimum wage) to the bonus payment of workers with wages between the minimum wage and 1 million pesos. On the other hand, to help formal workers whose contracts were suspended, the national government created the Support for Formal Employment Program: a monthly 160,000 pesos grant for the time the worker was in contractual suspension during April, May, and June 2020. Moreover, with this program the national government also committed to cofinance micro-, small-, and medium-sized firms' payrolls, initially for 3 months, granting 351,000 pesos per formal worker, conditional on the firm retaining all personnel (this transfer is exclusive for firms reporting a 20% or greater decrease in income).

To provide micro, small, and medium firms with liquidity, the government also stepped-up credit guarantees for loans required for payrolls (90% guaranteed by the government), working capital (80%), and independent workers (80%). To date, almost 100,000 firms have benefited from the Support to Formal Employment Program, and close to 2.4 million formal jobs were protected. Additionally, pension funds contributions were suspended for 3 months; income tax payment was postponed to the end of the year; employers were allowed to concede paid vacations without previous notice; and the government injected 70 trillion pesos into the National Guarantees Fund to enhance firms' access to loans.

The total emergency expenditure of these policies totals 2.7% of the national GDP and is expected to increase the government's deficit to 8.2% of the GDP (Cárdenas & Martínez, 2020). However, this is still a small package compared to the one implemented by similar countries. For example, Peru and Chile have increased their public expenditure by 4.8% and 5.7% of their GDP, respectively. The most probable reason for such timid intervention is the lack of fiscal space Colombia had before the pandemic, since its debt was close to 50% of its GDP. In fact, the initial source to fund the emergency expenditure was local debt to territorial entities. In one of its first decrees, number 444 of March 21, 2020, the national government took the territorial savings (FONPET, a public pension fund, and FAE, a savings and stabilization fund) adding up to 1.5% of the GDP, to fund the first national programs. This led to a serious complaint from the local governments since it left them without sufficient space to react to the crisis. Only big cities, including Bogotá, could use debt as an instrument to fund further stimulus to counteract the recession and complement the packages designed by the national government.

Local Government Policies

The District of Bogotá implemented complementary policies to alleviate the foreseeable consequences of the shock concerning income and consumption. On March 25th, the "Sistema Distrital Bogotá Solidaria en Casa" was established with an overall budget of 5.9 trillion pesos financed through the district's general budget, national contributions, and private donations (Alcaldía Mayor de Bogotá, 2020b). This policy was intended to aid the poor and vulnerable among the population, especially those whose wellbeing and quality of living were particularly imperiled by the pandemic and were not covered by national programs, using monetary transfers, redeemable bonds, and food subsidies. The "Sistema Distrital Bogotá Solidaria en Casa" (SBSC hereafter) was later developed with the establishment of the Solidary Lease program on April 25th and was accompanied by the creation of the District System for the Mitigation of the Economic Impact, the Economic Foment and Reactivation (SMEIEFR from this point forward) on April 8th. The former measure was aimed to preserve jobs and save small companies by granting credits and transfers. The latter sought to protect the vulnerable population living under leases from getting evicted and/or losing access to public services. Both SBSC and SMEIEFR were posteriorly subscribed as constitutive parts of the scheme of subsidies and contributions of a broader, more ambitious policy: The Strategy of Guaranteed Minimum Income (SGMI).

The SGMI, formally constituted on the 2020–2024 District Development Plan as a part of "Purpose 1: Make a new social contract with equality of opportunities for social, productive and political inclusion", is a public policy that seeks to

Table 18.3 Guaranteed Minimum Income Funding

Program	Value (Million Pesos)
Education for all program: Access and permanence with equity and rural education emphasis	2,628,927.00
Effective public management program	539,686.00
Youth with capacities program: Life projects for citizenship, innovation, and XXI century work	48,005.00
Integral social mobility program	1,284,297.00
Exclusion for ethnic, religious, social, political, and sexual orientation prevention program	22,081.00
District care system program	3,792,999.00
Subsidies and transfers for equity program	1,373,928.00
Total	9,689,923.00

Source: Alcaldía Mayor de Bogotá D.C

progressively ensure a minimum income for households residing in Bogotá. Such income may be given in the form of monetary transfers (both conditioned and unconditioned), redeemable bonds, and a variety of subsidies. The minimum income is calculated taking into account the district's tributes, the donations destined to the SGMI, and other contributions. The District Development Plan estimates a total budget of 9,989,923 million pesos for the SGMI, around a 9% of the total cost of the Development Plan (ídem). These resources proceed from previous social programs established to improve welfare and quality of life (Table 18.3).

The SGMI is divided in two programs. On the one hand, the SMEIEFR is a production-oriented approach to the crisis. Its main goal is to preserve jobs and business dynamism structure in the district, focusing primarily on micro-, small-, and medium-sized companies. This system, funded by the same sources as the SBSC plus resources from the union and private sectors, consists of three strategic axes: potentializing opportunity sectors, mitigating the impact of the pandemic, and reactivating the economy, and sectorial protocol for the operation of the economy given the different degrees of confinement. Additionally, the SMEIEFR includes actions that allow the city's productive apparatus to access credit and liquidity, dialogue with unions and the private sector, and fiscal policies that ensure the system's sustainability.

On the other hand, the SBSC appears as a more consumption-oriented strategy compounded by two main programs: The Solidarity Lease and the Guaranteed Minimum Income. The Solidarity Lease was a social assistance program led by the District Secretariat of Habitat with the purpose of attending to the dwelling needs of the population. Specifically, the Solidarity Lease was steered toward a low-income population living under a daily/weekly/monthly lease modality. It intended to relieve these citizens from the burden of the expense of leases by granting monthly nonconditional monetary transfers for up to 3 months. The selection of the beneficiaries prioritized households under especially fragile economic conditions, such as heads of households over 60 years old; female heads of household; and households with members under 18 years old, those over 60 years old, or with some sort of disability, among others. Similarly, the district forbade evictions of vulnerable lodging users due to nonpayment of lodging costs for as long the compulsory precautionary isolation measures remain active; and ensured asylum for those in the population at risk of becoming homeless.

Simultaneously, the Solidarity Lease was complemented by subsidies to public services. In this case, all households classified as stratum 4 or less living in the urban, peri-urban, or rural perimeter of Bogotá were targeted. Four subsidies were implemented: (1) the Additional Basic Unit of Consumption, consisting of 1.41 free cubic meters of water per month for up to 3 months; (2) the Reduction over the Value of the Bill, which implies a 10% discount on the monthly electricity bill; (3) the Cubic Meter Relief, working as a 10% discount over the nonsubsidized value of gas; and (4) the Relief over the Value of the Bill for public service cleaning, that grants a 10% discount on the total value of the bill once all subsidies have been applied.

In parallel, the SBSC also includes a minimum income program, more closely related to the SGMI presented in the District Development Plan. This policy, first implemented in early April, intended to aid all the 350,000 poor households and around 150,000 vulnerable households (while the assistance provided to the poor population was funded using the district's budget, that for the vulnerable relied on transfers from the national government and private donations). The monetary and in-kind transfers aimed to benefit inactive or informal workers classified as poor or vulnerable by the 2018 population census, the SISBEN IV, and the Multipurpose Poll. The district's identification process also appealed to social cartography and other specialized sources to include the poor population not registered in official databases. Finally, in case a needy household were to be omitted by all the previous sources, the City Hall habilitated an online platform called "Bogotá Cuidadora", where citizens can subscribe and voluntarily ask for assistance.

The transferred amounts were stipulated as follows. Each poor household was to receive a total of 423,000 pesos in the form of monetary transfers, redeemable bonds, or in-kind-subsidies, equivalent to 65% of a Bogotá's poor household expenditure for 23 days (this was the expected duration of the lockdown at the time). In the case of the vulnerable, the value of the transfers decreased to 178,000 pesos, corresponding to a minimum food basket for a low-income household for the same 23 days. However, if the household, poor or vulnerable, was already a beneficiary of any of the transfer programs of the national government, the district only transferred the extra amount required to reach the value of the corresponding minimum income. Moreover, the benefits of the guaranteed minimum income were only subject to two conditions: The household must obey the quarantine and remain free of domestic violence complaints.

Furthermore, since July 13th, the guaranteed minimum income began its second phase (third cycle of the overall district's transfers), now under the name of guaranteed basic rent. As the city entered into a novel phase of the quarantine measures, this time characterized by alternating, localized lockdowns, the district decided to provide financial assistance to nearly 550,000 poor and vulnerable families selected

Table 18.4 Minimum Income: Transfers to Households (Million Pesos)

Cycle		Households	Value (Million Pesos)
1st cycle	Total	309,990.00	72,033.00
2nd cycle	1st trans. In 2nd cycle	79,657.00	44,525.00
	2nd trans. In 2nd cycle	230,062.00	
	Total	309,719.00	
3rd cycle	1st trans. In 3rd cycle	2378.00	35,794.00
	2nd trans. In 3rd cycle	249,019.00	
	Total	251,397.00	
Total		871,106.00	152,352.00

Source: Bogotá Solidaria en Casa (2020)

using the same identification strategy as for the first round of transfers. While households with bank accounts were to receive 240,000 pesos transfers, those without an account would get the equivalent value in kind (approximately 150,000 families).

Currently, 577,842 families have received monetary transfers either from the district or the national government. The district provided the transfers in three cycles: the first cycle took place from March 29th to May 22nd and involved 72,033 million pesos transferred to 309,990 households; the second went from May 21st to July 12th involving a total of 44,525 million pesos transferred to 309,719 beneficiaries of which 79,657 had not received transfers in the first cycle. Finally, until now 251,397 households have received transfers in the third cycle, to a total cycle value of 35,794 million pesos (Bogotá Solidaria en Casa, 2020). Although it would be desirable to quantify the total expected social expenditure of the district, disaggregated according to the different programs, such a calculation is implausible for two reasons. First, the transfers of the Basic Rent program are not homogenous among families. Since the district only transfers the amount needed to make the total income that a given household receives, in the form of social programs' transfers (whether provided by the local or the national government), reach a certain threshold, there is no way to estimate the final Basic Rent expenditure per household. Second, a similar case occurs with the public services subsidies: not only does this vary with the total consumption of each household, but many of these district subsidies only apply to the value of the bill after subtracting national subsidies. Nonetheless, Table 18.4 does provide a helpful summary of the expenditure of the Minimum Income program per transfer cycle, and the resources assigned to the Solidarity Lease policy.

At first sight, the distribution of transfers suggests that the district's household identification strategy was mostly adequate (Fig. 18.10). Individuals cataloged in the top three strata only received 0.1% of the transfers; stratum 2 families (a total of 240,145 households) received 61.1% of the transferred resources; stratum 1 families (85,453), 21.8%; and just stratum 3 families (63,942), 16.2%. Moreover, 0.9% of the resources were received by nonclassified families, thus suggesting that the district effectively used the alternative identification methods mentioned earlier (ídem).

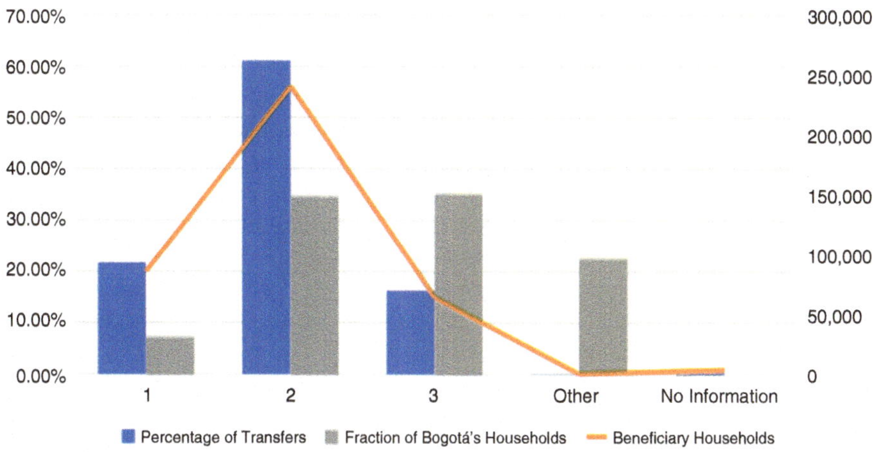

Fig. 18.10 District transfers distribution by strata
Source: Bogotá Solidaria en Casa (2020). Beneficieary Households graphed on secondary axis

A more detailed look at the district's social assistance programs reveals that by July 25th, 3117 households were beneficiaries of the Solidarity Lease transfers, which implied an overall expenditure of 614 million pesos. Additionally, over 55,492 public services had been reconnected or their disconnection had been overruled. At the same time, a total of 487,670 baskets of goods were delivered.

Finally, in mid-August, the district presented a new strategy summarized by what the city mayor referred to as the "Marshall Plan" for economic reactivation (clearly alluding to the original Marshall Plan executed by the United States during the post-war period). Bogotá's Marshall Plan consists of a compilation of tax incentives, new taxation schemes, incentives for formalization, and wider options for tax payments bestowed on both consumers and firms. Overall, with this proposal, the district seeks to relieve the tax burden of households and firms that have experienced a decrease in their income due to the pandemic, favor the recovery of employment, grant liquidity to the economic agents that allow them to continue their basic activities, reduce informality, and increase the aggregate demand and investment. Some of the measures undertaken are: the implementation of a novel monotax that simplifies taxation and enhances formalization and employment by reducing the transaction costs of the former; discounts and subsidies on a firm's registration costs; no-interest deferred payments on property taxes; and discounts on the industry and commerce tax proportional to the income lost during the pandemic, along with a temporary transition to a progressive scheme over the tariffs charged by such a tax that will last until 2028. As the implementation of Bogotá's Marshall Plan entails a fiscal expenditure that adds to the expenditure required by the social assistance programs that have been extensively addressed during this section, the district requested an additional debt budget of 11 trillion pesos to the council. This high amount of debt is possible to obtain given the ample fiscal space that we described in the previous section. Without such space, a fiscal response of this size would be unthinkable.

Final Discussion

The analyzed case of Bogotá is useful to provide a good example on how policies at the municipal level can successfully complement those policies implemented at the national level to ease the effects of the COVID-19 pandemic. On the one hand, these local policies can be adapted to the particular context of the city, in this case to the rampant informality of its labor market and the identification of poor and vulnerable households that are not in national databases. On the other hand, the designed policies can be more ambitious and revolutionary, since helping informal firms and establishing a basic income program would be too difficult to implement at a national level, both politically and financially. Trying such policies in a smaller context can allow posterior evaluations for their implementation at a national level. Moreover, the successful implementation of these policies would improve the long-term trajectory of the city. On the one hand, building a deeper social net to protect citizens from adverse shocks will improve the city's resilience to future crisis. On the other hand, inserting informal workers into the formal labor market will improve the chances of long-term gains in productivity.

Finally, this paper widens the scope of the recent fiscal policy literature. Although the importance of pre-existing fiscal space at the national level to soften the long-term impacts of a crisis had already been stressed (see Romer & Romer, 2017; Romer & Romer, 2019; Aizenman et al., 2019), less has been said regarding the central role that subnational entities can play in reactivating their local economies, and the subsequent relevance of promoting healthy fiscal behavior at the local level. Bogotá provides an excellent case for the benefits of having a good fiscal stance before the pandemic, since it allows large-scale programs without having consequences for medium-term fiscal sustainability. Furthermore, as argued by Shahrockh and Ravishankar (2013) for the cases of India, China, and Brazil, Bogotá also demonstrates how subnational entities may take advantage of their closeness to local realities in order to construct better-fitted policies that respond to the specific needs of the population under their jurisdiction and catalyze national policies and programs to deepen their impact and reach. Therefore, the present study contributes to a breaking with the common, centralized view of fiscal policy, to bestow a primary role to local governments. However, the main limitation of this paper is its inability to execute a judgment regarding the effectiveness of the policies implemented by the District of Bogotá to lessen the effects of the pandemic. More time will be needed to properly evaluate Bogotá's economic performance, the impact of the large variety of programs implemented, and the efficient usage of public resources. Nonetheless, this work serves as a cornerstone for such future research.

References

Aizenman, J., Jinjarak, Y., Nguyen, H., & Park, D. (2019, May). *Fiscal Epace and Increasing Fiscal Resilience*. ADB economics working paper series. https://www.adb.org/sites/default/files/publication/502236/ewp-582-fiscal-space-fiscal-resilience.pdf. Accessed Aug 2020.

Alcaldía Mayor de Bogotá D.C.. (2020a). *Conoce las normas que ha expedido el Distrito por coronavirus en Bogotá* [Discover the Norms Established by the District due to Coronavirus in Bogotá]. https://bogota.gov.co/mi-ciudad/gestion-juridica/normas-expedidas-por-el-distrito-por-el-coronavirus-en-bogota. Accessed 2 Aug 2020.

Alcaldía Mayor de Bogotá D.C. (2020b). *Plan De Desarrollo Económico, Social, Ambiental Y De Obras Públicas Del Distrito Capital 2020-2024 'Un Nuevo Contrato Social Y Ambiental Para La Bogotá Del Siglo XXI'* [Economic, social, environmental, and public work planning of the Capital District 2020–2024 'a new social and environmental contract for the XXI century Bogotá]. Colombia: Bogotá. http://www.sdp.gov.co/sites/default/files/edici_n_3001_pa_123_sd_de_2020.pdf. Accessed 2 Aug 2020.

Alvarez, A., Leon, D., Medellin, M., Zambrano, A., & Zuleta, H. (2020). *Coronavirus in Colombia: Vulnerability and policy options*. UNDP LAC COVID 19 policy document series no. 11.

Bogotá Solidaria en Casa. (2020). *Renta Básica Bogotá* [Basic Rent Bogotá] [Database]. https://bogotasolidariaencasa.gov.co/. Accessed 30 Jan 2021.

Cárdenas, M., & Martínez, H. (2020, July 24). *COVID-19 in Colombia: Impact and policy responses*. Center for Global Development. https://www.cgdev.org/publication/covid-19-colombia-impact-and-policy-responses. Accessed 2 Aug 2020.

Contraloría de Bogotá D.C. (2020). *Informes Obligatorios* [Mandatory reports] [Database]. http://www.contraloriabogota.gov.co/informes-obligatorios-0. Accessed 20 July 2020.

Cotelo, E. (2020, January 30). Análisis económico: ¿Cuáles son los departamentos que aportan más al PIB nacional? [Economic analysis: What departments contribute the Most to the national GDP?]. *En Perspectiva*. https://www.enperspectiva.net/en-perspectiva-programa/analisis-exante/analisis-economico-cuales-los-departamentos-aportan-mas-al-pib-nacional/. Accessed 2 Aug 2020.

DANE. (2018). *Proyecciones y Retroproyecciones de Población* [Projections and Retroprojections of the Population].. https://www.dane.gov.co/index.php/estadisticas-por-tema/demografia-y-poblacion/proyecciones-de-poblacion. Accessed 11 July 2020.

DANE. (2020). *Producto Interno Bruto de Bogotá D.C.* [Bogotá D.C. GDP].. https://www.dane.gov.co/index.php/estadisticas-por-tema/cuentas-nacionales/cuentas-nacionales-departamentales/cuentas-nacionales-departamentales-pib-trimestral-bogota-d-c. Accessed 11 July 2020.

Departamento Administrativo Nacional de Estadística [DANE]. (2020). *Boletín técnico. Mercado Laboral* [Technical Bulletin. Job Market]. https://www.dane.gov.co/files/investigaciones/boletines/ech/ech/anexo_empleo_may_20.xlsx. Accessed 6 July 2020.

Gobierno de Colombia. (2020). *Acciones tomadas por el Gobierno* [Actions Taken by the Government].. https://coronaviruscolombia.gov.co/Covid19/acciones-del-gobierno.html. Accessed 2 Aug 2020.

Grupo de Investigación en Macroeconomía de la Facultad de Economía Universidad de los Andes.. (2020). *Nota Macroeconómica No.23. El patrón socioconómico del COVID. El caso de Bogotá* [Macroeconomic Note No. 23. COVID's Socioeconomic Pattern. Bogotá's Case]. https://economia.uniandes.edu.co/components/com_booklibrary/ebooks/BM%2023.pdf. Accessed 2 Aug 2020.

Instituto Nacional de Estadística e Informática [INEI]. (2020). *Economía. Producto Interno Bruto por Departamento* [Economy. GDP by Department]. https://www.inei.gob.pe/estadisticas/indice-tematico/economia/. Accessed 2 Aug 2020.

Instituto Nacional de Estadística y Geografía [INEGI]. (2020). *Cuentas Nacionales* [National Accounts]. https://www.inegi.org.mx/sistemas/bie/?idserPadre=10200070#D10200070. Accessed 2 Aug 2020.

Instituto Nacional de Salud [INS]. (2020). *Coronavirus (COVID – 19) en Colombia* [Coronavirus (COVID-19) in Colombia]. https://www.ins.gov.co/Noticias/paginas/coronavirus.aspx. Accessed 2 Aug 2020.

Observatorio de Salud de Bogotá [SALUDATA]. (2020). *Datos de Salud. Demografía y Salud. Pobreza y Desigualdad en Bogotá D.C.* [Health Data. Demography and Health. Poverty and Inequality in Bogotá D.C.]. http://saludata.saludcapital.gov.co/osb/index.php/datos-de-salud/demografia/pobrezaygini/. Accessed 2 Aug 2020.

Puche, K., & Villa, V. (2018). *Evolución de las clases sociales en Colombia* [Evolution of Social Classes in Colombia]. http://www.fundesarrollo.org.co/wp-content/uploads/2020/01/Estudio-de-la-evoluci%C3%B3n-de-las-clases-sociales-en-Colombia.pdf.. Accessed 2 Aug 2020.

Redacción Bogotá. (2020, April 28). Crecimiento económico de Bogotá podría caer un 4,2% en 2020 por cuenta del Covid-19 [Economic Growth in Bogotá Might Drop 4.2% in 2020 due to COVID-19]. *El Espectador*. https://www.elespectador.com/noticias/bogota/crecimiento-economico-de-bogota-podria-caer-un-42-en-2020-por-cuenta-del-covid-10-articulo-916905/. Accessed 2 Aug 2020.

Romer, C. D., & Romer, D. H. (2017). *Why some times are different: Macroeconomic policy and the aftermath of financial crises* (NBER working paper 23931). https://doi.org/10.3386/w23931.

Romer, C. D., & Romer, D. H. (2019). *Fiscal space and the aftermath of financial crises: How it matters and why*. BPEA Conference Drafts. https://www.brookings.edu/wp-content/uploads/2019/03/Fiscal-Space-and-the-Aftermath-of-Financial-Crises.pdf

SALUDATA. (2020). *Datos de Salud. Enfermedades Transmisibles. Covid-19* [Health data. Transmissible disease. Covid-19]. http://saludata.saludcapital.gov.co/osb/index.php/datos-de-salud/enfermedades-trasmisibles/covid19/. Accessed 2 Aug 2020.

Shahrockh, F., & Ravishankar, V. J. (2013). Subnational Fiscal Policy in Large Developing Countries: Some Lessons from the 2008-09 Crisis for Brazil, China and India (April 1, 2013). World Bank Policy Research Working Paper No. 6409, Available at SSRN: https://ssrn.com/abstract=2251715

World Bank. (2020). *Indicators* [Database]. https://data.worldbank.org/indicator. Accessed 2 Aug 2020.

Chapter 19
Conclusions: COVID-19 and Cities: Experiences from Latin American and Asian Pacific Cities

Miguel A. Montoya, Daniel Lemus-Delgado, Johannes Rehner, and Aleksandra Krstikj

The emergence of the Sars-Cov-2 virus in December 2019 affected the various regions, countries, and communities around the world unequally. The novel coronavirus that originated in Asia soon spread throughout the planet, causing an unexpected pandemic for which most governments were unprepared. The effects were especially felt in the functioning of cities and in the daily life of citizens, at a magnitude that has not been seen since the deadly Spanish Flu of 1918. According to the World Health Organization (WHO), by the end of May 2021, 3.5 million deaths due to COVID-19 had been reported. However, some estimates indicate that the number of deaths could be considerably higher due to under-reporting, estimating that the actual number of fatalities could be approximately double the figure officially reported (Institute for Health Metrics and Evaluation [IHME], 2021).

As the pandemic spread, it generated at least three types of crises, affecting cities worldwide with different intensities depending on the place and time at which it occurred. In addition to the health crisis, the world witnessed economic recession and profound challenges in the political legitimacy of measures and governance processes. This led to tensions among members of the international community regarding the responsibilities countries assumed to contain the spread of the virus. Furthermore, doubts and mistrust arose around international organizations and the global health governance model. Specifically, some countries strongly questioned how the WHO

M. A. Montoya (✉)
School of Architecture, Art and Design, Tecnológico de Monterrey, Guadalajara, Mexico
e-mail: mmontoya@tec.mx

D. Lemus-Delgado
School of Social Science and Government, Tecnológico de Monterrey, Guadalajara, Mexico

J. Rehner
Institute of Geography, Pontificia, Universidad Católica de Chile, Santiago, Chile

A. Krstikj
School of Architecture, Art and Design, Tecnológico de Monterrey, Ciudad de Mexico, Mexico

© The Author(s), under exclusive license to Springer Nature Switzerland AG 2021

M. A. Montoya et al. (eds.), *COVID-19 and Cities*, The Urban Book Series,
https://doi.org/10.1007/978-3-030-84134-8_19

had acted during the pandemic, and geopolitical and commercial tensions intensified, for instance, between the USA and China (Boylan et al., 2021). Moreover, some scholars have shown how, in the context of the pandemic, old patterns of racism and xenophobia, especially against the Chinese community, have reappeared and increased (Chan & Montt Strabucchi, 2021). At the same time, with an unprecedented effort, the emergence of COVID-19 was an opportunity for the international scientific community to develop a vaccine and make other scientific advances to contain the pandemic as quickly and efficiently as possible, providing 17 different vaccines as of June 2021. In many ways, the health emergency caused by COVID-19 gave the opportunity for human beings to show the best and worst that they are capable of.

Today more than ever, it is clear that humanity will continue to be challenged by pandemics and their impacts on society. Tedros Adhanom Ghebreyesus, the director-general of the WHO, warned against getting complacent as the world fights the surge of COVID-19. During an annual address to the UN Assembly in May 2021, he said COVID-19 could be just a taster for the future of worldwide airborne viruses: "Make no mistake, this will not be the last time the world faces the threat of a pandemic… It's an evolutionary certainty that there will be another virus with the potential to be more transmittable and more deadly than this one" (WHO, 2021).

Therefore, addressing the current pandemic should be understood as a step toward more resilient cities, rather than only focusing on the emergency response and managing a particular crisis. More resilient systems should be more capable of responding to future pandemics or other massive public health issues, and the post-pandemic "new normal" could be more sustainable if urban systems incorporate improvements and learn from this crisis.

COVID-19 and Urban Resilience

The pandemic caused a moment of doubt for cities and their inhabitants, but also left important lessons to be learnt. The health actions to contain the outbreak included measures such as mass confinements, QR codes to track individuals that could spread the disease, and the mandatory use of masks in public places and meetings as well as on transport systems. These actions confronted paradigmatic visions of the value of individual freedom with the state's responsibility to ensure the common good and public health. At the same time, teleworking and online classes showed new possibilities for work, collaboration, and learning. The way cities and citizens met the challenges revealed inequalities regarding the possibilities of access to technology and the appropriate places for work or distance learning. It soon became apparent that although cities faced the same sea of uncertainty, not all people traveled in the same boat.

During the pandemic, despite similarities in government measures (lockdowns, mobility restrictions, etc.) and recommendations for individual protection, it became clear that cities had been impacted to different degrees, and it can be assumed that those who built prior capacities to be resilient could more effectively tackle the crisis. Furthermore, advances in making cities more inclusive, safe, and sustainable as a response to pandemics have the potential of bringing them a step forward on the path to resilience, not only regarding future pandemics, but mostly in confronting perpetual structural challenges and pressures; but how to achieve that? To shed light on this problem, the contributors of this volume asked several questions aimed at discussing the capacity of cities and the tools needed for evolutionary transformation toward better resilience. This book is an analysis of experiences, responses, and uncertainties faced by cities in Asia Pacific and Latin America, collected from different authors and perspectives in a transdisciplinary manner, which has allowed us to draw some lessons about advancing the building of resilience in cities.

City Planning, Mobility, and the Lockdown

Firstly, several chapters make contributions to the relationship between city planning and resilience in the light of the pandemic, clarifying that resilience is not an abstract concept. The essays of Hisako Koura from Japan and Yuan Ren from China both identify changes in working style, density, and mobility as crucial aspects to an alternative planning approach for advancing resilience agendas. There is some concurrence in the conclusions, despite the fundamentally different development stages, governance approaches, and contextual needs between cities in China and Japan. While Hisako Koura identifies changing work patterns, under increasing online working, as possible catalysts for strengthening new living localities and local cohesion in the context of Japan's shrinking cities, Yuan Ren states that "temporary mobility management" and the use of big data and monitoring are important for strengthening risk management and enhancing urban governance in mega-cities within the context of rapid urbanization in China (Ren, this volume). Thus, smart mobility and local diversity in the sphere of daily life improve spatial redundancy as a crucial aspect of resilience (Koura, this volume).

Security of food provision, and maintaining food supply, as well as supply of other basic goods under lockdown conditions, have also been challenges for cities, but the sector appears to have been able to adapt and to quickly expand online shopping and delivery systems. Furthermore, the operations of supermarkets, fresh goods markets ("farmers markets"/"wet markets"/"ferias"/"tianguis"), and other providers of essential goods in the cases studied were either uninterrupted or only briefly interrupted. Rather than there being a problem with general food security, the lockdown has produced a significant loss of jobs and informal income sources in this sector, including from restaurants and other providers of prepared food (Boza, this volume).

Urban Design and Form

Second, from the perspective of the internal structure of cities: What type of proposals can be identified for the short-, mid-, and long-term improvements of resilience that builds up the city's capacity for evolving toward a better systemic design? The relocation and migration toward rural areas has been shrinking cities in Japan, a phenomenon supported by the enhancement of ICT infrastructure under the pandemic conditions can be seen as favorable signs for the reorganization of urban functions toward a polycentric structure (Koura, this volume). However, the studies of Mangi et al. (this volume), Krstikj et al. (this volume), and Girotti Sperandio et al. (this volume) address issues of urban form as a key aspect of designing resilient cities. They highlight important challenges of such a task for the cities in Latin America. The particular spatial setting of the gated communities, which have surged in both continents under the influence of urban fragmentation and social inequity, was found to be generally more resilient against acute shocks in Shanghai compared with Bogotá. The Shanghai gated community model can be considered more balanced in terms of providing quality living for residents and reducing the need for daily mobility (Mangi et al., this volume). This brings about an important insight: The examples from Shanghai, considered to be a "city of islands", outperform other types of segregated settlements, which is especially relevant when temporary isolation becomes an unavoidable necessity. However, the quality and the size of such "islands", both directly linked to urban design and form, are even more important in order to ensure continuity of critical services during a period of lockdown. The spatial distribution of services and public space was found to be a considerable dimension for the future planning of resilient cities in Latin America (Krstikj et al., this volume). This is considering that spatial equity of services, rather than density, plays a role in resilience when facing large-scale health crises, since they are essential for enduring prolonged periods of reduced mobility. Therefore, the determination to include equity as a fundamental pillar in future urban planning of services could determine the success of resilience agendas in cities with pronounced socio-spatial segregation, such as in the majority of cities in the Latin American region. Thus, the resilience perspective contributes directly to the UN's "Sustainable Development Goals and Agenda 2030".

While these lessons focus on mid- and long-term solutions to improve resilience, short-term adaptive strategies and actions also need to be considered, and context-based and thoughtful local urban improvements should be observed. Active mobility initiatives, reframing the use of public spaces, and the implementation of urban community gardens bring to light possible forms of urban planning as a driver of healthy and resilient cities (Girotti Sperandio et al., this volume). Such short-term locally based improvements could be a better fit for areas that do not have the resources (or the luxury) to wait for the large-scale one-model-fits-all type of solution.

There are also contributions that address issues of design and planning on an even smaller scale. It is shown how the internal design and organization of nursing homes, their "space syntax", can prevent the propagation of airborne diseases such as COVID-19 (Martín López & Durán López, this volume). On the same scale, but with reference to private housing environments, Cobreros et al. (this volume) discuss how biophilic design contributes to personal wellbeing that is particularly important during lockdowns. The authors approach these issues based on the subjective experiences of inhabitants and offer conceptual and practical guidance when discussing the importance of relating to nature in housing spaces while under confinement. Even though the results are deliberately biased toward housing conditions, and in highly segregated and unequal conditions, limited to certain material conditions, in future research these might be combined with experiences from Asian metropolises where design based on personal experience is particularly important in conditions of extremely high urban density.

Emergence of New Pathways for Inclusion vs. Deepening the Gaps

The third question that we were looking to answer was to what degree and by which means do the described processes, measures, or politics aim to recover a previous state of the urban system, or do they look for different development pathways along which the city can evolve? The difficult circumstances caused by the pandemic forced us to reconsider the limits and possibilities of urban spaces as a means for human flourishing. In a time of crisis, fear, hope, and uncertainty, the pandemic also provided an opportunity to imagine better cities and aim for more sustainable development paths, instead of only looking for a recovery to a previous state. Prepandemic inequity, poverty, and deficient access to services make a large part of the Latin American urban population more vulnerable. Informal settlements with overcrowded living conditions, where inhabitants rely on urban life for daily survival, frequently only offer informal services and lack basic amenities such as clean water. These parts of Latin American cities have been particularly hit by the pandemic (Azparren Almeira, this volume; Schmidt et al., this volume). Trying to overcome the crisis without a structural change may lead to a "K-shaped recovery" that would deepen existing inequality and contradictions (Matos de Oliviera & Emídio, this volume). Grassroots initiatives to feed the most vulnerable during the COVID-19 crisis are presented as an expression of resistance to unjust cities and to the "landscape of authoritarianism, individualism and despair" (Leetoy & Gravante, this volume).

Despite the widely accepted Agenda 2030 and the significant progress presented through the Human Development Indicators in Latin America and several Asian countries during the last decade, the precarious economic situation of a large part of society meant that they could not maintain social distancing and limit their economic activities, especially in low- and middle-income countries. For example, in Mexico, of the 220,000 deaths due to the new coronavirus, according to a study prepared by the National Autonomous University of Mexico (UNAM), 94% of the deceased people were workers, housewives, drivers, street vendors, and retirees with adverse economic conditions. In addition, half of them only had primary school education (Forbes, 2021). Likewise, 7 out of 10 jobs lost during the pandemic were those of women (El País, 2021). Thus, the COVID-19 pandemic is no "equalizer" (Matos de Oliviera & Emídio, this volume) but tends to deepen existing social gaps, affecting not only economic variables but also life trajectories. This is especially detrimental for the Latin American region where the pandemic is expected to have long-term impacts on poverty, inequality, and the implementation of the 2030 Agenda.

New infectious diseases can expand quicker in overcrowded areas with unhealthy private and public spaces. Schmidt et al. (this volume) claim that not only are fast containment strategies important, but long-term investment in access to sanitation helps build resilient cities and puts them in a better position to fight new pandemics. Thus, a successful containment of a pandemic will be determined by both technical- and governance-related preparedness reflected in the design of urban spaces, public services, and infrastructure. For example, to improve the baseline water security so that citizens can benefit in both periods of crisis and in "normal" times is not only a technical task, but also a challenge to governance (Schmidt et al., this volume). Investing in improved infrastructure from a long-term perspective is a key task and requires funding programs that guarantee the essential infrastructure of the city, especially in the most vulnerable areas where access to water and sanitation services is often precarious. Moreover, specific measures designed to buffer negative economic impacts are also needed to make the confinement a realistic goal. A guaranteed minimum income requires elevated fiscal stability and resources, allowing the financing of programs with responsible levels of debt (Arboleda & Zembrano, this volume).

Thus, the pandemic has been an opportunity to think about resilient, creative, and innovative cities with better governance models, safer public spaces, and improved infrastructures. The pandemic constitutes a reminder of the importance of being better connected in order to flexibly adapt to challenges of organizing work in an innovative manner. Nevertheless, it is also essential to think about how cities can generate more inclusive opportunities for their inhabitants. As established in 1 of the 17 Sustainable Development Goals (SDGs) of the 2030 Agenda for Sustainable Development, authentic development includes making cities inclusive, safe, resilient, and sustainable. With the SDGs, the global community aims to share a blueprint for peace and prosperity for people and the planet, now and in the future. Therefore, most of the processes, measures, and politics involved in the handling of the crisis recognized that the capacity to respond to the pandemic in urban settlements was related to pre-existing socioeconomic inequalities and were looking for a way to imagine a better tomorrow for all.

Innovations and Restructuring

Furthermore, we asked: What kind of innovation or profound restructuring has been observed or can be proposed? The construction of resilient cities brought about the necessity for architectural interventions that will allow the reconstruction of vulnerable urban areas. Likewise, the pandemic can change the trend in the design of closed spaces in offices and public buildings, even affecting the design of residential care institutions for the elderly and the health infrastructure (Martín López & Durán

López, this volume), as well as leisure, recreation, and other spaces (Cobreros et al., this volume). These interventions may contribute to a paradigmatic change from object to people-driven design through concepts such as biophilia and empathy. Among other things, cities should be planned considering shared spaces and community-based services as fundamental tools for reducing inequalities (Azparren Almeira, this volume; Boza, this volume; Leetoy & Gravante, this volume). However, the design of spaces for individual use is also an opportunity for change and innovation in terms of standards in planning housing spaces, considering issues of personal wellbeing (Cobreros et al., this volume) that do not necessarily require important investment or technological innovation. The promotion of resilience can be envisioned through any city planning aspect, even the promotion of sustainable cultural tourism, which also implies a redesign of spaces and capacity for sporting events and shows (Giorgi et al., this volume).

Perhaps the most evident impact in terms of adapting through technology was the rapid increase in online sales, including traditional retail and supermarkets. The pandemic set the basis for the expansion of online service companies through their mobile applications (such as Amazon, Uber, Rappi, Alibaba, JD.com, etc.). This operational change will most likely improve existing inefficiencies and lead to an important restructuring of the food supply service sector (Boza, this volume).

At the same time, the pandemic showed how universities and cities could be profoundly affected by limited international student mobility (Likhovtseva, this volume), which affected life, identity, and urban development. The universities, like other educational institutions, had to suddenly recognize that their physical teaching spaces and infrastructure were not adequate to contain the spread of the virus. Classrooms and other buildings in schools and universities are prone to the spread of contagious diseases transmitted by air due to the number of students, teachers, and administrative staff who share enclosed spaces during prolonged periods. A long-lasting transition to online learning would have important impacts as universities have multiple linkages to urban systems, such as the urban economy, local innovation, and the international exchange of ideas and knowledge—being an important support in fighting the pandemic itself (Likhovtseva, this volume). Recovering academic life in postpandemic cities implies a gradual transformation of architectural spaces.

Interactions, Governance, and Decision-Making

Finally, we asked: Through which specific interactions, and among what types of individuals and organizations, and by what kind of decision, can such improvements be achieved? Are these allowing for relevant and long-lasting improvements as a response to the pandemic? These topics were emphasized by a concern with the appropriate scale for responding to a crisis and the need for long-lasting improvements. Although there is a need for national policies, financial response, and administrative crisis management, cities manage less extensive territories and have more direct dialogue with citizens, which results in flexibility and institutional and spatial proximity between actors—aspects that can be utilized by city governments for more effectively managing crisis situations.

When comparing the nation-state with cities in the management of the crisis, the experiences of the Latin American and Asian cities demonstrated that city leaders can take faster action according to the circumstances around them. Even though publicly financed specific aid policies (oriented to small businesses, low-income households, etc.) are mostly designed and executed on a national level, implementing ambitious local programs, such as a guaranteed basic income and incentives for formality, is more accessible if implemented by the city rather than by the national government (Arboleda & Zembrano, this volume). As evidenced by various authors in their contributions to this book, cities that succeeded in containing the virus have responded in an agile, flexible, and appropriate way to the challenges posed by COVID-19. In this context, the leading role of city governance should be recognized as crucial for future pathways along which the city can evolve.

Some contributions discuss the outstanding role of community-based initiatives within cities, aiming, for instance, to address basic food needs and fill in where the state is failing and the market is not offering viable solutions (Azparren Almeira, this volume; Leetoy & Gravante, this volume). This discussion is linked to the role of Community Resilience Initiatives (CRIs; Fransen et al., 2021), particularly highlighting the way grassroots initiatives tried to cope with the emergency alone by offering services that cover dramatic needs due to inefficient central governance or shortcomings of top-down emergency measures. Although such grassroots initiatives, such as soup kitchens that serve the heavily affected and marginalized poor, may be seen as an emergent and ephemeral phenomenon that will disappear in a postpandemic recovery, Leetoy and Gravante (this volume) highlight in their essay the persistent and transforming value of such initiatives as they promote an ethical understanding of citizenship based on kindness, reciprocity, and compassion.

In addition, city authorities can take advantage of pre-existing cooperation networks with other cities, such as networks to promote specific agendas related to the mitigation of climate change or the sister cities scheme, to forge international collaboration networks for fighting the crisis. These networks help share knowledge and receive medical delegations of experts to advise on measures to contain the spread of the virus. They also have been useful for receiving help with medical equipment, such as masks and indispensable mechanical respirators, during the most critical moments of the pandemic. The importance of cities in the context of International Development Cooperation was increasing during recent years, and the pandemic is likely to strengthen this trend (Cerda Dueñas & Lemus Delgado, this volume). Nevertheless, to face the enormous challenges of the twenty-first century, it seems crucial for cities to act as part of networks and to seek multilateral (instead of just bilateral) partnerships.

On the other hand, in terms of the COVID-19 crisis management and inter-scalar governance mechanisms, the reaction of different state entities, such as the health sector, the federal or central government, and, on some occasions, cities (as in the case of Mexico City), has been lacking coherent communication and strategies, causing delay and contradictions, leading to confusion (Gil Robles & Sanchez-Jimenez, this volume). Others highlight coordination problems and contradicting policies as in the case of Brazil (Schmidt et al., this volume). In this sense, it is essential to re-evaluate the structures and processes of governance in cities, particularly in their relation to national governance mechanisms. Especially, but not exclusively, during periods of social crisis, governance becomes a critical factor in responding to challenges and building the resilience of the city. This requires not only efficient communication, but also dialogue and collaboration between all levels of government, civil society, and other stakeholders. Cities can be particularly efficient in design policies that can be adjusted to the local context and complement existing strategies at the national level.

Nevertheless, other authors make a claim for centrally managed mobility control and lockdowns. These actions are legitimized by the need for clear action, although the negative impact on urban life and on the economy is recognized (Ren, this volume). The comparison between Latin American and Chinese experiences reflects the differences in governance structures. They also highlight the possibility of infrastructure enhancement and investment to foster economic recovery which will neither necessarily be possible nor lead to the same results in Latin America due to the very different governance process and shortcomings in public finances (Giorgi et al., this volume).

Final Remarks

This book presents a series of contributions, both essays and empirically based case studies from Latin America and Asia (mostly China), on the challenges that the novel coronavirus pandemic in 2020 and 2021 posed on urban systems. The multidisciplinary contributions are placed in different political, social, and economic contexts and are founded in their respective disciplinary, epistemological, and methodological context. Nevertheless, they all contribute to the discussion of urban resilience of cities under the influence of a global crisis.

Although not all national or local authorities acted efficiently during the pandemic, it is possible to affirm that cities can be the propitious space to weave networks of collaboration, to promote projects and programs, to generate forms of interaction, and to strengthen community resilience as a way to overcome the various crises. The experience during the pandemic of Latin American and Asian Pacific cities provides essential lessons on crisis management during the emergence of COVID-19. The way governments and citizens coped with the pandemic shows that, despite institutional weaknesses, structural deficiencies, or the pandemic's unexpectedness, the crises generated by this new disease can be solved more efficiently by cities due to active civil agency, innovativeness, governance flexibility, and the ability to react. However, as the authors themselves attest throughout this book, many aspects of cities need to be improved. Reconstruction of vulnerable areas with infrastructure developments, redesigning residential models with more effective service provisions, improving the spatial equity of services and public spaces, and integrating wellbeing in all private and public spaces through biophilia and empathy are just some of the proposals that this book brings about. Imagination, political will, and new forms of governance can support this indispensable transformation of cities aimed at promoting inclusion, equity, and urban health.

Finally, there is a fundamental need to alter the way we develop our urban society if we are to survive: from the present shortsighted vision based only on the needs of the living to a future-oriented preparedness-based smart planning for those to come. There is no better place to perform that transformation than the city—the hub of innovation, talent, and opportunity. The city has once again proven during the COVID-19 pandemic that it is the perfect place to prepare for the unknown challenges of the future. The key is to make cities resilient and equitable. Only then, will it be possible to offer places for a safer and dignified life.

References

Boylan, B. M., McBeath, J., & Wang, B. (2021). US–China relations: Nationalism, the trade war, and COVID-19. *Fudan Journal of the Humanities and Social Sciences, 14*, 23–40. https://doi.org/10.1007/s40647-020-00302-6.

Chan, C., & Montt Strabucchi, M. (2021). Many-faced orientalism: Racismand xenophobia in a time of the novel coronavirus in Chile. *Asian Ethnicity, 22*(2), 374–394. https://doi.org/10.1080/14631369.2020.1795618.

El País. (2021, May 17). *Siete de cada 10 desempleados por la pandemia en México son mujeres.* https://elpais.com/mexico/economia/2021-05-17/siete-de-cada-10-desempleados-por-la-pandemia-en-mexico-son-mujeres.html. Accessed 30 May 2021.

Forbes. (2021, May 23). *El 94% de mexicanos muertos por Covid eran obreros y amas de casa: UNAM.* https://www.forbes.com.mx/el-94-de-mexicanos-muertos-por-covid-eran-obreros-y-amas-de-casa/. Accessed 30 May 2021.

Fransen, J., Peralta, D. O., Vanelli, F., Edelenbos, J., & Calzada Olvera, B. (2021). The emergence of Urban Community resilience initiatives during the COVID-19 pandemic: An international exploratory study. *European Journal of Development Research.* https://doi.org/10.1057/s41287-020-00348-y.

Institute for Health Metrics and Evaluation [IHME]. (2021, May 13). *Estimation of total mortality due to COVID-19.* http://www.healthdata.org/special-analysis/estimation-excess-mortality-due-covid-19-and-scalars-reported-covid-19-deaths. Accessed 30 May 2021.

World Health Organization [WHO]. (2021, May 24). *Director-General's opening remarks at the World Health Assembly - 24* May 2021. https://www.who.int/director-general/speeches/detail/director-general-s-opening-remarks-at-the-world-health-assembly%2D%2D-24-may-2021. Accessed 30 May 2021.

Papers Included in this Volume

Arboleda, D., & Zembrano, A. (this volume). Vulnerability after COVID-19 and the response of a developing City: The case of Bogota, Colombia.

Azparren Almeira, A. L. (this volume). The impact of COVID-19 on informal settlements in Buenos Aires, Argentina.

Boza, S. (this volume). Feeding cities during COVID-19 lockdowns: Responses from China and Latin America.
Cerda Dueñas, C., & Lemus Delgado, D. R. (this volume). Cities, COVID-19, and international development cooperation: Challenges and opportunities.
Cobreros, C., Flores-Garcia, M., Biondi, S., Maya, M., & Ontiveros-Ortiz, E. N. (this volume). Re-signifying domestic space in times of confinement based on Biophilic design.
Gil Robles, M. A., & Sanchez-Jimenez, B. A. (this volume). City governance and resilience during the COVID-19 emergency: A case study of Mexico City.
Giorgi, E., Valderrey, F., & Montoya, M. A. (this volume). Cultural tourism and the economic recovery of cities post-COVID-19.
Girotti Sperandio, A. M., Torezan Silingardi, A. A., Gastaldo Cifoni, G., de Souza Salomão, R. (this volume). Cities' health dimension post-pandemic: *Brazil urban planning aspects*.
Koura, H. (this volume). Diversification of urbanism in the process of City region transformation.
Krstikj, A., Contreras Ruiz Esparza, M. G., Wang, M., & Pérez-Paredes, E. A. (this volume). Planning the Equitable Distribution of Services in Emerging Regions: Atizapán de Zaragoza, Mexico and Yinchuan, China.
Leetoy, S., & Gravante, T. (this volume). Feeding, solidarity and care: The grassroots experiences of Latin American soup kitchens in a global pandemic.
Likhovtseva, E. (this volume). "Universities in lockdown": The impact of reduced international student mobility upon cities in the post-COVID 19 era.
Mangi, E., Cheshmehzangi, A., & Botti, G. (this volume). COVID-19, gated communities and urban resilience: A comparative analysis between China and Colombia.
Martín López, L., & Durán López, R. (this volume). A typological analysis of nursing home environments during the COVID-19 pandemic: Risks and potential.
Matos de Oliviera, A. L., & Emídio, A. P. (this volume). "The Great Equalizer"? The Long-Term Effects of the COVID-19 Pandemic on Poverty, Inequality and the 2030 Agenda in Latin America.
Ren, Y. (this volume). Appropriate population mobility management in an epidemic.
Schmidt, A. F. J., Tjong, E., Hase Ueta, M., Weins, N. W., & do Carmo, R. L. (this volume). Building strategies and resilience in the face of a pandemic in urban China and Brazil: COVID-19, access to water and inequality.

Index

© The Author(s), under exclusive license to Springer Nature Switzerland AG 2021

M. A. Montoya et al. (eds.), *COVID-19 and Cities*, The Urban Book Series,
https://doi.org/10.1007/978-3-030-84134-8

Printed by Printforce, the Netherlands